STEM CELLS AND REGENERATIVE MEDICINE

STEM CELLS AND REGENERATIVE MEDICINE

VOLUME VII

DISEASES AND THERAPY

STEM CELLS AND REGENERATIVE MEDICINE

Additional books in this series can be found on Nova's website
under the Series tab.

Additional E-books in this series can be found on Nova's website
under the E-book tab.

STEM CELLS AND REGENERATIVE MEDICINE

VOLUME VII

DISEASES AND THERAPY

PHILIPPE TAUPIN

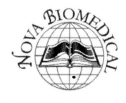

Nova Science Publishers, Inc.
New York

Copyright © 2012 by Nova Science Publishers, Inc.

All rights reserved. No part of this book may be reproduced, stored in a retrieval system or transmitted in any form or by any means: electronic, electrostatic, magnetic, tape, mechanical photocopying, recording or otherwise without the written permission of the Publisher.

For permission to use material from this book please contact us:
Telephone 631-231-7269; Fax 631-231-8175
Web Site: http://www.novapublishers.com

NOTICE TO THE READER

The Publisher has taken reasonable care in the preparation of this book, but makes no expressed or implied warranty of any kind and assumes no responsibility for any errors or omissions. No liability is assumed for incidental or consequential damages in connection with or arising out of information contained in this book. The Publisher shall not be liable for any special, consequential, or exemplary damages resulting, in whole or in part, from the readers' use of, or reliance upon, this material. Any parts of this book based on government reports are so indicated and copyright is claimed for those parts to the extent applicable to compilations of such works.

Independent verification should be sought for any data, advice or recommendations contained in this book. In addition, no responsibility is assumed by the publisher for any injury and/or damage to persons or property arising from any methods, products, instructions, ideas or otherwise contained in this publication.

This publication is designed to provide accurate and authoritative information with regard to the subject matter covered herein. It is sold with the clear understanding that the Publisher is not engaged in rendering legal or any other professional services. If legal or any other expert assistance is required, the services of a competent person should be sought. FROM A DECLARATION OF PARTICIPANTS JOINTLY ADOPTED BY A COMMITTEE OF THE AMERICAN BAR ASSOCIATION AND A COMMITTEE OF PUBLISHERS.

Additional color graphics may be available in the e-book version of this book.

Library of Congress Cataloging-in-Publication Data

ISSN: 2159-8754

ISBN: 978-1-61209-931-6

Published by Nova Science Publishers, Inc. † New York

Contents

Introduction	Adult Neurogenesis and Neural Stem Cells: Developmental and Therapeutic Potential	**vii**
Chapter I	Enhanced Neurogenesis Following Neurological Disease	**1**
Chapter II	Alzheimer's Disease: Increased Neurogenesis and Possible Disease Mechanisms Related to Neurogenesis	**17**
Chapter III	Neurogenesis, NSCs, Pathogenesis and Therapies for Alzheimer's Disease	**33**
Chapter IV	Adult Neurogenesis and Drug Therapy	**55**
Chapter V	Neurogenic Factors Are Targets in Depression	**65**
Chapter VI	Pharmacology of Adult Neurogenesis: Compensatory and Regenerative Processes	**73**
Chapter VII	Adult Neurogenesis, Neuroinflammation, and Therapeutic Potential of Adult Neural Stem Cells	**87**
Chapter VIII	A Dual Activity of ROS and Oxidative Stress on Adult Neurogenesis and Alzheimer's Disease	**111**
Chapter IX	Adult Neurogenesis and Neural Stem Cells as a Model for the Discovery and Development of Novel Drugs	**123**
Chapter X	Neurogenic Drugs and Compounds	**133**
Chapter XI	Very Small Embryonic-like Stem Cells for Regenerative Medicine	**143**
Chapter XII	Transplantation of Cord Blood Stem Cells for Treating Hematologic Diseases and Strategies to Improve Engraftment	**149**
Chapter XIII	Transplantation of Two Populations of Stem Cells to Improve Engraftment	**171**
Chapter XIV	Ex Vivo Fucosylation of Stem Cells to Improve Engraftment	**179**

Chapter XV	Thirteen Compounds Promoting Oligodendrocyte Progenitor Cell Differentiation and Remyelination for Treating Multiple Sclerosis	**187**
Chapter XVI	Antibodies against CD20 (Rituximab) for Treating Multiple Sclerosis	**199**
Conclusion 1	Neurogenic Drugs for Treating Neurological Diseases and Disorders	**205**
Conclusion 2	Aneuploidy and Adult Neurogenesis in Alzheimer's Disease: Therapeutic Strategies	**211**
Conclusion 3	Ex Vivo Fucosylation to Improve the Engraftment Capability and Therapeutic Potential of Human cord Blood Stem Cells	**215**
Index		**219**

Introduction

Adult Neurogenesis and Neural Stem Cells: Developmental and Therapeutic Potential

Neural stem cells (NSCs) are the self-renewing multipotent cells that generate the main phenotypes of the nervous system; namely, neuronal, astroglial and oligodendroglial. As such, they hold the potential to treat a broad range of neurological diseases and injuries, including Alzheimer's and Parkinson's diseases, age-related macular degeneration, cerebral strokes, and brain and spinal cord injuries. It is now well accepted that neurogenesis occurs in the adult mammalian (including the human) brain. Newly generated neuronal cells in the adult brain originate from residual stem cells. In support of this contention, self-renewing multipotent neural progenitor and stem cells have been isolated and characterized from the adult brain. This reveals that the adult brain has the capacity to self-repair.

Novel strategies are being devised to treat and cure neurological diseases and injuries. One such strategy involves stimulation of endogenous neural progenitor or stem cells and the transplantation of neural progenitor and stem cells, derived from the adult central nervous system (CNS), to repair and restore the degenerated or injured nerve pathways. Neurogenesis occurs in discrete regions of the adult brain, primarily the dentate gyrus of the hippocampus and the subventricular zone. This raises the question of the mechanisms underlying adult neurogenesis and the function of newly generated neuronal cells in the adult brain. Cellular and molecular microenvironments, or niches, that control neurogenesis have been identified and characterized in the adult brain. Niches for neurogenesis therefore hold the key to the developmental and therapeutic potential of adult NSCs. Newly generated neuronal cells in the adult brain may be involved in physio- and patho-logical processes, such as learning and memory and Alzheimer's disease and depression. Determining the relative contribution of adult neurogenesis to these processes, and the plasticity of the adult CNS will lead to a better understanding of the functioning of the nervous system.

Much remains to be elucidated and determined in this field of research. Adult NSCs remain to be unequivocally identified and characterized and the mechanisms of adult neurogenesis (the developmental and therapeutic potential of adult NSCs) are still to be fully understood and unraveled. Research conducted in adult neurogenesis and NSC research will have tremendous impacts not only for cellular therapy but also for our understanding of the physiopathology of the nervous system.

Acknowledgments

Reproduced from: Taupin P. Adult neurogenesis and neural stem cells: developmental and therapeutic potential. Drug Discovery Today (2009) 4(1): Editorial. Copyright (2009), with permission from Elsevier.

Chapter I

Enhanced Neurogenesis following Neurological Disease

Abstract

Neurological diseases are disorders of the nervous system that have biological origins, and impair one's ability to live a normal life. Neurological diseases originate from neurochemical alterations or the loss of specific cell populations of the nervous system. The causes for these disorders remain poorly understood. Their symptoms span from psychiatric to neurological to physical impairments. For decades, finding a cure for neurological diseases was synonymous with compensating for the neurochemical loss, by stimulating endogenous cells, replacing the dysfunctional or degenerated cells, or by preventing the degeneration of cell populations in neurodegenerative diseases, to restore brain functions. There is still no cure for neurological diseases, albeit in some cases treatments are available to alleviate some of the symptoms. With recent evidences that neurogenesis occurs in the adult brain and that neural stem cells (NSCs) reside in the adult brain, new theories have emerged regarding the possible involvement of newly generated neuronal cells in neurological diseases, and the potential of NSCs for the treatment of neurological diseases. Studies have shown that adult neurogenesis is increased in neurological diseases. Hence, researchers are now integrating these new data to understand the contribution of adult neurogenesis in neurological diseases, its significance, and potential for functional recovery. In this chapter, we will review the literature on adult neurogenesis in neurological diseases. This chapter discusses the functions of adult neurogenesis in the diseased brain, and its potential for the treatment of neurodegenerative diseases. Although, many questions regarding the involvement of this plasticity in neurological diseases remain unanswered, these developments point to new hypotheses and concepts regarding neurological diseases, their origins, developments, and treatments.

Adult Neurogenesis in Alzheimer's Disease and in Neurodegenerative Diseases of the Brain

Alzheimer's disease (AD) is a progressive, neurodegenerative disease characterized by amyloid plaque deposits and neurofibrillary tangles [1,2]. AD is associated with a loss of nerve cells in areas of the brain that are vital to memory and other mental abilities, such as the hippocampus. It is a slowly progressing disease, starting with mild memory problems and ending with severe brain damage. AD is the most common form of dementia among older people. The disease usually begins after age 60, and risk increases with age. On an average, patients with AD live for 8–10 yr after they are diagnosed, although the disease can last for as many as 20 yr. Three genes, presenilin 1 (PS 1), presenilin 2 (PS 2), and amyloid precursor protein (APP), have been discovered that cause early onset of the disease, that is, familial form of AD. Other genetic mutations that cause excessive accumulation of amyloid protein are associated with age-related form of the disease, that is, sporadic form of AD. There are several animal models that have been devised to study the genes known to be involved in AD, such as gene-altered mice, knockout, or expressing mutant forms of PS 1 [3,4] or APP [5–7].

Recent investigations of autopsies of AD brain patients have reported an increase in the expression of markers for immature neuronal cells, such as doublecortin, polysialylated nerve cell adhesion molecule (PSA-NCAM), neurogenic differentiation factor, and turned on after division (TOAD-64, also known as TUC-4), in the subgranular zone and the granular layer of the dentate gyrus (DG), as well as in the CA1 region of Ammon's horn, suggesting that neurogenesis is increased in the hippocampus of patients suffering from AD [8]. These data conflict with previous reports aiming at characterizing adult neurogenesis in animal models of AD mutant [9,10] and knockout [4] for PS 1 and mutant for APP [6]. These studies, where neurogenesis was assessed by bromodeoxyuridine (BrdU) staining, showed decrease in neurogenesis in the DG and subventricular zone (SVZ). They also showed decrease in the number of differentiated neurons in the hippocampus, as detected by immunoreactivity for β-tubulin, a neuronal marker. Such discrepancies between the studies could be explained by the limitation of the transgenic animal models as representative of AD. Both are single gene-deficient transgenic mice models, thus they neither fully reproduce the features of familial AD, nor the sporadic form of AD. To this aim, studies from other models such as transgenic mice co-expressing a mutant τ protein, involved in neurofibrillary tangles formation and progressive motor disturbance, and a mutant form of APP [5], may provide better systems for studying adult neurogenesis in AD. A more recent study reports an increase in neurogenesis in the DG and SVZ of transgenic mouse models [11], which express the Swedish and Indiana APP mutations [7]. Although the observed increase in neurogenesis correlates the observation made from human tissues [8], concerns have been raised regarding the validity of such models, as representative of AD [12]. These data show the difficulties encountered in using animal models for studying neurological diseases and disorders, and particularly AD [13,14]. Further analysis of the adult SVZ in the APP transgenic mice reports a thinning of the ventricular zone [15], suggesting a decrease in the number of progenitor cells during early neurogenesis, resulting in a partial depletion of the neural progenitor cell population in the adult. This depletion of the neural progenitor cell population may underlie the decrease in neurogenesis observed in the adult transgenic mice for PS 1 and APP. The authors observed that the rate of proliferation of the newly generated neuronal cells in the adult mutants is similar to the wild type, suggesting that PS 1 and APP are not involved in the regulation of neural progenitor proliferation, but rather in the regulation of neuronal survival, migration, or differentiation. The involvement of PS 1 and APP in adult neurogenesis is further highlighted by the expression of PS 1 in newly generated neuronal cells in the adult DG [16], and by the involvement of APP in the regulation of adult neurogenesis in vitro, and in vivo [17,18]. However, the function of these molecules in adult neurogenesis is at present unclear, and remains to be investigated.

Huntington's Disease

Huntington's disease (HD) results from genetically programmed degeneration of neuronal cells in certain areas of the brain [19]. The caudate nucleus is the part of the brain that is, most severely, and preferentially affected in HD. This degeneration causes uncontrolled movements, loss of intellectual faculties, and emotional disturbance. HD is a familial disease, passed from parent to child through a mutation; a polyglutamine repeat (poly Gln, polyQ, or p[CAG]n) expansion that lengthens a glutamine (CAG) segment in the novel huntingtin protein [20]. Actual treatments for HD consist of controlling emotional and movement problems associated with the disease. Models such as transgenic HD mice for the 5′-end of the human HD gene carrying CAG repeat expansions (R6/1) [21], and quinolinic acid lesion-induced striatal cell loss rat model of HD have been devised.

In the SVZ close to the caudate nucleus of adult human post-mortem samples, confocal immunofluorescence analysis for molecular markers, such as the cell cycle marker proliferating cell nuclear antigen (PCNA), the neuronal marker β-tubulin, and the glial cell marker glial fibrillary acidic protein, has shown that progenitor cell proliferation and neurogenesis are increased in the SVZ of HD brains [22]. Furthermore, the authors correlated the degree of cell proliferation with pathological severity and length of polyglutamine repeats in the HD gene. Studies from R6/1 transgenic mouse model of HD reported that the level of PCNA mRNA is increased approximately twofold in the striatum of 12-wk-old mice [23], and a decrease in neurogenesis in the DG [24]. However, these data are difficult to extrapolate to adult neurogenesis in HD, as it has been reported that mutated forms of huntingtin affect brain development [25]. Thus, the consequence of the mutation of huntingtin during brain development could underlie the decrease in neurogenesis observed in the adult transgenic mice. More recently, Tattersfield et al. reported that quinolinic acid striatal lesioning of the adult brain increases SVZ neurogenesis, leading to the putative migration of neuroblasts to damaged areas of the striatum, and the formation of new neurons [26], as previously observed in patients with HD [22]. Further confirming that adult neurogenesis is increased in HD.

Parkinson's Disease

Parkinson's disease (PD) is a chronic and progressive neurodegenerative disease of the brain primarily associated with the loss of a specific type of dopamine neurons in the substantia nigra (SN) [27]. The SN is in the ventral midbrain and contains neurons that use dopamine as a neurotransmitter and send their axons to the striatum. It is believed that a gradual decline in the number of nigral dopamine neurons occurs with normal aging in humans, and that PD is caused by an abnormally rapid rate of cell death. PD belongs to a group of conditions called motor system disorders. The four primary symptoms of PD are tremor or trembling in hands, arms, legs, jaw, and face; rigidity or stiffness of the limbs and trunk; bradykinesia, or slowness of movement; and postural instability, or impaired balance and coordination. The disease is considerably more common in the age group of over 50 yr. PD is not usually inherited. A variety of medications provide dramatic relief from the symptoms. However, no drug yet can stop the progression of the disease, and in many cases medications lose their benefit over time. In such cases, surgery may be considered. There are several animal models of PD. Among them, are the 1-methyl-4phenyl-1,2,3,6-tetrahydropyridine and 6-hydroxydopamine-lesioned models, known to kill significant proportion of the nigral dopaminergic nerve cell population [28].

In a recent study that reports the generation of new dopaminergic neuronal cells in the adult rat SN [29], the authors have also investigated how the generation of new dopaminergic neuronal cells would be affected following lesion of the SN. They showed that the rate of neurogenesis, as measured by BrdU labeling, is increased twofold 3 wk following lesion induced by a systemic dose of 1-methyl-4-phenyl-1,2,3,6-tetrahydropyridine. However, a more recent study finds no evidence of new dopaminergic neurons in the SN of 6-hydroxydopamine-lesioned hemi-Parkinsonian rodents [30], contradicting these results. Thus, the generation of new dopaminergic neurons following lesion of the SN, as well as in the adult SN, remains a source of controversy [30–32], and needs to be further confirmed.

Adult Neurogenesis in Epilepsy

Epilepsy is a brain disorder in which populations of neurons signal abnormally. In the affected individual, this translates into a variety of seizures that range from mild behavioral changes to more severe symptoms, such as convulsions, muscles spasms, and loss of consciousness. Long-term abnormalities in learning, memory, and behavior have been reported [33]. This ailment is one of the most prevalent neurological disorders, affecting approx 1% of Americans. Treatments are available for patients with epilepsy, and seizures can be controlled in most cases by modern medicine and surgical techniques. It is hypothesized that abnormal brain wiring and/or neurotransmitter imbalance are underlying factors in epilepsy. The hippocampal formation is a critical area in the pathology of epilepsy; it has been suggested that the DG may function as a gate with respect to controlling the propagation of seizures [33,34]. Granule cells can regulate the through-put of epileptiform activity transiting through the hippocampal formation, by virtue of specific feed-forward inhibitory pathways [35]. One of the most common forms of epilepsy is the temporal lobe epilepsy (TLE). TLE often has its onset during childhood or is associated with a prolonged seizure episode early in life that is followed, after a variable latent period, by the development of epilepsy. In patients suffering from TLE, dispersed granular cell layer was reported [36,37]. Neuronal cell death has been reported in both the granular and pyramidal layers, with granule cell loss occurring at a lesser rate than in other hippocampal areas [37]. Ectopic granule-like neuronal cells, as defined by their expression of calcium-binding protein calbindin D28K, are found in the hilus and inner molecular layer [36]. The dentate granule cells give rise to abnormal axonal projections, a process described as mossy fiber (MF) sprouting, to the supragranular inner molecular layer of the DG, and the basal dendrites of CA3 pyramidal cells in stratum oriens [38–40]. There are several models that reproduce some of the traits of epileptic seizures observed in human, including the kainic model of epilepsy [41–43], the electrical kindling [44], and the pilocarpine seizure model [45,46]. Systemic kainic acid and pilocarpine injection produce seizures with many similarities to TLE, including an initial episode of prolonged status epilepticus (SE), followed by a latent period and spontaneously recurrent seizures, and temporal lobe pathology similar to that seen in humans. In both models, as in TLE, limbic seizures cause apoptosis of granule and pyramidal cells, with granule cell loss occurring at a lesser rate than in other hippocampal areas [47–51]. In these models, ectopic granule-like cells in the hilus and inner molecular layer, as well as aberrant growth (sprouting) of granule cell axons (MFs) in the supragranular dentate inner molecular layer, and the basal dendrites of CA3 pyramidal cells in stratum oriens have been reported [49,52–55], as in patients with epilepsy [38–40]. MF sprouting begins during week 2 after SE, and peaks after 2 mo [45,49].

It is postulated that a reduction in inhibition by loss of interneurons [48] and/or the development of recurrent excitatory circuitry by the sprouting of MF into ectopic positions after loss of their normal targets, and subsequent hippocampal hyperexcitability, are the determining events in the pathogenesis of limbic epilepsy [40,52,53]. Alternatively, it has also been proposed that aberrant granule cell axonal projections stabilize the network by preferentially innervating inhibitory neurons, and thereby restoring recurrent inhibition [55]. The implication of MF sprouting in seizures has been challenged by recent data showing that spontaneous recurrent seizures are still observed when MF sprouting is prevented by pre-treatment with cycloheximide, a protein synthesis inhibitor, in pilocarpine- or kainate-treated animals [56,57]. Therefore, the origin, precise mechanisms, and relative contribution of cell death, ectopic granule-like cells, and MF sprouting in epileptic seizures remain to be defined.

Recently, a number of investigators used the BrdU paradigm to study the effect of experimentally induced seizures on adult neurogenesis. They have reported an increase in dentate granule cell neurogenesis following limbic-induced seizures in adult rodents. The first investigation relating neurogenesis and seizure activity in adult rodents was reported by Parent et al. in the DG of pilocarpine-treated rats [58]. The authors reported ectopic granule-like BrdU-immunolabeled cells in the hilus, as far as the CA3 cell layer, and a marked increase in dentate granule cell neurogenesis following seizure activity. The number of BrdU-immunolabeled cells in the hilus/CA3 layer was reported to increase with time after BrdU administration, showing that ectopic granule-like cells in the hilus derived from newly generated neuronal cells that are born after seizures, and can migrate into the hilus, as far as the CA3 cell layer. In the subgranular zone, cell proliferation was reported to increase within 3 d, and persists for at least 2 wk after pilocarpine treatment. The increase of neurogenesis observed in the DG, and the subsequent differentiation of the newly generated neuronal cells induced by the seizure activity, follows the same time-course than the MF remodeling [45,49], taking into account the additional time required for the differentiation of these cells into mature neurons [59]. Thus, the authors hypothesized that MF remodeling derives from newly born granule neurons rather than from pre-existing, mature dentate granule cells, as previously suggested [38–40,49,52–55]. The authors further supported their hypothesis by reporting that MF-like processes immunostained for TOAD-64, a marker for newly generated neuronal cells, were detected in the granule cell layer of the stratum oriens of CA3 area and the inner molecular layer of the DG. These data suggest that hippocampal network plasticity associated with chronic seizures originate from newly generated cells in the DG. It remains to be determined whether the newly generated granule cells account for all the "ectopic" granule cells observed in SE, and whether seizure-induced MF remodeling arises primarily from the developing axons of newly generated dentate granule cells.

Further studies have confirmed increased neurogenesis in dentate granule cell layer, and the presence of newly generated dentate granule-like cells in ectopic locations, such as the hilus, the inner molecular layer of the DG, and the hilar/CA3 border, following seizure activity in different models of epilepsy—the kainic model of epilepsy [60–64], the electrical kindling [60,65,66], pilocarpine seizure model [62,64], and in other models [67,68]. It was further reported that (1) unilaterally induced seizures (such as intracerebroventricular kainic acid injection induce bilateral granule cell progenitor proliferation) [61], (2) SE not only stimulates neurogenesis in the DG, but also in the SVZ [69], (3) seizures preferentially stimulate proliferation of radial glia-like astrocytes in the adult DG [70], (4) a population of cells in the developing CNS reported to have neural stem cell (NSC) capabilities [71,72], and (5) the severity of SE affect the outcome of the newly generated cells in the DG, with the most severe SE leading to the death of most of the newly generated neuronal cells within 4 wk post-SE [73].

In a follow-up study, Parent et al. aimed to examine whether seizure-induced MF remodeling arises primarily from the developing axons of newly generated dentate granule cells and/or from mature granule cells [74]. The authors applied low-dose, whole-brain X-ray irradiation, to inhibit dentate granule cell neurogenesis, in adult rats after pilocarpine-induced SE. The authors reported that low-dose radiation treatment reduces dentate granule cell neurogenesis, and had no effect on seizure-induced MF sprouting. Thus, MF reorganization after pilocarpine-induced SE occurs even in the absence of dentate granule cell neurogenesis, suggesting that sprouting arises also from the mature granule cells, and not primarily from newly generated neuronal cells as previously suggested [58]. The effect of low-dose radiation treatment on dentate granule cell neurogenesis [75] and seizure activity was further confirmed in recent studies [76]. Altogether, these data show that adult neurogenesis is increased following seizures in animal models and that the newly generated neuronal cells elicit the two main features of epilepsy: formation of aberrant axonal projections and migration to ectopic locations. These data also show that although increased hippocampal dentate granule cell neurogenesis, ectopic granule-like cell migration, and abnormal synaptogenesis are prominent features of animal models of TLE, they might represent independent events. Thus, it remains to be determined, what are the function(s) of the newly generated cells in SE. Furthermore, these investigations and analysis remain to be validated in human patients with epilepsy.

Altogether, these studies show that adult neurogenesis is increased in neurological diseases, albeit there is no functional recovery. Why if new neurons are generated is there no functional recovery? What are the function(s) of the newly generated cells in neurodegenerative diseases and how functional recovery could be promoted remain to be determined?

Function of the Newly Generated Neuronal Cells in Neurological Diseases

In the adult CNS, the function(s) of the newly generated neuronal cells remains the center of intense research. Recent evidence suggests that newly generated neuronal cells in the adult DG are involved in memory [77,78], stress [79], and depression [80,81], whereas, newly generated neuronal cells in the olfactory bulb are involved in odor perception and memory [82]. However, the function of the newly generated neuronal cells in the diseased brain remains to be determined. There are few speculations and hypotheses that can be raised in the context of their attributes in neurological diseases.

The increase in neurogenesis, observed in neurological diseases and in models of neurological diseases, may represent a mechanism directed toward the replacement of dead or damaged neurons. Such an increase has also been reported in other pathological conditions, such as stroke [83] and traumatic brain injury [84], and may represent attempts by the CNS to self-repair. However, notwithstanding that neurogenesis appears to be increased in the brains of patients and animal models of neurological diseases, progressive cell losses are still occurring and no functional recovery is achieved. Thus, the increase of neurogenesis in itself is insufficient to promote functional recovery in neurological diseases. Several hypotheses can be raised to explain the limited capacity of the CNS to self-repair. First, the number of new neurons generated is too low to compensate for the neuronal loss. Second, the neurons that are produced may be non-functional because they do not develop into fully mature neurons, they do not develop into the right type of neurons, or they are incapable of integrating into the surviving brain circuitry. Third, the microenvironment of the diseased or injured brain may be toxic for the newly generated neuronal cells. Thus, neurogenesis in the adult CNS elicits only a limited repair capacity in neurological diseases. But the data presented show that the diseased brain has the potential for self-repair even in humans. This has important implications for cellular therapy applied to the adult CNS, and for designing new strategies to treat neurological diseases.

Recent evidence suggests that self-repair mechanisms may operate in the adult rodents' SN [29], the area of the CNS affected in PD, although these data remain the source of controversies [30–32]. If such turnover of dopaminergic neuronal cells was confirmed, progression of the disease would then be determined not only by the rate of degeneration of SN neurons, but also by the efficacy in the formation of new dopamine neurons. Thus, disturbances of the equilibrium between cell genesis and cell death could result in neurodegenerative disorders. Therefore, in PD, neurogenesis might not only be a process for functional recovery, but it may also play a key role in the pathology of the disease. In contrast, a recent study reported that the induction of recurrent seizures following irradiation treatment prevents the seizure-induced increase of neurogenesis in the DG [74]. These data provide a strong argument against a critical role of adult neurogenesis in epileptogenesis. They particularly suggest that newly generated granule-like cells at the hilar/CA3 border are not critical to limbic seizures in pilocarpine-treated rats, although the newly generated granule cells elicit the prominent features of the response to seizures, such as ectopic granule-like cell migration, and abnormal synaptogenesis. Nonetheless, they could be a contributing factor, when present. These data argue against a critical role for neurogenesis in SE. Thus, neurogenesis may have different levels of involvement in neurological diseases. This remains to be thoroughly investigated, as a prerequisite for designing strategy to treat and cure neurological diseases.

Stimulation of neurogenesis might not only serve neuronal regeneration, but might be an attempt by the CNS to compensate for other neuronal functions associated with the disease. For example, in conditions such as AD and epilepsy, which are associated with memory impairment [85,86], the ability of the diseased brain to mobilize new neurons in the hippocampus could have especially important consequences regarding memory function. In both AD and epilepsy, the hippocampus is the most affected brain area, and it has recently been suggested that memory function may depend on hippocampal neurogenesis [77,78]. Thus, the increase of neurogenesis in neurological diseases might also serve cognitive function recovery. Also, patients with neurological diseases, such as AD, epilepsy, HD, and PD, but also those recovering from stroke and injury, are at a greater risk of depression [87–89]. Stress [79] and depression [80,81] reduce granule cell neurogenesis in adult rodents, whereas ischemia stimulates neurogenesis [83]. Thus, the increase in neurogenesis in neurological diseases may also be an attempt by the organism to compensate for these symptoms.

Therapy

In neurodegenerative diseases, dysfunction or loss of specific cells causes patients to present with psychiatric or neurological symptoms. With recent evidence that neurogenesis occurs in the adult brain and that cells with NSC properties can be isolated from the adult brain and cultured in vitro, new opportunities to treat neurodegenerative diseases have emerged. Cell therapeutic interventions might involve both the stimulation of the endogenous neural progenitor cells and cell transplantation.

Stimulation of Endogenous Neural Progenitor Cells

Although the brain does not regenerate following injury and in neurodegenerative diseases, the findings that neurogenesis is stimulated in neurological diseases show that the diseased brain has the potential to self-repair. The process of neurogenesis is regulated by a variety of intrinsic and extrinsic stimuli, including steroid hormones, trophic factors, aging, stresses, and environmental enrichment [79,90–96]. It may be possible to stimulate neurogenesis in the diseased brain in the aim of promoting functional recovery or slowing the disease course. Several studies have reported that environmental enrichment has a beneficial effect in the diseased [97,98] and injured brain [99]. Pharmacological agents and compounds, such as lithium [100], would provide means to stimulate neurogenesis, alone or in combination with trophic factors, steroids, and environmental enrichment [90–96]. Although no data have been reported suggesting that adequate numbers of cells can be generated to repopulate a diseased/injured area and promote functional recovery, strategies designed to enhance neurogenesis could have therapeutic value in neurological diseases.

Transplantation

Cell therapy is a prominent area of investigation in the biomedical field, particularly for the treatment of otherwise incurable neurodegenerative diseases. In this view, both fetal derived cells and NSCs are being proposed as elective sources of brain cells for transplantation. Recent data suggest that the use of fetal cells presents some limitation for transplantation [101], leaving the NSC a model of choice for future therapy. Neural progenitor and stem cells have been transplanted in animal models, and show potent engraftment, proliferation, migration, and neural differentiation [102–106]. Classical neural transplantation approach consists in grafting cells in the proximity of the site of the degeneration or lesion, or into its target area, such as in PD or in focal injuries. In other neurodegenerative diseases, such as AD, HD, and multiple sclerosis, where the degenerative area is widespread, such strategy is not applicable. Because of the property of neural progenitor and stem cells to migrate to tumor sites [107,108] and diseased areas [109], NSC therapy offers a much broader potential to cure neurodegenerative diseases. A recent study has reported that the systemic injection of neural progenitors and stem cells may provide significant clinical benefit in an animal model of multiple sclerosis [109]. Thus, NSCs may provide a therapeutic tool for the treatment of a broad range of neurodegenerative diseases.

Conclusions

The promise of adult stem cell research is as important therapeutically, as for our understanding and knowledge of developmental biology. The recent development in adult neurogenesis and NSCs has directed researchers to investigate whether newly generated neuronal cells were involved in neurological diseases. Taken together, the data reviewed here show that neurogenesis is stimulated in neurological diseases, albeit there is no functional recovery, and progressive cell losses and damages are still occurring. These studies have forced us to rethink and redefine the origins, mechanisms, and treatments for neurological diseases, and it has also forced us to re-evaluate CNS plasticity.

However, the main issues remain to be addressed:

1. Are the newly generated cells induced to proliferate in neurological diseases from the same pool as in adult neurogenesis?
2. What are the mechanisms underlying the increase of neurogenesis in neurological diseases?
3. What are the functions of these newly generated neuronal cells in the diseased and injured brain?
4. How can we promote functional recovery?

The field of adult neurogenesis and NSCs is a challenging one. Future studies will bring new developments and NSC research closer to therapy.

Acknowledgments

Reproduced from: Taupin P. Enhanced neurogenesis following neurological disease. Cell cycle in the central nervous system. Humana Press (2006), pp 195-206, chpt. 15. Copyright (2006), with kind permission from Springer Science+Business Media.

References

[1]   Fukutani Y, Kobayashi K, Nakamura I, Watanabe K, Isaki K, Cairns NJ. Neurons, intracellular and extracellular neurofibrillary tangles in subdivisions of the hippocampal cortex in normal ageing and Alzheimer's disease. *Neurosci Lett* 1995;200:57–60.

[2]   Hardy J, Selkoe DJ. The amyloid hypothesis of Alzheimer's disease: progress and problems on the road to therapeutics. Science 2002;297:353–356. Erratum in: *Science* 2002;297:2209.

[3]   Borchelt DR, Thinakaran G, Eckman CB, et al. Familial Alzheimer's disease-linked presenilin 1 variants elevate Abeta1-42/1-40 ratio in vitro and in vivo. *Neuron* 1996;17:1005–1013.

[4]   Feng R, Rampon C, Tang YP, et al. Deficient neurogenesis in forebrain-specific presenilin-1 knockout mice is associated with reduced clearance of hippocampal memory traces. Neuron 2001;32:911–926. Erratum in: *Neuron* 2002;33:313.

[5]   Lewis J, Dickson DW, Lin WL, et al. Enhanced neurofibrillary degeneration in transgenic mice expressing mutant tau and APP. *Science* 2001;293:1487–1491.

[6]   Haughey NJ, Nath A, Chan SL, Borchard AC, Rao MS, Mattson MP. Disruption of neurogenesis by amyloid beta-peptide, and perturbed neural progenitor cell homeostasis, in models of Alzheimer's disease. *J Neurochem* 2002;6:1509–1524.

[7]   Hsia AY, Masliah E, McConlogue L, et al. Plaque-independent disruption of neural circuits in Alzheimer's disease mouse models. *Proc Natl Acad Sci USA* 1999;96:3228–3233.

[8]   Jin K, Peel AL, Mao XO, et al. Increased hippocampal neurogenesis in Alzheimer's disease. *Proc Natl Acad Sci USA* 2004;101:343–347.

[9]   Wen PH, Shao X, Shao Z, et al. Overexpression of wild type but not an FAD mutant presenilin-1 promotes neurogenesis in the hippocampus of adult mice. *Neurobiol Dis* 2002;10:8–19.

[10] Wen PH, Hof PR, Chen X, et al. The presenilin-1 familial Alzheimer disease mutant P117L impairs neurogenesis in the hippocampus of adult mice. *Exp Neurol* 2004;188:224–237.

[11] Jin K, Galvan V, Xie L, et al. Enhanced neurogenesis in Alzheimer's disease transgenic (PDGF-APPSw, Ind) mice. *Proc Natl Acad Sci USA* 2004;101:13,363–13,367.

[12] Schwab C, Hosokawa M, McGeer PL. Transgenic mice overexpressing amyloid beta protein are an incomplete model of Alzheimer disease. *Exp Neurol* 2004;188:52–64.

[13] Janus C, Westaway D. Transgenic mouse models of Alzheimer's disease. *Physiol Behav* 2001;73: 873–86.

[14] Dodart JC, Mathis C, Bales KR, Paul SM. Does my mouse have Alzheimer's disease? *Genes Brain Behav* 2002;1:142–155.

[15] Haughey NJ, Liu D, Nath A, Borchard AC, Mattson MP. Disruption of neurogenesis in the subventricular zone of adult mice, and in human cortical neuronal precursor cells in culture, by amyloid beta-peptide: implications for the pathogenesis of Alzheimer's disease. *Neuromol Med* 2002;1:125–135.

[16] Wen PH, Friedrich VL, Jr, Shioi J, Robakis NK, Elder GA. Presenilin-1 is expressed in neural progenitor cells in the hippocampus of adult mice. *Neurosci Lett* 2002;318:53–56.

[17] Caille I, Allinquant B, Dupont E, et al. Soluble form of amyloid precursor protein regulates proliferation of progenitors in the adult subventricular zone. *Development* 2004;131:2173–2181.

[18] Yasuoka K, Hirata K, Kuraoka A, He JW, Kawabuchi M. Expression of amyloid precursor protein-like molecule in astroglial cells of the subventricular zone and rostral migratory stream of the adult rat forebrain. *J Anat* 2004;205:135–146.

[19] Sawa A, Tomoda T, Bae BI. Mechanisms of neuronal cell death in Huntington's disease. *Cytogenet Genome Res* 2003;100:287–295.

[20] Li SH, Li XJ. Huntingtin-protein interactions and the pathogenesis of Huntington's disease. *Trends Genet* 2004;20:146–154.

[21] Mangiarini L, Sathasivam K, Seller M, et al. Exon 1 of the HD gene with an expanded CAG repeat is sufficient to cause a progressive neurological phenotype in transgenic mice. *Cell* 1996;87:493–506.

[22] Curtis MA, Penney EB, Pearson AG, et al. Increased cell proliferation and neurogenesis in the adult human Huntington's disease brain. *Proc Natl Acad Sci USA* 2003;100:9023–9027.

[23] Luthi-Carter R, Strand A, Peters NL, et al. Decreased expression of striatal signaling genes in a mouse model of Huntington's disease. *Hum Mol Genet* 2000;9:1259–1271.

[24] Lazic SE, Grote H, Armstrong RJ, et al. Decreased hippocampal cell proliferation in R6/1 Huntington's mice. *Neuroreport* 2004;15:811–813.

[25] White JK, Auerbach W, Duyao MP, et al. Huntingtin is required for neurogenesis and is not impaired by the Huntington's disease CAG expansion. *Nat Genet* 1997;17:404–410.

[26] Tattersfield AS, Croon RJ, Liu YW, Kells AP, Faull RL, Connor B. Neurogenesis in the striatum of the quinolinic acid lesion model of Huntington's disease. *Neuroscience* 2004;127:319–332.

[27] Fernandez-Espejo E. Pathogenesis of Parkinson's disease: prospects of neuroprotective and restorative therapies. *Mol Neurobiol* 2004;29:15–30.

[28] Beal MF. Experimental models of Parkinson's disease. *Nat Rev Neurosci* 2001;2:325–334.

[29] Zhao M, Momma S, Delfani K, et al. Evidence for neurogenesis in the adult mammalian substantia nigra. *Proc Natl Acad Sci USA* 2003;100:7925–7930.

[30] Frielingsdorf H, Schwarz K, Brundin P, Mohapel P. No evidence for new dopaminergic neurons in the adult mammalian substantia nigra. Proc *Natl Acad Sci USA* 2004;101:10,177–10,182.

[31] Lie DC, Dziewczapolski G, Willhoite AR, Kaspar BK, Shults CW, Gage FH. The adult substantia nigra contains progenitor cells with neurogenic potential. *J Neurosci* 2002;22:6639–6649.

[32] Lindvall O, McKay R. Brain repair by cell replacement and regeneration. *Proc Natl Acad Sci USA* 2003;100:7430–7431.

[33] Majak K, Pitkanen A. Do seizures cause irreversible cognitive damage? Evidence from animal studies. *Epilepsy Behav* 2004;5:S35–S44.

[34] Heinemann U, Beck H, Dreier JP, Ficker E, Stabel J, Zhang CL. The dentate gyrus as a regulated gate for the propagation of epileptiform activity. *Epilepsy Res* 1992;7:273–280.

[35] Sloviter RS. Feedforward and feedback inhibition of hippocampal principal cell activity evoked by perforant path stimulation: GABA-mediated mechanisms that regulate excitability in vivo. *Hippocampus* 1991;1:31–40.

[36] Houser CR. Granule cell dispersion in the dentate gyrus of humans with temporal lobe epilepsy. *Brain Res* 1990;535:195–204.

[37] de Lanerolle NC, Kim JH, Robbins RJ, Spencer DD. Hippocampal interneuron loss and plasticity in human temporal lobe epilepsy. *Brain Res* 1989;495:387–95.

[38] Sutula T, Cascino G, Cavazos J, Parada I, Ramirez L. Mossy fiber synaptic reorganization in the epileptic human temporal lobe. *Ann Neurol* 1989;26:321–330.

[39] Represa A, Tremblay E, Ben-Ari Y. Sprouting of mossy fibers in the hippocampus of epileptic human and rat. *Adv Exp Med Biol* 1990;268:419–424.

[40] Babb TL, Kupfer WR, Pretorius JK, Crandall PH, Levesque MF. Synaptic reorganization by mossy fibers in human epileptic fascia dentata. *Neuroscience* 1991;42:351–363.

[41] Ben-Ari Y, Tremblay E, Riche D, Ghilini G, Naquet R. Electrographic, clinical and pathological alterations following systemic administration of kainic acid, bicuculline or pentetrazole: metabolic mapping using the deoxyglucose method with special reference to the pathology of epilepsy. *Neuroscience* 1981;6:1361–1391.

[42] Nadler JV. Kainic acid as a tool for the study of temporal lobe epilepsy. *Life Sci* 1981;29:2031–2042.

[43] Ben-Ari Y. Limbic seizure and brain damage produced by kainic acid: mechanisms and relevance to human temporal lobe epilepsy. *Neuroscience* 1985;14:375–403.

[44] Represa A, Le Gall La Salle G, Ben-Ari Y. Hippocampal plasticity in the kindling model of epilepsy in rats. *Neurosci Lett* 1989;99:345–350.

[45] Cavalheiro EA, Leite JP, Bortolotto ZA, Turski WA, Ikonomidou C, Turski L. Long-term effects of pilocarpine in rats: structural damage of the brain triggers kindling and spontaneous recurrent seizures. *Epilepsia* 1991;32:778–782.

[46] Turski L, Ikonomidou C, Turski WA, Bortolotto ZA, Cavalheiro EA. Cholinergic mechanisms and epileptogenesis. The seizures induced by pilocarpine: a novel experimental model of intractable epilepsy. *Synapse* 1898;3:154–171.

[47] Sloviter RS. "Epileptic" brain damage in rats induced by sustained electrical stimulation of the perforant path. I. Acute electrophysiological and light microscopic studies. *Brain Res Bull* 1983;10:675–697.

[48] Sloviter RS. Decreased hippocampal inhibition and a selective loss of interneurons in experimental epilepsy. *Science* 1987;235:73–76.

[49] Mello LE, Cavalheiro EA, Tan AM, et al. Circuit mechanisms of seizures in the pilocarpine model of chronic epilepsy: cell loss and mossy fiber sprouting. *Epilepsia* 1993;34:985–995.

[50] Cavazos JE, Das I, Sutula TP. Neuronal loss induced in limbic pathways by kindling: evidence for induction of hippocampal sclerosis by repeated brief seizures. *J Neurosci* 1994;14:3106–3121.

[51] Sloviter RS, Dean E, Sollas AL, Goodman JH. Apoptosis and necrosis induced in different hip-pocampal neuron populations by repetitive perforant path stimulation in the rat. *J Comp Neurol* 1996;366:516–533.

[52] Tauck DL, Nadler JV. Evidence of functional mossy fiber sprouting in hippocampal formation of kainic acid-treated rats. *J Neurosci* 1985;5:1016–1022.

[53] Cronin J, Dudek FE. Chronic seizures and collateral sprouting of dentate mossy fibers after kainic acid treatment in rats. *Brain Res* 1988;474:181–184.

[54] Represa A, Ben-Ari Y. Kindling is associated with the formation of novel mossy fibre synapses in the CA3 region. *Exp Brain Res* 1992;92:69–78.

[55] Sloviter RS. Possible functional consequences of synaptic reorganization in the dentate gyrus of kainate-treated rats. *Neurosci Lett* 1992;137:91–96.

[56] Longo BM, Mello LE. Blockade of pilocarpine- or kainate-induced mossy fiber sprouting by cycloheximide does not prevent subsequent epileptogenesis in rats. *Neurosci Lett* 1997;226:163–166.

[57] Longo BM, Mello LE. Supragranular mossy fiber sprouting is not necessary for spontaneous seizures in the intrahippocampal kainate model of epilepsy in the rat. *Epilepsy Res* 1998;32:172–182.

[58] Parent JM, Yu TW, Leibowitz RT, Geschwind DH, Sloviter RS, Lowenstein DH. Dentate granule cell neurogenesis is increased by seizures and contributes to aberrant network reorganization in the adult rat hippocampus. *J Neurosci* 1997;17:3727–3738.

[59] Cameron HA, Woolley CS, McEwen BS, Gould E. Differentiation of newly born neurons and glia in the dentate gyrus of the adult rat. *Neuroscience* 1993;56:337–344.

[60] Bengzon J, Kokaia Z, Elmer E, Nanobashvili A, Kokaia M, Lindvall O. Apoptosis and proliferation of dentate gyrus neurons after single and intermittent limbic seizures. *Proc Natl Acad Sci* USA 1997;94:10,432–10,437.

[61] Gray WP, Sundstrom LE. Kainic acid increases the proliferation of granule cell progenitors in the dentate gyrus of the adult rat. *Brain Res* 1998;790:52–59.

[62] Scharfman HE, Goodman JH, Sollas AL. Granule-like neurons at the hilar/CA3 border after status epilepticus and their synchrony with area CA3 pyramidal cells: functional implications of seizure-induced neurogenesis. *J Neurosci* 2000;20:6144–6158.

[63] Nakagawa E, Aimi Y, Yasuhara O, et al. Enhancement of progenitor cell division in the dentate gyrus triggered by initial limbic seizures in rat models of epilepsy. *Epilepsia* 2000;41:10–18.

[64] Covolan L, Ribeiro LT, Longo BM, Mello LE. Cell damage and neurogenesis in the dentate granule cell layer of adult rats after pilocarpine- or kainate-induced status epilepticus. *Hippocampus* 2000;10:69–80.

[65] Parent JM, Janumpalli S, McNamara JO, Lowenstein DH. Increased dentate granule cell neurogenesis following amygdala kindling in the adult rat. *Neurosci Lett* 1998;247:9–12.

[66] Scott BW, Wang S, Burnham WM, De Boni U, Wojtowicz JM. Kindling-induced neurogenesis in the dentate gyrus of the rat. *Neurosci Lett* 1998;248:73–76.

[67] Jiang W, Wan Q, Zhang ZJ, et al. Dentate granule cell neurogenesis after seizures induced by pentylenetrazol in rats. *Brain Res* 2003;977:141–148.

[68] Ferland RJ, Gross RA, Applegate CD. Increased mitotic activity in the dentate gyrus of the hip-pocampus of adult C57BL/6J mice exposed to the flurothyl kindling model of epileptogenesis. *Neuroscience* 2002;115:669–683.

[69] Parent JM, Valentin VV, Lowenstein DH. Prolonged seizures increase proliferating neuroblasts in the adult rat subventricular zone-olfactory bulb pathway. *J Neurosci* 2002;22:3174–3188.

[70] Huttmann K, Sadgrove M, Wallraff A, et al. Seizures preferentially stimulate proliferation of radial glia-like astrocytes in the adult dentate gyrus: functional and immunocytochemical analysis. *Eur J Neurosci* 2003;18:2769–2778.

[71] Hartfuss E, Galli R, Heins N, Gotz M. Characterization of CNS precursor subtypes and radial glia. *Dev Biol* 2001;229:15–30.

[72] Anthony TE, Klein C, Fishell G, Heintz N. Radial glia serve as neuronal progenitors in all regions of the central nervous system. *Neuron* 2004;41:881–890.

[73] Mohapel P, Ekdahl CT, Lindvall O. Status epilepticus severity influences the long-term outcome of neurogenesis in the adult dentate gyrus. *Neurobiol Dis* 2004;15:196–205.

[74] Parent JM, Tada E, Fike JR, Lowenstein DH. Inhibition of dentate granule cell neurogenesis with brain irradiation does not prevent seizure-induced mossy fiber synaptic reorganization in the rat. *J Neurosci* 1999;19:4508–4519.

[75] Tada E, Parent JM, Lowenstein DH, Fike JR. X-irradiation causes a prolonged reduction in cell proliferation in the dentate gyrus of adult rats. *Neuroscience* 2000;99:33–41.

[76] Ferland RJ, Williams JP, Gross RA, Applegate CD. The effects of brain-irradiation-induced decreases in hippocampal mitotic activity on flurothyl-induced epileptogenesis in adult C57BL/6J mice. *Exp Neurol* 2003;179:71–82.

[77] Gould E, Beylin A, Tanapat P, Reeves A, Shors TJ. Learning enhances adult neurogenesis in the hippocampal formation. *Nat Neurosci* 1999;2:260–265.

[78] Shors TJ, Miesegaes G, Beylin A, Zhao M, Rydel T, Gould E. Neurogenesis in the adult is involved in the formation of trace memories. Nature 2001;410:372–376. Erratum in: *Nature* 2001;414:938.

[79] Gould E, McEwen BS, Tanapat P, Galea LA, Fuchs E. Neurogenesis in the dentate gyrus of the adult tree shrew is regulated by psychosocial stress and NMDA receptor activation. *J Neurosci* 1997;17:2492–2498.

[80] Jacobs BL, Praag H, Gage FH. Adult brain neurogenesis and psychiatry: a novel theory of depression. *Mol Psychiat* 2000;5:262–269.

[81] Santarelli L, Saxe M, Gross C, et al. Requirement of hippocampal neurogenesis for the behavioral effects of antidepressants. *Science* 2003;301:805–809.

[82] Rochefort C, Gheusi G, Vincent JD, Lledo PM. Enriched odor exposure increases the number of newborn neurons in the adult olfactory bulb and improves odor memory. *J Neurosci* 2002;22:2679–2689.

[83] Liu J, Solway K, Messing RO, Sharp FR. Increased neurogenesis in the dentate gyrus after transient global ischemia in gerbils. *J Neurosci* 1998;18:7768–7778.

[84] Dash PK, Mach SA, Moore AN. Enhanced neurogenesis in the rodent hippocampus following traumatic brain injury. *J Neurosci Res* 2001;63:313–319.

[85] Wang R, Dineley KT, Sweatt JD, Zheng H. Presenilin 1 familial Alzheimer's disease mutation leads to defective associative learning and impaired adult neurogenesis. *Neuroscience* 2004;126:305–312.

[86] Kotloski R, Lynch M, Lauersdorf S, Sutula T. Repeated brief seizures induce progressive hippocampal neuron loss and memory deficits. *Prog Brain Res* 2002;135:95–110.

[87] Gilliam FG, Santos J, Vahle V, Carter J, Brown K, Hecimovic H. Depression in epilepsy: ignoring clinical expression of neuronal network dysfunction? *Epilepsia* 2004;45:28–33.

[88] Sawabini KA, Watts RL. Treatment of depression in Parkinson's disease. *Parkinsonism Relat Disord* 2004;10:S37–S41.

[89] Perna RB, Rouselle A, Brennan P. Traumatic brain injury: depression, neurogenesis, and medication management. *J Head Trauma Rehabil* 2003;18:201–203.

[90] Cameron HA, Gould E. Adult neurogenesis is regulated by adrenal steroids in the dentate gyrus. *Neuroscience* 1994;61:203–209.

[91] Craig CG, Tropepe V, Morshead CM, Reynolds BA, Weiss S, van der Kooy D. In vivo growth factor expansion of endogenous subependymal neural precursor cell populations in the adult mouse brain. *J Neurosci* 1996;16:2649–2658.

[92] Kuhn HG, Winkler J, Kempermann G, Thal LJ, Gage FH. Epidermal growth factor and fibroblast growth factor-2 have different effects on neural progenitors in the adult rat brain. *J Neurosci* 1997;17:5820–5829.

[93] Taupin P, Ray J, Fischer WH, et al. FGF-2-responsive neural stem cell proliferation requires CCg, a novel autocrine/paracrine cofactor. *Neuron* 2000;28:385–397.

[94] Kuhn HG, Dickinson-Anson H, Gage FH. Neurogenesis in the dentate gyrus of the adult rat: age-related decrease of neuronal progenitor proliferation. *J Neurosci* 1996;16:2027–2033.

[95] Kempermann G, Kuhn HG, Gage FH. More hippocampal neurons in adult mice living in an enriched environment. *Nature* 1997;386:493–495.

[96] van Praag H, Kempermann G, Gage FH. Running increases cell proliferation and neurogenesis in the adult mouse dentate gyrus. *Nat Neurosci* 1999;2:266–270.

[97] Auvergne R, Lere C, El Bahh B, et al. Delayed kindling epileptogenesis and increased neurogenesis in adult rats housed in an enriched environment. *Brain Res* 2002;954:277–85.

[98] Faverjon S, Silveira DC, Fu DD, et al. Beneficial effects of enriched environment following status epilepticus in immature rats. *Neurology* 2002;59:1356–1364.

[99] Will B, Galani R, Kelche C, Rosenzweig MR. Recovery from brain injury in animals: relative efficacy of environmental enrichment, physical exercise or formal training (1990–2002). *Prog Neurobiol* 2004;72:167–182.

[100] Chen G, Rajkowska G, Du F, Seraji-Bozorgzad N, Manji HK. Enhancement of hippocampal neuro-genesis by lithium. *J Neurochem* 2000;75:1729–1734.

[101] Olanow CW, Goetz CG, Kordower JH, et al. A double-blind controlled trial of bilateral fetal nigral transplantation in Parkinson's disease. *Ann Neurol* 2003;54:403–414.

[102] Suhonen JO, Peterson DA, Ray J, Gage FH. Differentiation of adult hippocampus-derived progenitors into olfactory neurons in vivo. *Nature* 1996;383:624–627.

[103] Fricker RA, Carpenter MK, Winkler C, Greco C, Gates MA, Bjorklund A. Site-specific migration and neuronal differentiation of human neural progenitor cells after transplantation in the adult rat brain. *J Neurosci* 1999;19:5990–6005.

[104] Armstrong RJ, Tyers P, Jain M, et al. Transplantation of expanded neural precursor cells from the developing pig ventral mesencephalon in a rat model of Parkinson's disease. *Exp Brain Res* 2003;151:204–217.

[105] Uchida N, Buck DW, He D, et al. Direct isolation of human central nervous system stem cells. *Proc Natl Acad Sci USA* 2000;97:14,720–14,725.

[106] Fricker-Gates RA, Winkler C, Kirik D, Rosenblad C, Carpenter MK, Bjorklund A. EGF infusion stimulates the proliferation and migration of embryonic progenitor cells transplanted in the adult rat striatum. *Exp Neurol* 2000;165:237–247.

[107] Aboody KS, Brown A, Rainov NG, et al. Neural stem cells display extensive tropism for pathology in adult brain: evidence from intracranial gliomas. Proc Natl Acad Sci USA 2000;97:12,846–12,851. *Erratum in: Proc Natl Acad Sci USA* 2001;98:777.

[108] Brown AB, Yang W, Schmidt NO, et al. Intravascular delivery of neural stem cell lines to target intracranial and extracranial tumors of neural and non-neural origin. *Hum Gene Ther* 2003;14: 1777–1785.

[109] Pluchino S, Quattrini A, Brambilla E, et al. Injection of adult neurospheres induces recovery in a chronic model of multiple sclerosis. *Nature* 2003;422:688–694.

Chapter II

Alzheimer's Disease: Increased Neurogenesis and Possible Disease Mechanisms Related to Neurogenesis

Alzheimer's disease (AD) is a neurodegenerative disease for which there is no cure. Aging is the major contributing factor for the increased risk of developing AD. The risk of developing AD doubles every 5 years after the age of 65 and the disease affects more 30% of individuals of over the age of 80 (Ferri et al. 2006). There are two forms of the disease, the late-onset AD (LOAD) and the early-onset AD (EOAD). LOAD is diagnosed after the age of 65 and most cases of LOAD are sporadic forms of the disease. LOAD is most common form of the disease, it accounts for over 93% of all cases of AD (Burns, Byrne, and Maurer 2002). EOAD is diagnosed at younger than 65 and most cases of EOAD are inherited forms of AD or familial Alzheimer's disease (FAD). It is a rare form of the disease. Genetic, acquired, and environmental risks factors are believed to be causative factors for LOAD, whereas genetic inherited mutations are causal factors for EOAD (Zilka, Ferencik, and Hulin 2006). Among the genetic factors that are established risk factors for LOAD is the presence of certain alleles of the apolipoprotein E gene (ApoE) in the genetic makeup of the individual. These risk factors increase the probability of developing AD. Mutations causative for EOAD concern a number of genes, some of which have been characterized. These genes are referred to as familial Alzheimer genes, among which is the gene of beta-amyloid precursor protein (APP). About 200 families in the world carry genetic mutations that lead to the development of the disease. Rare cases of sporadic form of EOAD occur, with no family history and no identified causal genetic mutations. The diagnosis of AD is primarily performed by symptoms, like cognitive impairments and behavioral changes, and by the assessments of risk factors (Dubois et al. 2007; Patterson et al. 2008). The average life expectancy of patients diagnosed with AD is 8.5 years. Current treatments consist in drug and occupational therapies (Scarpini, Scheltens, and Feldman 2003). Recent advances in adult neurogenesis and neural stem cell (NSC) research open new opportunities for our understanding of and for developing new treatments and cures for AD.

Neurogenesis, the generation of nerve cells, occurs in the adult brain and NSCs reside in the adult central nervous system (CNS) of mammals, including in humans (Gage 2000).

NSCs are the self-renewing multipotent cells that have the ability to give rise to the main phenotypes of the nervous system, nerve cells, astrocytes, and oligodendrocytes. In the adult brain, neurogenesis occurs primarily in two regions, the dentate gyrus (DG) of the hippocampus and the subventricular zone (SVZ) along the ventricles (Eriksson et al. 1998; Taupin 2006; Curtis et al. 2007). In the DG, newly generated neuronal cells in the subgranular zone (SGZ) migrate to the granule cell layer, where they differentiate into granule-like cells and extend axonal projections to the CA3 region of the Ammon's horn (Gould et al. 1998; Taupin 2009, "Characterization"). Newly generated neuronal cells in the anterior part of the SVZ migrate through the rostro-migratory stream to the olfactory bulb, where they differentiate into interneurons (Lois and Alvarez-Buylla 1994; Doetsch and Alvarez-Buylla 1996). It is postulated that newly generated neuronal cells in the adult brain originate from NSCs. Because of their potential to generate the main phenotypes of the nervous system, NSCs represent a promising model for cellular therapy for treating a vast array of neurological diseases and injuries, and particularly neurodegenerative disease like AD (Taupin 2008, "Adult neural stem cells"). The stimulation locally endogenous neural progenitor or stem cells in the adult brain or the transplantation of neural progenitor and stem cells, isolated from the adult brain and propagated *in vitro*, are proposed to repair and restore the degenerated or injured nerve pathways.

The confirmation that adult neurogenesis occurs in the adult brain and NSCs reside in the adult CNS, reveals that the adult brain may be amenable to repair. The contribution of adult neurogenesis and newly generated neuronal cells to the physiopathology and functioning of the nervous system remains the source and center of intense interest and research. Reports show that neurogenesis is enhanced in the brain of patients with AD (Jin, Peel, et al. 2004). Aneuploidy would underlie the process of neurodegeneration and amyloid formation. The process of adult neurogenesis holds the potential to generate populations of cells that are aneuploids, particularly in the hippocampus. Do adult neurogenesis and NSCs contribute to the pathology of neurological diseases like AD? Do adult neurogenesis and newly generated neuronal cells of the adult brain contribute to pathogenesis of AD? In the following sections, we will review and discuss the potential involvement of adult neurogenesis and newly generated neuronal cells of the adult brain in the pathology and pathogenesis of AD.

Etiology and Pathology of Alzheimer's Disease

Alzheimer's disease is a neurodegenerative disease. It is associated initially with the loss of nerve cells in areas of the brain that are vital to memory and other mental abilities, like the enthorhinal cortex, hippocampus, and neocortex. As the disease advances, other regions of the brain are affected, including the medial temporal area, lateral hemisphere, basal forebrain, and locus coeruleus, leading to severe incapacities (Burns et al. 2002). As the disease and neurodegeneration further progress, so do the disabilities and impairments, leading ultimately to death. AD was described by Alois Alzheimer in 1906, who reported first the histopathological features of AD: the presence of amyloid plaques and neurofibrillary tangles in the brain of patients with severe dementia (Alzheimer 1906).

Amyloid Plaques and Neurofibrillary Tangles

Amyloid plaques and neurofibrillary tangles are the hallmarks of AD. Amyloid plaques are extracellular deposits of proteins surrounded by degenerating nerve cells, in the brain of patients with AD (Anderson et al. 2004). They are composed of amyloid fibrils. Amyloid fibrils are aggregates of protein beta-amyloid. Protein beta-amyloid is a 40 amino acid beta-peptide. It is synthesized and secreted by nerve cells, by post-transcriptional maturation of APP (Kang et al. 1987). APP is processed by alpha-, beta- and gamma-secretase enzymes.

Protein beta-amyloid is an amyloidogenic protein. These proteins are soluble in their physiological state. Under pathological conditions, they form insoluble extracellular aggregates or deposits of amyloid fibrils (Serpell, Sunde, and Blake 1997). In physiological conditions, APP is cleaved by the alpha- and gamma-secretase enzymes into a 40 amino acid beta-peptide. Certain pathological conditions, like the presence or expression of amyloid-promoting factors or certain gene mutations, including in *APP*, cause excessive cleavage of APP by the beta- and gamma-secretase enzymes, resulting in an increase production of a 42 amino acid beta-amyloid peptide. This latter form of protein beta-amyloid aggregates into insoluble amyloid deposits particularly in the brain, forming aggregates and deposits of amyloid fibrils.

Amyloid plaques are thought to be the first histological change that occurs in the brain of patients with AD (St. George-Hyslop 2000). The density of amyloid plaques increases as the disease advances. They are distributed throughout the brain of those patients, particularly in the region of degeneration, like the entorhinal cortex, hippocampus, temporal, frontal, and inferior parietal lobes. The role and contribution of amyloid plaques in the pathology of AD remain unclear and the source of controversies. On the one hand, it is proposed that deposits of protein beta-amyloid may be a causative factor of AD. According to according to this hypothesis, referred as amyloid hypothesis, as the amyloid deposits in the brain, brain cells start dying, and the signs and symptoms of the disease begin (Hardy and Selkoe 2002; Meyer-Luehmann et al. 2006). On the other hand, the correlation between the density of amyloid plaques and the severity of the dementia is not clearly established (Terry 1996). The deposit of protein beta-amyloid would be a consequence rather than a cause of AD.

Neurofibrillary tangles are deposits of proteins present inside neuronal cells in the brain of patients with AD. They are composed of hyperphosphorylated tau proteins (Fukutani et al. 1995). Tau protein is a microtubule-associated phosphoprotein. It is involved in the formation of microtubules (Kim, Jensen, and Rebhun 1986). The hyperphosphorylation of tau proteins result in their aggregation and in the breakdown of microtubules (Iqbal et al. 1998). This leads to the formation of neurofibrillary tangles and cell death (Alonso et al. 2001). As the disease advances, the regions of the brain affected expand, leading to severe incapacity and death (Brun and Gustafson 1976).

Genetic Factors and Mutations

There are two forms of the diseases, sporadic and inherited. Most cases of LOAD are sporadic forms of the disease and are diagnosed after the age of 65. EOAD is diagnosed at younger age than 65 and most cases of EOAD are inherited forms of AD. LOAD is believed to be caused by genetic, acquired, and environmental factors, among them the presence of certain alleles in the genetic makeup of the individuals, hypertension and diabetes, and neuroinflammation and oxidative stress (Cankurtaran et al. 2008). The presence of the apolipoprotein E varepsilon 4 allele (ApoE4) is the best established genetic risk factor for LOAD. ApoE is a plasma protein; it participates in the transport of cholesterol and other lipids in the blood (Mahley 1988). There are four major isoforms of the gene coding for ApoE encoded by different alleles in humans, *ApoE*, *ApoE2*, *ApoE3* and *ApoE4*. *ApoE* accounts for the vast majority of causes and risks to develop LOAD: up to 50% of people who have AD have at least one *ApoE4* allele. Neuronal sortilin-related receptor (SORL1) belongs to a family of proteins termed retromer (Raber, Huang, and Ashford 2004). Retromers are involved in intracellular trafficking. Reduced expression of the gene coding for SORL1 (SORL1) is associated with an increase in density of amyloid plaques in the brain and increased risk for LOAD. The variants of *SORL1* may promote AD by suppressing the activity of the gene. This may affect the processing of APP and increase its production (Rogaeva et al. 2007). Other genes have been linked with the occurence of LOAD, among them variants for the genes coding for alpha2-macroglobulin, monoamine oxidase A, myeloperoxidase and cystatin C (*CST3*) (Finckh et al. 2000). These risk factors increase the probability of developing the disease.

So far, three genes have been identified as carrying genetic mutations underlying the development of EOAD. These genes are also known as FAD genes. These genes are the *APP* gene, the presenilin-1 gene (*PSEN1*) and the presenilin-2 gene (*PSEN2*) (Schellenberg 1995). APP is a 695-770 amino acid protein coding for the protein beta-amyloid. The PSEN proteins are components of the gamma-secretase complex. These enzymes play a role in the maturation of APP into the 42 protein beta-amyloid (Nishimura, Yu, and St. George-Hyslop 1999). Mutations in *PSEN1* and *PSEN2* lead to excessive cleavage by gamma-secretase enzyme, resulting in increased production and aggregation of protein beta-amyloid (Newman, Musgrave, and Lardelli 2007). Mutations in these genes almost always result in the individual developing the disease (Hardy 2001).

Aneuploidy

Aneuploidy is an abnormal number of chromosomes in the cells of the body. It is a common cause of genetic disorders. Several studies report that cells of patients with AD elicit aneuploidy, particularly for chromosome 21, 13, and 18. Lymphocytes of patients with LOAD present an elevation in aneuploidy for chromosomes 13 and 21 (Migliore et al. 1999). Preparations of lymphocytes of patients with sporadic and inherited forms of AD elicit a two-fold increase in the incidence of aneuploidy for chromosomes 18 and 21 (Geller and Potter 1999). In regions of degeneration 4–10% of neurons, like the hippocampus, are aneuploids and express proteins of the cell cycle in the brain of patients with AD (Busser, Geldmacher, and Herrup 1998; Yang, Geldmacher, and Herrup 2001). The adult brain contains a substantial number of cells that are aneuploids; estimated at 5–7% of the cells in the brain of adult mice (Rehen et al. 2005). The genetic imbalance in aneuploid cells signifies that they are fated to die (Herrup et al. 2004). The relatively high percentage of aneuploid cells in regions of degeneration in AD brains suggests that they undergo a slow death process. These cells may live in this state for months, possibly up to 1 year (Herrup and Arendt 2002; Yang, Mufson, and Herrup 2003). This supports their involvement in the slow and progressive neurodegenerative process of AD. Cyclin B, the marker of the phase G2 of the cell cycle, is also expressed in neurons in regions of degeneration, particularly the hippocampus, in patients with AD (Vincent, Rosado, and Davies 1996).

In the adult brain, most nerve cells are post-mitotic cells. The characterization of aneuploidy and cyclin B in nerve cells in region of degeneration reveal that cell cycle re-entry and DNA duplication, without cell division, precedes neuronal death in the brain of patients with AD. The deregulation and/or re-expression of proteins of the cell cycle in nerve cells triggering cycle re-entry, with blockage in phase G2, and aneuploidy would underlie the neurodegenerative process and pathogenesis of AD.

Enhanced Neurogenesis

The expression of markers of immature neuronal cells, like doublecortin and polysialylated nerve cell adhesion molecule, is enhanced in the hippocampus, particularly the DG, in the brain of AD patients, most likely with LOAD (Jin, Peel, et al. 2004). In animal models, neurogenesis is decreased in the DG of adult mice deficient for PSEN1 and/or APP, in the DG of adult transgenic mice over expressing variants of APP or PSEN1, and in the DG of adult PDAPP transgenic mice, a mouse model of AD with age-dependent accumulation of protein beta-amyloid (Wen et al. 2002; Donovan et al. 2006; Verret et al. 2007; Zhang et al. 2007; Rodríguez et al. 2008). It is increased in the DG of adult transgenic mice that express the Swedish and Indiana APP mutations (Jin, Galvan, et al. 2004). Mice deficient for or over expressing variants of *APP* or *PSEN*1, and transgenic mice that express the Swedish and Indiana APP mutations, a mutant form of human APP, are transgenic mice that express variants of FAD genes. Transgenic mice deficient for APP and PSEN1 provide information on the activities and functions of the proteins involved in EOAD. They are not representative of complex diseases, like LOAD. They do not represent the disease. The aggregation of protein beta-amyloid affects adult neurogenesis (Heo et al. 2007). It may have adverse effects on neurogenesis during development in transgenic mice for APP, affecting the adult phenotype. In all, the discrepancies of the data observed on adult neurogenesis in autopsies and animal models of AD may originate from the validity of the animal models used in those studies, as representative of AD and to study adult phenotypes (German and Eisch 2004).

The discrepancies of the data observed on adult neurogenesis may also originate from the validity of the protocols used as a paradigm to study adult neurogenesis, like the immunohistochemistry for markers of the cell cycle and for the thymidine analog bromodeoxyuridine (BrdU). Most of the studies conducted in autopsies and animal models of neurological diseases and disorders use either immunoshistochemistry for markers of the cell cycle or the BrdU labeling paradigm, to study and quantify adult neurogenesis *in situ*. Proteins of the cell cycle, like cyclin B-the marker of the phase G2-are expressed in neurons in regions in where neurodegeneration occurs. Some at-risk neurons in regions of degeneration are aneuploids in the brain of patients with AD (Busser, Geldmacher, and Herrup 1998; Yang, Geldmacher, and Herrup 2001). Cell cycle re-entry and DNA duplication, without cell division, precedes neuronal death in degenerating regions of the CNS. This suggests that when using immunohistochemistry for proteins of the cell cycle, to study adult neurogenesis, this paradigm does not allow discriminate between cells undergoing DNA duplication, without cell division, as part of their pathological fate and newly generated neuronal cells (Taupin 2007). BrdU is used for birth dating and monitoring cell proliferation (Miller and Nowakowski 1998). There are pitfalls and limitations over the use of thymidine analogs, and particularly BrdU, for studying neurogenesis (Nowakowski and Hayes 2000; Gould and Gross 2002). BrdU is a thymidine analog. It is not a marker of cell proliferation; it is a marker for DNA synthesis. Studying and quantifying neurogenesis with BrdU require distinguishing cell proliferation and neurogenesis from other events involving DNA synthesis, like DNA repair, abortive cell cycle re-entry and cell cycle re-entry and gene duplication, without cell division, leading to aneuploidy (Taupin 2007). In addition, BrdU has a number of side effects. It is a toxic and mutagenic substance. It alters DNA stability and lengthens the cell cycle. BrdU has mitogenic, transcriptional, and translational effects on cells that incorporate it. It triggers cell death and the formation of teratomes. Hence, data involving the use of immunohistochemistry for proteins of the cell cycle and BrdU labeling, as paradigms for studying adult neurogenesis in neurological diseases and disorders, and particularly in AD, must be carefully assessed, analyzed, and discussed.

In all, AD is a neurodegenerative disease that affect mostly individual over 65 years of age. There are two forms of the disease, sporadic and inherited. It is characterized by widespread neurodegeneration, amyloid deposits and neurofi brillary tangles, aneuploidy and enhanced neurogenesis, though this latter observation remains to be fully established. It is proposed that enhanced neurogenesis may be a result, rather than a cause, of the illness (Taupin 2008, "Adult neurogenesis pharmacology"; Taupin 2008, "Adult neurogenesis and drug therapy"). Enhanced neurogenesis in the DG of the brain with neurological diseases and disorders, particularly neurodegenerative diseases, may contribute to a regenerative attempt, to compensate for the neuronal loss.

Possible Mechanisms Related to Adult Neurogenesis

The confirmation that adult neurogenesis occurs in the adult brain and NSCs reside in the adult CNS not only brings new opportunities for the treatment of AD, but also raises the question of the involvement of adult neurogenesis and newly generated neuronal cells of the adult brain in the etiology and pathogenesis of the disease. Amyloid plaques, neurofibrillary tangles, aneuploidy and enhanced neurogenesis are landmarks of the pathology of AD, but their role and contribution to AD remain to be fully elucidated and established, this particularly in light of and relation to recent developments in adult neurogenesis and NSC research.

Aneuploidy in AD Patients

Aneuploidy may originate from the nondisjunction of chromosomes during mitosis or meiosis. It may originate from cell cycle re-entry with cells undergoing DNA duplication without cell division and from cell fusion (Alvarez-Dolado et al. 2003; Torres, Williams, and Amon 2008). Cells that are the most likely to develop aneuploidy are dividing cells. Lymphocytes of patients with EOAD and LOAD elicit an elevation in aneuploidy for chromosomes for chromosome 13, 18 and 21 (Geller and Potter 1999; Migliore et al. 1999). Hence, the nondisjunction of chromosomes, particularly of chromosomes 13, 18 and 21, in stem cells and/or populations of somatic cells that retain their ability to divide is at the origin of aneuploidy in patients with AD (Potter 1991).

In the adult brain, most nerve cells are post-mitotic. The characterization of cyclin B and aneuploidy in neurons suggests that cells re-entered the cell cycle and underwent DNA replication, but did not complete the cell cycle, in regions of degeneration in the brain of patients with AD (Vincent, Rosado, and Davies 1996; Busser, Geldmacher, and Herrup 1998; Yang, Geldmacher, and Herrup 2001). AD is associated with the loss of nerve cells initially in areas of the brain, like the enthorhinal cortex, hippocampus, and neocortex. As the disease advances, other regions of the brain are affected by neurodegeneration, including the medial temporal area, lateral hemisphere, basal forebrain, and locus coeruleus. The genetic imbalance in aneuploid cells signifies that they are fated to die and that they undergo a slow death process (Yang, Mufson, and Herrup 2003; Herrup et al. 2004). Cell cycle re-entry and DNA replication, without mitosis, is at the origin of aneuploidy in nerve cells of the adult brain. It is an underlying factor in the neurodegenerative process and pathogenesis of AD.

Aneuploidy for Chromosome 21 and Amyloid Deposits

Amyloid plaques are deposits of protein amyloid (Anderson et al. 2004). Deposit of protein amyloid is one of the histopathological features of AD and one the probable cause for the pathogenesis of AD. The gene for APP is located on chromosome 21 (21q21) (Goldgaber et al. 1987; Schellenberg et al. 1992). Cells of patients with AD elicit aneuploidy, particularly for chromosome 21 (Geller and Potter 1999; Migliore et al. 1999). Aneuploidy for chromosome 21 would result in the overexpression of APP and promote the formation of amyloid plaques. In patients with FAD, with mutation of the APP gene, it would result in the overexpression of mutant form of amyloid protein in aneuploid cells and amyloid formation. In patients with the sporadic form of AD, it would result in the overexpression of wild type amyloid protein in aneuploid cells and amyloid formation, under certain conditions or risk factors. According to the amyloid hypothesis, aneuploidy for chromosome 21 would underlie cell death and the pathogenesis of AD.

In support of this contention, Down's syndrome has for pathogenic cause trisomy for the chromosome 21. Patients with Down's syndrome develop, during their thirties and forties, dementia and neuropathology that share some characteristics with AD, particularly with regard to amyloid formation and deposits (Glenner and Wong 1984). Aneuploidy for chromosome 21 would underlie the pathogenesis and pathology of the dementia that occurs in patients with Down's syndrome and AD. Aneuploidy for chromosome 21 has been proposed as one of the mechanisms underlying the formation of amyloid deposits and the pathogenesis of AD and Down's syndrome (Potter 1991). Protein beta-amyloid induces cell cycle re-entry and neuronal death (Chen et al. 2000). Hence, aneuploidy for chromosome 21 in neurons in regions of degeneration would underlie the pathogenesis of AD, not only by promoting the formation of amyloid plaques, but also by promoting cell cycle re-entry and DNA duplication, without cell division, leading to aneuploidy and neuronal cell death.

Aneuploidy for Chromosome 17 and Neurofibrillary Tangles Formation

Neurofibrillary tangles are one of the histopathological features of AD and one the probable cause for cell death in AD. Neurofibrillary tangles are deposits of proteins present inside neuronal cells (Alonso et al. 2001). They are composed of hyperphosphorylated tau proteins (Fukutani et al. 1995). The tau gene is located on chromosome 17 (17q21.1) (Iqbal et al. 1989). Aneuploidy for chromosome 17 would result in the overexpression of tau protein. It would underlie the pathogenesis of AD, by promoting the formation of neurofibrillary tangles and cell death.

Aneuploidy for Chromosomes 1, 14 and 19 and Pathogenesis of AD

The *PSEN1* and *PSEN2* genes carry genetic mutations underlying the development of EOAD (Schellenberg 1995). The PSEN proteins, components of the gamma-secretase complex, play a role in the maturation of APP into protein beta-amyloid (Nishimura, Yu, and St. George-Hyslop 1999). Mutations in *PSEN1* and *PSEN2* lead to excessive cleavage by the gamma-secretase enzyme. This results in increased production and aggregation of protein beta-amyloid, leading to the development of the EOAD (Newman, Musgrave, and Lardelli 2007). The *PSEN1* and *PSEN2* genes are located on chromosome 14 (14q24.3) and 1 (1q31–q42), respectively (Nishimura et al. 1999). The presence the *ApoE4* allele is a genetic risk factor for LOAD. The ApoE gene is located on chromosome 19q13.2. Aneuploidy for chromosomes 1, 14 and 19, and more generally for chromosomes carrying genes involved in the development of AD, including *SORL1* and *CST3* genes, would contribute to the pathogenesis of the disease, EOAD or LOAD, depending on the gene involved in the disease. In support of this contention, people who have two *ApoE4* alleles have a higher risk of being diagnosed with AD, after age of 65 (Strittmatter et al. 1993).

Aneuploidy and Adult Neurogenesis

Neurogenesis occurs in the adult brain and NSCs reside in the adult CNS. In the adult mammalian brain, neurogenesis occurs primarily in the DG and SVZ. The process of adult neurogenesis holds the potential to generate populations of cells that are aneuploids particularly in the neurogenic areas. The nondisjunction of chromosomes during the process of cell division of newly generated progenitor cells of the adult brain could lead to newly generated neuronal cells that are aneuploids or to aneuploid cells that would not proceed with their developmental program (Taupin 2009, "Adult neurogenesis, neural stem cells"; Taupin 2009, "Adult neurogenesis in the pathogenesis") (see figure 4.1).

Hence, neurogenesis could also be a contributing factor of aneuploidy in AD. In the adult brain aneuploidy may therefore originate both from cycle re-entry and DNA duplication, without cell division, in regions of degeneration including the hippocampus, and from the nondisjunction of chromosomes in neural progenitor and stem cells of the adult brain, and their progenies, that retain their ability to divide in neurogenic areas particularly in the hippocampus. This reveals that adult neurogenesis could be an underlying factor in the neurodegenerative process and therefore pathogenesis of AD.

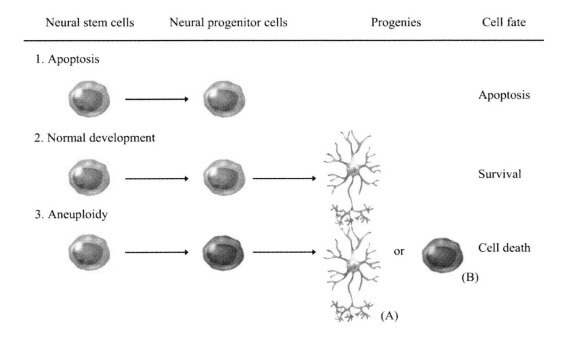

Figure 1. Fate of newly generated neural progenitor and neuronal cells in the adult brain. Neurogenesis occurs in the adult brain, primarily in the DG of the hippocampus and SVZ. Adult NSCs represent a promising model for cellular therapy for treating a vast array of neurological diseases and injuries, and particularly neurodegenerative diseases like AD. The role and contribution of adult neurogenesis and newly generated neuronal cells of the adult brain to the physiopathology and functioning of the nervous system remain to be elucidated. NSCs are the self-renewing multipotent cells that have the ability to give rise to the main phenotypes of the nervous system; they generate of a large number of progenies through an intermediate population of the cells, the neural progenitor cells (in orange). (1.Apoptosis) Cell death is a normally occurring process in the neurogenic zones, as a significant proportion of newly generated cells are believed to undergo apoptosis rather than achieving maturity. (2. Normal development) Newly generated neuronal cells that survive, survive for extended period of time, at least 2 years in humans, and extend functional projections. They may be involved in plasticity and contribute to regenerative attempts in the diseased and injured nervous system, particularly in AD. (3.Aneuploidy) Aneuploidy is landmark of the pathology of AD and contributes to the pathogenesis of the disease. The process of adult neurogenesis holds the potential to generate populations of neural progenitor cells that are aneuploids (in green). The nondisjunction of chromosomes during the process of cell division of newly generated neural progenitor cells of the adult brain could lead to newly generated neuronal cells that are aneuploids (A) or to newly generated neural progenitor cells that are aneuploids and would not proceed with their developmental program (B). The genetic imbalance in aneuploid cells signifies that they are fated to die. Newly generated neuronal cells that are aneuploids and newly generated neural progenitor cells that are aneuploids and would not proceed with their developmental program in the adult brain may contribute to the pathogenesis of AD. They may contribute to the process of neurodegeneration, amyloid deposits and neurofibrillary tangles formation, particularly in the hippocampus. This reveals that adult neurogenesis would not only be beneficial for the adult brain, it may also be involved in the pathogenesis of neurological diseases, particularly in AD.

It is estimated that 0.004% of the granule cell population is generated per day in the DG of adult macaque monkeys (Kornack and Rakic 1999). Despite neurogenesis being an event with relatively low frequency in the adult mammalian brain, the fact that cells that are the most likely to develop aneuploidy are dividing cells and that neurogenesis occurs in the adult hippocampus, a region of the brain particularly and among the first affected in AD, suggests that aneuploidy originating from adult neurogenesis may play a critical role in the process of degeneration and pathogenesis in AD. Such aneuploidy, particularly for chromosomes 17 and 21 and other genes involved in AD, would further contribute to the pathogenesis of AD, by promoting the formation of amyloid deposits and neurofibrillary tangles in the neurogenic areas, particularly the hippocampus. In all, adult neurogenesis may play a critical role in the pathogenesis of AD, in the process of neurodegeneration, amyloid deposits and neurofibrillary tangles formation.

Factors Promoting Aneuploidy in Alzheimer's Disease

Hyperphosphorylation of Tau Protein

Hyperphosphorylated tau protein is a component and promotes the formation of neurofibrillary tangles (Alonso et al. 2001). Tau is a microtubule-associated protein, involved in the formation of microtubules (Kim, Jensen, and Rebhun 1986). The hyperphosphorylation of tau by kinases leads to the dissociation of tau and tubulin, and to the breakdown of microtubles (Iqbal et al. 1998). This causes the disruption in the mitotic spindle, promoting aneuploidy during mitosis. Hyperphosphorylated tau protein may contribute to the pathogenesis of AD, not only by the polymerization and aggregation of tau proteins, resulting in the formation of neurofibrillary tangles and cell death, but also by promoting the nondisjunction of chromosomes and aneuploidy in dividing cells. Hyperphosphorylated tau protein could be a contributing factor in the generation of newly generated neuronal cells that are aneuploids or to newly generated neural progenitor cells that are aneuploids and would not proceed with their developmental program in the adult brain, particularly in the hippocampus (Taupin 2009, "Adult neurogenesis, neural stem cells").

Mutation in PSEN1

The PSEN1 proteins are components of the gamma-secretase complex and play a role in the maturation of APP into protein beta-amyloid (Nishimura, Yu, and St. George-Hyslop 1999). Mutated forms of PSEN1 are detected in the centrosomes and interphase kinetochores of dividing cells. Mutated PSEN1 proteins may be involved in the segragation and migration of chromosomes during cells division (Li et al. 1997). Mutated PSEN1 proteins may contribute to the pathogenesis of EOAD, not only by promoting the formation of deposits of amyloid fibrils, but also by promoting the nondisjunction of chromosomes and aneuploidy in dividing cells (Boeras et al. 2008). Mutated PSEN1 proteins could be a contributing factor in the generation of aneuploid newly generated neuronal cells or to aneuploid newly generated neural progenitor cells that would not proceed with their developmental program in the adult brain, particularly in the hippocampus (Taupin 2009, "Adult neurogenesis, neural stem cells").

Modulation of Adult Neurogenesis

Neurogenesis is modulated in the adult brain, particularly in the hippocampus, by a broad range of environmental, physio- and pathological stimuli and processes, trophic factors/cytokines and drugs (Taupin 2007). The stimulation of neurogenesis in the adult brain may contribute to the generation of newly generated neuronal cells that are aneuploids or to newly generated neural progenitor cells that are aneuploids and would not proceed with their developmental program in the neurogenic regions of the adult brain, particularly the hippocampus. It is reported that neurogenesis is enhanced in the hippocampus, particularly the DG, in the brain of patients with AD (Jin, Peel, et al. 2004). Enhanced neurogenesis in the DG of the brain with neurological diseases and disorders, particularly neurodegenerative diseases, may contribute to a regenerative attempt to compensate for the neuronal loss (Taupin 2008, "Adult neurogenesis pharmacology"). Hence, enhanced neurogenesis in the DG of the brain of patients with AD could be a contributing factor in the generation of newly generated neuronal cells that are aneuploids or of newly generated neural progenitor cells that are aneuploids and would not proceed with their developmental program in the adult brain and therefore could be a contributing factor to the pathogenesis of AD (Taupin 2009, "Adult neurogenesis, neural stem cells").

Oxidative Stress

Oxidative stress is an environmental risk factor for LOAD. Oxidative stress induces cell cycle re-entry and neuronal death (Langley and Ratan 2004). It promotes aneuploidy, particularly for chromosome 17 that carries the tau gene (Ramírez et al. 2000). Oxidative stress may promote the pathogenesis of LOAD, not only by promoting cell cycle re-entry and DNA duplication, without cell division, in the brain, leading to neuronal death and the process neurodegeneration, but also by promoting the generation of aneuploid cells fated to die and the formation of neurofibrillary tangles, leading to cell death (Taupin 2009, "Adult neurogenesis, neural stem cells").

Conclusion and Perspectives

The confirmation, that adult neurogenesis occurs in the adult brain and NSCs reside in the adult CNS of mammals reveals that the adult brain has the potential for self repair. It opens new opportunities for the treatment of a broad range of neurological diseases and injuries, including neurodegenerative diseases like AD, cerebral strokes, and spinal cord injuries. The role and contribution of adult neurogenesis and newly generated neuronal cells to the physio- and pathology of the adult brain remain to be elucidated, particularly in neurodegenerative diseases like AD. Neurogenesis is enhanced in the hippocampus of patients with AD. Though these data remain to be confirmed and validated, it suggests that adult neurogenesis would contribute to a regenerative attempt to compensate for the neuronal loss in AD. Aneuploidy is a landmark of the pathology of AD and contributes to the pathogenesis of the disease. Aneuploidy contributes directly and indirectly to the processes of amyloid deposits, neurofibrillary tangles formation and neurodegeneration in the brain. Cells that are the most likely to develop aneuploidy are dividing cells. Hence, the process of adult neurogenesis holds the potential to generate populations of aneuploid cells particularly in the hippocampus, a region where neurogenesis occurs in the adult brain and that is primarily affected in AD. Newly generated neuronal cells of the adult brain that are aneuploids or newly generated neural progenitor cells that are aneuploids and would not proceed with their developmental program may contribute to the pathogenesis of AD, in the process of neurodegeneration, amyloid deposits, and neurofibrillary tangles formation. This reveals that adult neurogenesis would not only elicit a beneficial effect for the adult brain, but it may also be involved in the pathogenesis of neurological diseases and disorders, particularly in AD. Adult neurogenesis may be the target of new drugs aimed at treating AD, by promoting neuroregeneration and decreasing the risk of the generation of newly generated neuronal cells of the adult brain that are aneuploids or of newly generated neural progenitor cells that are aneuploids and would not proceed with their developmental program in the adult hippocampus. Future studies will aim at characterizing the role and contribution of adult neurogenesis and NSCs in the pathogenesis and pathology of AD and other neurological diseases. Results from such studies will lead to a better understanding of neurological diseases and disorders, and to novel and more effective treatments and cures for these diseases, particularly AD.

Acknowledgments

Reproduced from: Taupin P. Alzheimer's disease: increased neurogenesis and possible disease mechanisms related to neurogenesis. Dementia: Volume II: Science and biology. Praeger Publishers (2011), pp 115-133, chpt. 4. Copyright 2011, with kind permission from Praeger Publishers.

References

Alonso, A., T. Zaidi, M. Novak, I. Grundke-Iqbal, and K. Iqbal. 2001. Hyperphosphorylation induces self-assembly of tau into tangles of paired helical filaments/straight filaments. *Proc Natl Acad Sci USA* 98: 6923–6928.

Alvarez-Dolado, M., R. Pardal, J. M. Garcia-Verdugo, J. R. Fike, H. O. Lee, K. Pfeffer, C. Lois, S. J. Morrison, and A. Alvarez-Buylla. 2003. Fusion of bone-marrow-derived cells with Purkinje neurons, cardiomyocytes and hepatocytes. *Nature* 425: 968–973.

Alzheimer, A. 1906. Uber einen eigenartigen schweren erkrankungsprozeb der hirnrinde. *Neurologisches cenrealblatt* 23: 1129–1136.

Anderson, D. H., K. C. Talaga, A. J. Rivest, E. Barron, G. S. Hageman, and L. V. Johnson. 2004. Characterization of beta amyloid assemblies in drusen: The deposits associated with aging and age-related macular degeneration. *Exp Eye Res* 78: 243–256.

Boeras, D. I., A. Granic, J. Padmanabhan, N. C. Crespo, A. M. Rojiani, and H. Potter. 2008. Alzheimer's presenilin 1 causes chromosome missegregation and aneuploidy. *Neurobiol Aging* 29: 319–328.

Brun, A., and L. Gustafson. 1976. Distribution of cerebral degeneration in Alzheimer's disease: A clinico-pathological study. *Arch Psychiatr Nervenkr 223*: 15–33.

Burns, A., E. J. Byrne, and K. Maurer. 2002. Alzheimer's disease. *Lancet* 360: 163–165.

Busser, J., D. S. Geldmacher, and K. Herrup. 1998. Ectopic cell cycle proteins predict the sites of neuronal cell death in Alzheimer's disease brain. *J Neurosci* 18: 2801–2807.

Cankurtaran, M., B. B. Yavuz, E. S. Cankurtaran, M. Halil, Z. Ulger, and S. Ariogul. 2008. Risk factors and type of dementia: Vascular or Alzheimer? *Arch Gerontol Geriatr* 47: 25–34.

Chen, Y., D. L. McPhie, J. Hirschberg, and R. L. Neve. 2000. The amyloid precursor protein-binding protein APP-BP1 drives the cell cycle through the S-M checkpoint and causes apoptosis in neurons. *J Biol Chem* 275: 8929–8935.

Curtis, M. A., M. Kam, U. Nannmark, M. F. Anderson, M. Z. Axell, C. Wikkelso, S. Holtas, et al. 2007. Human neuroblasts migrate to the olfactory bulb via a lateral ventricular extension. *Science* 315: 1243–1249.

Doetsch, F., and A. Alvarez-Buylla. 1996. Network of tangential pathways for neuronal migration in adult mammalian brain. *Proc Natl Acad Sci USA* 93: 14895–14900.

Donovan, M. H., U. Yazdani, R. D. Norris, D. Games, D. C. German, and A. J. Eisch. 2006. Decreased adult hippocampal neurogenesis in the PDAPP mouse model of Alzheimer's disease. *J Comp Neurol* 495: 70–83.

Dubois, B., H. H. Feldman, C. Jacova, S. T. DeKosky, P. Barberger-Gateau, J. Cummings, A. Delacourte, et al. 2007. Research criteria for the diagnosis of Alzheimer's disease: Revising the NINCDS–ADRDA criteria. *Lancet Neurol* 6: 734–746.

Eriksson, P. S., E. Perfi lieva, T. Bjork-Eriksson, A. M. Alborn, C. Nordborg, D. A. Peterson, and F. H. Gage. 1998. Neurogenesis in the adult human hippocampus. *Nat Med* 4: 1313–1317.

Ferri, C. P., M. Prince, C. Brayne, H. Brodaty, L. Fratiglioni, M. Ganguli, K. Hall, et al. 2006. The role of oxidative stress in the pathogenesis of Alzheimer's disease. *Bratisl Lek Listy* 107: 384–394.

Finckh, U., H. von der Kammer, J. Velden, T. Michel, B. Andresen, A. Deng, J. Zhang, et al. 2000. Genetic association of a cystatin C gene polymorphism with late-onset Alzheimer disease. *Arch Neurol* 57: 1579–1583.

Fukutani, Y., K. Kobayashi, I. Nakamura, K. Watanabe, K. Isaki, and N. J. Cairns. 1995. Neurons, intracellular and extra cellular neurofi brillary tangles in subdivisions of the hippocampal cortex in normal ageing and Alzheimer's disease. Neurosci Lett 200: 57–60.

Gage, F. H. 2000. Mammalian neural stem cells. *Science* 287: 1433–1438.

Geller, L. N., and H. Potter. 1999. Chromosome missegregation and trisomy 21 mosaicism in Alzheimer's disease. *Neurobiol Dis* 6: 167–179.

German, D. C., and A. J. Eisch. 2004. Mouse models of Alzheimer's disease: Insight into treatment. *Rev Neurosci* 15: 353–369.

Glenner, G. G., and C. W. Wong. 1984. Alzheimer's disease and Down's syndrome: Sharing of a unique cerebrovascular amyloid fi bril protein. *Biochem Biophys Res Commun* 122: 1131–1135.

Goldgaber, D., M. I. Lerman, O. W. McBride, U. Saffi otti, and D. C. Gajdusek. 1987. Characterization and chromosomal localization of a cDNA encoding brain amyloid of Alzheimer's disease. *Science* 235: 877–880.

Gould, E., and C. G. Gross. 2002. Neurogenesis in adult mammals: Some progress and problems. *J Neurosci* 22: 619–623.

Gould, E., P. Tanapat, B. S. McEwen, G. Flugge, and E. Fuchs. 1998. Proliferation of granule cell precursors in the dentate gyrus of adult monkeys is diminished by stress. *Proc Natl Acad Sci USA* 95: 3168–3171.

Hardy, J. 2001. The genetic causes of neurodegenerative diseases. *J Alzheimers Dis* 3: 109–116.

Hardy, J., and D. J. Selkoe. 2002. The amyloid hypothesis of Alzheimer's disease: Progress and problems on the road to therapeutics. Science 297: 353–356. Erratum in: *Science* 297: 2209.

Heo, C., K. A. Chang, H. S. Choi, H. S. Kim, S. Kim, H. Liew, J. A. Kim, E. Yu, J. Ma, and Y. H. Suh. 2007. Effects of the monomeric, oligomeric, and fibrillar Abeta42 peptides on the proliferation and differentiation of adult neural stem cells from subventricular zone. *J Neurochem* 102: 493–500.

Herrup, K., and T. Arendt. 2002. Re-expression of cell cycle proteins induces neuronal cell death during Alzheimer's disease. *J Alzheimers Dis* 4: 243–247.

Herrup, K., R. Neve, S. L. Ackerman, and A. Copani. 2004. Divide and die: Cell cycle events as triggers of nerve cell death. *J Neurosci* 24: 9232–9239.

Iqbal, K., A. C. Alonso, C. X. Gong, S. Khatoon, J. J. Pei, J. Z. Wang, and I. Grundke-Iqbal. 1998. Mechanisms of neurofi brillary degeneration and the formation of neurofibrillary tangles. *J Neural Transm Suppl* 53: 169–180.

Iqbal, K., I. Grundke-Iqbal, A. J. Smith, L. George, Y. C. Tung, and T. Zaidi. 1989. Identifi cation and localization of a tau peptide to paired helical filaments of Alzheimer disease. *Proc Natl Acad Sci USA* 86: 5646–5650.

Jin, K., V. Galvan, L. Xie, X. O. Mao, O. F. Gorostiza, D. E. Bredesen, and D. A. Greenberg. 2004. Enhanced neurogenesis in Alzheimer's disease transgenic (PDGF-APPSw, Ind) mice. *Proc Natl Acad Sci USA* 101: 13363–13367.

Jin, K., A. L. Peel, X. O. Mao, L. Xie, B. A. Cottrell, D. C. Henshall, and D. A. Greenberg. 2004. Increased hippocampal neurogenesis in Alzheimer's disease. *Proc Natl Acad Sci USA* 101: 343–347.

Kang, J., H. G. Lemaire, A. Unterbeck, J. M. Salbaum, C. L. Masters, K. H. Grzeschik, G. Multhaup, K. Beyreuther, and B. Müller-Hill. 1987. The precursor of Alzheimer's disease amyloid A4 protein resembles a cell-surface receptor. *Nature* 325: 733–736.

Kim, H., C. G. Jensen, and L. I. Rebhun. 1986. The binding of MAP-2 and tau on brain microtubules in vitro: Implications for microtubule structure. *Ann NY Acad Sci* 466: 218–239.

Kornack, D. R., and P. Rakic. 1999. Continuation of neurogenesis in the hippocampus of the adult macaque monkey. *Proc Natl Acad Sci USA* 96: 5768–5773.

Langley, B., and R. R. Ratan. 2004. Oxidative stress-induced death in the nervous system: Cell cycle dependent or independent? *J Neurosci Res* 77: 621–629.

Li, J., M. Xu, H. Zhou, J. Ma, and H. Potter. 1997. Alzheimer presenilins in the nuclear membrane, interphase kinetochores, and centrosomes suggest a role in chromosome segregation. *Cell* 90: 917–927.

Lois, C., and A. Alvarez-Buylla. 1994. Long-distance neuronal migration in the adult mammalian brain. *Science* 264: 1145–1148.

Mahley, R. W. 1988. Apolipoprotein E: Cholesterol transport protein with expanding role in cell biology. *Science* 240: 622–630.

Meyer-Luehmann, M., J. Coomaraswamy, T. Bolmont, S. Kaeser, C. Schaefer, E. Kilger, A. Neuenschwander, et al. 2006. Exogenous induction of cerebral beta-amyloidogenesis is governed by agent and host. *Science* 313: 1781–1784.

Migliore, L., N. Botto, R. Scarpato, L. Petrozzi, G. Cipriani, and U. Bonuccelli. 1999. Preferential occurrence of chromosome 21 malsegregation in peripheral blood lymphocytes of Alzheimer disease patients. *Cytogenet Cell Genet* 87: 41–46.

Miller, M. W., and R. S. Nowakowski. 1988. Use of bromodeoxyuridine-immunohistochemistry to examine the proliferation, migration and time of origin of cells in the central nervous system. *Brain Res* 457: 44–52.

Newman, M., F. I. Musgrave, and M. Lardelli. 2007. Alzheimer disease: Amyloidogenesis, the presenilins and animal models. *Biochim Biophys Acta* 1772: 285–297.

Nishimura, M., G. Yu, P. H. St. George-Hyslop. 1999. Biology of presenilins as causative molecules for Alzheimer disease. *Clin Genet* 55: 219–225.

Nowakowski, R. S., and N. L. Hayes. 2000. New neurons: Extraordinary evidence or extraordinary conclusion? *Science* 288: 771.

Patterson, C., J. W. Feightner, A. Garcia, G. Y. Hsiung, C. MacKnight, and A. D. Sadovnick. 2008. Diagnosis and treatment of dementia: 1. Risk assessment and primary prevention of Alzheimer disease. *CMAJ* 178: 548–556.

Potter, H. 1991. Review and hypothesis: Alzheimer disease and Down syndrome-chromosome 21 nondisjunction may underlie both disorders. *Am J Hum Genet* 48: 1192–1200.

Raber, J., Y. Huang, and J. W. Ashford. 2004. ApoE genotype accounts for the vast majority of AD risk and AD pathology. *Neurobiol Aging* 25: 641–650.

Ramírez, M. J., S. Puerto, P. Galofré, E. M. Parry, J. M. Parry, A. Creus, R. Marcos, and J. Surrallés. 2000. Multicolour FISH detection of radioactive iodineinduced 17cen-p53 chromosomal breakage in buccal cells from therapeutically exposed patients. *Carcinogenesis* 21: 1581–1586.

Rehen, S. K., Y. C. Yung, M. P. McCreight, D. Kaushal, A. H. Yang, B. S. Almeida, M. A. Kingsbury, et al. 2005. Constitutional aneuploidy in the normal human brain. *J Neurosci* 25: 2176–2180.

Rodríguez, J. J., V. C. Jones, M. Tabuchi, S. M. Allan, E. M. Knight, F. M. LaFerla, S. Oddo, and A. Verkhratsky. 2008. Impaired adult neurogenesis in the dentate gyrus of a triple transgenic mouse model of Alzheimer's disease. *PLoS ONE* 3: e2935.

Rogaeva, E., Y. Meng, J. H. Lee, Y. Gu, T. Kawarai, F. Zou, T. Katayama, et al. 2007. The neuronal sortilin-related receptor SORL1 is genetically associated with Alzheimer disease. *Nat Genet* 39: 168–177.

Scarpini, E., P. Scheltens, and H. Feldman. 2003. Treatment of Alzheimer's disease: Current status and new perspectives. *Lancet Neurol* 2: 539–547.

Schellenberg, G. D. 1995. Genetic dissection of Alzheimer disease, a heterogeneous disorder. *Proc Natl Acad Sci* USA 92: 8552–8559.

Schellenberg, G. D., T. D. Bird, E. M. Wijsman, H. T. Orr, L. Anderson, E. Nemens, J. A. White, et al. 1992. Genetic linkage evidence for a familial Alzheimer's disease locus on chromosome 14. *Science* 258: 668–671.

Serpell, L. C., M. Sunde, and C. C. Blake. 1997. The molecular basis of amyloidosis. *Cell Mol Life Sci* 53: 871–887.

St. George-Hyslop, P. H. 2000. Piecing together Alzheimer's. Sci Am 283: 76–83.

Strittmatter, W. J., A. M. Saunders, D. Schmechel, M. Pericak-Vance, J. Enghild, G. S. Salvesen, and A. D. Roses. 1993. Apolipoprotein E: High-avidity binding to beta-amyloid and increased frequency of type 4 allele in late-onset familial Alzheimer disease. *Proc Natl Acad Sci USA* 90: 1977–1981.

Taupin, P. 2006. Neural progenitor and stem cells in the adult central nervous system. Ann *Acad Med Singapore* 35: 814–817.

Taupin, P. 2007. BrdU immunohistochemistry for studying adult neurogenesis: Paradigms, pitfalls, limitations, and validation. *Brain Res Rev* 53: 198–214.

Taupin, P. 2008. Adult neural stem cells: A promising candidate for regenerative therapy in the CNS. *Intl J Integ Biol* 2: 85–94.

Taupin, P. 2008. Adult neurogenesis pharmacology in neurological diseases and disorders. *Expert Rev Neurother* 8: 311–320.

Taupin, P. 2008. Adult neurogenesis and drug therapy. *Cent Nerv Syst Agents Med Chem 8:* 198–202.

Taupin, P. 2009. Characterization and isolation of synapses of newly generated neuronal cells of the adult hippocampus at early stages of neurogenesis. *J Neurodegener Regen* 2: 9–17.

Taupin, P. 2009. Adult neurogenesis, neural stem cells and Alzheimer's disease: Developments, limitations, problems and promises. *Curr Alzheimer Res* 6: 461–470.

Taupin, P. 2009. Adult neurogenesis in the pathogenesis of Alzheimer's disease. *J Neurodegener Regen* 2: 6–8.

Taupin, P. 2010. A dual activity of ROS and oxidative stress on adult neurogenesis and Alzheimer's disease. *Cent Nerv Syst Agents Med Chem* 10: 16–21.

Terry, R. D. 1996. The pathogenesis of Alzheimer disease: An alternative to the amyloidhypothesis. *J Neuropathol Exp Neurol* 55: 1023–1025.

Torres, E. M., B. R. Williams, and A. Amon. 2008. Aneuploidy: Cells losing their balance. *Genetics* 179: 737–746.

Verret, L., J. L. Jankowsky, G. M. Xu, D. R. Borchelt, and C. Rampon. 2007. Alzheimer's-type amyloidosis in transgenic mice impairs survival of newborn neurons derived from adult hippocampal neurogenesis. *J Neurosci* 27: 6771–6780.

Vincent, I., M. Rosado, and P. Davies. 1996. Mitotic mechanisms in Alzheimer's disease? *J Cell Biol* 132: 413–425.

Wen, P. H., X. Shao, Z. Shao, P. R. Hof, T. Wisniewski, K. Kelley, V. L. Friedrich Jr., et al. 2002. Overexpression of wild type but not an FAD mutant presenilin-1 promotes neurogenesis in the hippocampus of adult mice. *Neurobiol Dis* 10: 8–19.

Yang, Y., D. S. Geldmacher, and K. Herrup. 2001. DNA replication precedes neuronal cell death in Alzheimer's disease. *J Neurosci* 21: 2661–2668.

Yang, Y., E. J. Mufson, and K. Herrup. 2003. Neuronal cell death is preceded by cell cycle events at all stages of Alzheimer's disease. *J Neurosci* 23: 2557–2563.

Zhang, C., E. McNeil, L. Dressler, and R. Siman. 2007. Long-lasting impairment in hippocampal neurogenesis associated with amyloid deposition in a knock-in mouse model of familial Alzheimer's disease. *Exp Neurol* 204: 77–87.

Zilka, N., M. Ferencik, and I. Hulin. 2006. Neuroinflammation in Alzheimer's disease: Protector or promoter? *Bratisl Lek Listy* 107: 374–383.

Chapter III

Neurogenesis, NSCs, Pathogenesis and Therapies for Alzheimer's Disease

Abstract

Neurogenesis occurs in the adult brain and neural stem cells (NSCs) reside in the adult central nervous system (CNS) of mammals. Adult NSCs offer tremendous potential for cellular therapy for the treatment of neurological diseases and injuries, particularly of Alzheimer's disease (AD). The contribution of newly generated neuronal cells of the adult brain to the functioning of the nervous system remains to be elucidated. Neurogenesis is enhanced in the brain of patients with AD. Enhanced neurogenesis would contribute to regenerative attempts in AD, to compensate for the neuronal loss. Adult neurogenesis holds the potential to generate aneuploid cells, a landmark of AD pathology. Aneuploid newly generated neuronal cells in the adult brain would contribute to the pathogenesis of AD. Adult neurogenesis would not only be beneficial, but also detrimental for patients with AD. We will review and discuss the potential of adult NSCs for the treatment of AD and their contribution to the pathogenesis of the disease, as well as the development of novel drugs and therapies for treating AD.

Abbreviations

AD: Alzheimer's disease;
ApoE4:   apolipoprotein E varepsilon 4 allele;
APP: amyloid precursor protein;
BrdU: Bromodeoxyuridine;
CNS: central nervous system;
DG: dentate gyrus;
EOAD: early onset AD;
FAD: familial Alzheimer's disease;
EOAD: early onset AD;
NSCs: neural stem cells;

PSEN-1:   presenilin-1;
PSEN-2:   presenilin-2;
RMS: rostro-migratory stream;
SGZ: subgranular zone;
SVZ: subventricular zone

Introduction

Neurogenesis occurs in discrete regions of the adult mammalian brain, in various species including humans [1-3]. Newly generated neuronal would originate for a pool of residual stem cells [4]. The confirmation that neurogenesis occurs in the adult brain and NSCs reside in the adult CNS has tremendous implications for our understanding of the development and of the physio- and pathology of the nervous system, and for therapy. The adult brain has the potential for self-repair [5]. The contribution of adult neurogenesis and newly generated neuronal cells of the adult brain to the physio- and pathology remains to be elucidated and adult NSCs have yet to be brought to therapy.

AD is the most common form of senile dementia. It is a neurodegenerative disease characterized by memory and cognitive deficits, amyloid deposits, neurofibrillary tangles, neurodegeneration and aneuploidy, leading to severe incapacity and death [6]. Reports show that neurogenesis is enhanced in the brain of patients with AD [7]. It is proposed that enhanced neurogenesis in the brain of AD patients would represent a regenerative attempt to compensate for the neuronal loss. The process of adult neurogenesis holds the potential to generate populations of cells that are aneuploid, particularly in the neurogenic regions [8]. Aneuploid newly generated neuronal cells in the adult brain would contribute to the pathogenesis of AD. Hence, adult neurogenesis might have a dual role in AD. This has tremendous implication for our understanding of AD and for therapy.

Adult Neurogenesis and Neural Stem Cells

Neurogenesis in the Adult Brain of Mammals

Neurogenesis occurs throughout adulthood in the mammalian brain, primarily in the subventricular zone (SVZ) along the ventricles and in the dentate gyrus (DG) of the hippocampus, in various species including humans [1-5]. Newly generated neuronal cells, in the anterior part of the SVZ, migrate through the rostro-migratory stream (RMS) to the olfactory bulb, where they differentiate into olfactory interneurons [9, 10]. In the DG, newly generated neuronal cells in the subgranular zone (SGZ), a layer beneath the granular layer, migrate to the granule cell layer, where they differentiate into neuronal cells of the granular layer and extend axonal projections to the CA3 region of the Ammon's horn [11-13]. Newly generated neuronal cells in the DG establish synaptic contacts and functional connections with neighboring and target cells [14-16]. It is estimated that, in rodents (mice), it takes approximately 15 days for neural progenitor cells of the SVZ to migrate through the RMS, a distance of 3 to 5 mm, and to differentiate into olfactory interneurons, and approximately 4 weeks for newly generated neuronal cells of the SGZ to migrate to the granule cell layer of the DG and to differentiate into granule-like cells [10, 12]. Newly generated neuronal cells in the adult hippocampus survive for extended period of time, at least 2 years in humans [1].

The SVZ harbors the largest pool of dividing neural progenitor cells of the adult brain [17, 18]. The number of newly generated neuronal cells per day in the adult brain is relatively low, particularly in the DG. In mice, the number of newly generated neuronal cells per day in the DG is estimated at 9,000 new neuronal cells, or about 0.1 percent of the granule cell population [19, 20]. In adult macaque monkey, the number of newly generated neuronal cells per day in the DG is estimated at 0.004 percent of the granule cell population [21]. Neurogenesis has been reported to occur in other areas of the adult brain, like the CA1 region of the hippocampus, neocortex, striatum, albeit at lower level [22-24].

Hence, neurogenesis occurs in the adult brain. It is a functional neurogenesis and a rare event. Newly generated neuronal cells of the adult brain that survive and extend axonal projections to their target cells may replace nerve cells born during development.

Neural Progenitor and Stem Cells *In Vitro*

NSCs are the self-renewing multipotent cells that generate, through a transient amplifying population of cells, the main cell types of the nervous system: nerve cells, astrocytes and oligodendrocytes [4, 5]. Self-renewing multipotent NSCs have been isolated and characterized *in vitro*, from various regions of the adult brain, including the SVZ, hippocampus and spinal cord, and from various mammalian species, including from human biopsies and *post-mortem* tissues [25-29]. The isolation and characterization of neural and progenitor cells from the adult brain reveal that NSCs reside in the adult CNS and that it has the potential for self-repair. Adult-derived neural progenitor and stem cells also provide a source of tissue that may be used for cellular therapy, for transplantation.

Stem cells are defined by the following main attributes: i) self-renewal over an extended period of time, ii) generation of a large number of differentiated progenies and iii) regeneration of the tissue following injury. Progenitor cells are cells that do not fulfill the attributes of stem cells [30]. One of the limitations of the established protocols to derive self-renewing multipotent NSCs *in vitro* is that they lead to heterogeneous cultures of neural progenitor and stem cells. After 4 days *in vitro*, 62 percent of the adult derived-neural progenitor and stem cells in culture originate from 23 percent of the plated cells, revealing the existence of different populations of cells with different properties of growth in the culture. Overtime the fast-dividing neural progenitor and stem cells represent a majority of the cells in culture reflecting the heterogeneity of adult derived-neural progenitor and stem cells *in vitro* [31]. A second limitation of neural progenitor and stem cells *in vitro*, but also *in vivo*, is the lack of specific markers of NSCs. Molecular markers, like the intermediate filament nestin, the transcription factors sox-2, oct-3/4 and the RNA binding protein Musashi 1, are expressed by neural progenitor and stem cells of the adult brain *in vitro* and *in vivo*. However, they are also expressed by other cell types in the brain, like glial cells and reactive astrocytes, and in gliomas [32-37]. Hence, adult NSCs remain elusive and the heterogeneity of the established protocols to derive self-renewing multipotent NSCs *in vitro* limits their potential therapeutic use.

Modulation of Adult Neurogenesis *In Vivo*

Neurogenesis is modulated in the adult brain, particularly in the hippocampus. It is modulated by a broad range of environmental stimuli, physio- and pathological conditions, trophic factors/cytokines, neurotransmitters and drugs, including enriched environment, learning and memory tasks, physical activity, AD and epilepsy [38]. Environmental enrichment, learning and memory tasks and physical activity stimulate hippocampal neurogenesis in adult rodents [19, 39-41]. Neurogenesis is enhanced in the adult hippocampus of animal models of epilepsy [42], strokes [43] and traumatic brain injuries [44]. It is enhanced in the SVZ and hippocampus in the brain of patients with Huntington's disease and AD, respectively [7, 45]. This suggests that neurogenesis in the adult brain is involved in various physio- and pathological conditions and processes of the nervous system, including neurological diseases and pharmacology [46]. The role and contribution of newly generated neuronal cells of the adult brain to these processes remains to be elucidated. Newly generated neuronal cells of the adult brain would contribute to the plasticity of the nervous system and regenerative attempts after injuries [47, 48].

Bromodeoxyuridine (BrdU)-labeling and immunohistochemistry for markers of the cell cycle are the main methods used for studying cell division and neurogenesis in the adult brain of rodents and primates. BrdU is a thymidine analog used for birth dating and monitoring cell proliferation [49]. It is a mutagenic and toxic substance. As a thymidine analog, it is a marker of DNA synthesis, not of cell proliferation. Drug treatments and various physio- and pathological conditions affect the cerebral flow and the permeability of the blood-brain barrier and the availability of BrdU in the brain [50-52]. Markers of the cell cycle, like proliferating nuclear antigen, Ki-67 and phosphorylated histone H3, reveal that quiescent cells have re-entered the cell cycle and resumed DNA synthesis, but does reveal whether they have completed the cell cycle. Hence, there are limitations and pitfalls over the use of BrdU-labeling and immunohistochemistry for markers of the cell cycle to study cell proliferation and neurogenesis [53, 54]. Studying neurogenesis with BrdU-labeling and immunohistochemistry for markers of the cell cycle requires distinguishing cell proliferation and neurogenesis from other events involving DNA synthesis and cell cycle re-entry, like abortive cell cycle re-entry, leading to apoptosis, and gene duplication, without cell division, leading to aneuploidy [55]. Therefore, studies involving BrdU-labeling and immunohistochemistry for markers of the cell cycle, for studying adult neurogenesis must be carefully analyzed and discussed.

Cellular Therapy

Cellular therapy is the replacement of tissues by new ones. Because of their potential to generate the main phenotypes of the nervous system, NSCs hold the potential to treat and cure a broad range of neurological diseases and injuries, particularly neurodegenerative diseases, like AD and Parkinson's disease, cerebral strokes and spinal cord injuries. The confirmation that adult neurogenesis occurs in the adult brain and NSCs reside in the adult CNS opens new opportunities to repair and restore the damaged or degenerated nervous system: the stimulation of endogenous neural progenitor or stem cells and the transplantation of adult-derived neural progenitor and stem cells [3, 4, 5, 48] (Table 1).

Table 1. Potential therapeutic approaches for the treatment of Alzheimer's disease

Cellular therapy	Stimulation/Transplantation	Therapy
Endogenous neural progenitor or stem cells	Local	Regeneration
	SVZ	Regeneration/Reverse deficits
	Hippocampus	Reverse deficits
Adult-derived neural progenitor and stem cells	Intracerebral	Regeneration
	Intracerebral	Regeneration
Pharmacology	Target	Therapy
Drugs	Newly generated neuronal cells	Reverse deficits/Regeneration
	Aneuploid newly generated neuronal cells	Prevent deleterious effects

The confirmation that adult neurogenesis occurs in the adult brain and NSCs reside in the adult CNS opens new opportunities to repair and restore the damaged or degenerated nervous system: the stimulation of endogenous neural progenitor or stem cells and the transplantation of adult-derived neural progenitor and stem cells. Neural progenitor and stem cells of the SVZ may be stimulated to repair and restore distant brain regions through their migration to the sites of degenerations and injuries. The modulation of adult neurogenesis may be applied to promote the regenerative and recovery processes, as well as to reverse deficits, associated particularly with the hippocampus. Adult-derived neural progenitor and stem cells may be transplanted in local areas of the adult brain. Intravenous injection provides a strategy for delivering neural progenitor and stem cells in the adult CNS applicable for neurological diseases and injuries, with widespread neurodegeneration or damages, like in AD. Adult neurogenesis and newly generated neuronal cells of the adult brain are the target of drugs used for treating neurological diseases and disorders and contribute to their activities. Drugs targeting the newly generated neuronal cells of the adult brain and adult neurogenesis carry the risk of promoting the generation of aneuploid neuronal cells in the adult brain. Therapeutic strategies will aim at discovering and developing novel drugs that specifically target the newly generated neuronal cells of the adult brain to compensate or reverse deficits, particularly associated with the hippocampus. Such strategy will involve limiting the potential deleterious effects of the generation of aneuploid neuronal cells, without disrupting the regenerative capacity of adult neurogenesis.

Neural progenitor and stem cells of the adult brain may be stimulated locally, by trophic factors or cytokines, to repair and restore the degenerated or injured nerve pathways. Alternatively, new neuronal cells are generated at sites of degeneration in the diseased brain and after CNS injuries, like in Huntington's disease and in experimental models of cerebral strokes. They originate from the SVZ. They migrate partially through the RMS to the sites of degenerations and injuries [56, 57]. Neural progenitor and stem cells of the SVZ may be stimulated to repair and restore distant brain regions through their migration to the sites of degenerations and injuries. Adult neurogenesis is modulated in discrete regions of the adult brain, the hippocampus and SVZ, by a broad range of environmental, physio- and pathological stimuli and processes, by trophic factors/cytokines and drugs [38]. The modulation of adult neurogenesis may be applied to promote the regenerative and recovery processes, as well as to reverse deficits, associated with those areas of the brain, particularly the hippocampus (Table 1).

Adult-derived neural progenitor and stem cells may be transplanted in local areas of the adult brain, to repair and restore the degenerated or injured nerve pathways. Alternatively, adult-derived neural progenitor and stem cells administered intravenously migrate to diseased and injured sites of the brain [58, 59]. Intravenous administration of neural progenitor and stem cells is a non-invasive procedure for transplantation, particularly promising to deliver neural progenitor and stem cells in the CNS, for the treatment of brain diseases and tumors. The intracerebral transplantation of neural progenitor and stem cells may be applicable to treat neurological diseases and injuries for which the neurodegeneration or the damages are not widespread, like Parkinson's disease. It may not be applicable for the treatment of neurological diseases and injuries, with multiples site of neurodegeneration or damages, like AD. In contrast, intravenous injection provides a strategy for delivering neural progenitor and stem cells in the adult CNS applicable for neurological diseases and injuries, with widespread neurodegeneration or damages, like in AD and multiple sclerosis [59].

Adult NSCs that have limited ethical and political constraints offer a promising model and a model of choice for cellular therapy. However, there are limitations over the use of adult NSCs for cellular therapy. First, the heterogeneity of established protocols to isolate and propagate, *in vitro*, neural progenitor and stem cells from the adult brain is a factor limiting their therapeutic potential. Second, stem cells reside in specialized microenvironments or "niches" [60, 61]. An astroglial and an angiogenic niche for neurogenesis have been identified and characterized in the adult brain [62, 63]. The microenvironment controls the developmental potential of stem cells and their proliferation and maturation. As such, it plays a key role in the therapeutic potential of stem cells, whether endogenous or transplanted. Future investigations will aims at establishing homogeneous population of self-renewing multipotent NSCs *in vitro* and unraveling the molecular and cellular mechanisms underlying the developmental potential of NSCs in the adult brain [64].

Alzheimer's Disease

A Senile Dementia and Neurodegenerative Disease

AD was first described by Alois Alzheimer in 1906 [65]. It is the most common form of senile dementia. AD is characterized by memory and cognitive deficits, but also anosmia [66, 67]. Age is the principal risk factor for AD and the incidence of the disease doubles every 5 years after age 65 [68]. AD is a neurodegenerative disease. It is initially associated with the loss of nerve cells in areas of the brain that are vital to memory and other cognitive abilities, like the enthorhinal cortex, hippocampus and neocortex. As the disease progresses, other regions of the brain are affected, leading to severe incapacity and death [69]. Beside, neurodegeneration, AD is characterized in the brain by the presence of amyloid plaques, neurofibrillary tangles and aneuploidy [6, 65, 69]. Amyloid plaques and neurofibrillary tangles are the histopathological hallmarks of AD.

There are two forms of the disease. The early onset form of AD (EOAD) is a rare form of the disease. It is diagnosed before age 65. EOAD is primarily an inherited disease. It runs is about 200 families in the world. The late onset form of AD (LOAD) is diagnosed after the age of 65. Most cases of LOAD are sporadic forms of the disease. LOAD is the most common form of the disease, accounting for over 93 percent of all cases of AD [6, 69]. Doctors diagnose AD primarily by symptoms of cognitive impairments, behavioural changes and risk factor assessments [71, 71]. There is no cure for AD which leads to death within 3 to 9 years after being diagnosed [68, 69]. The disease affects more than 35 million of individuals worldwide.

Amyloid Plaques and Neurofibrillary Tangles

Amyloid plaques are distributed throughout the brain of patients with AD, particularly in the regions of degeneration, like the entorhinal cortex, hippocampus and temporal, frontal and inferior parietal lobes [72]. Their density increases as the disease advances. Amyloid plaques are thought to be the first histological change to occur in the brain of patients with AD [6]. They are composed of extracellular deposits of amyloid fibrils or protein beta-amyloid and of alpha 1-antichymotrypsin, in the brain of AD patients [73]. Alpha 1-antichymotrypsin is a serine protease inhibitor.

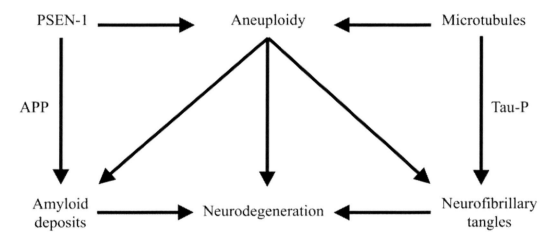

Figure 1. Neurogenetic events in Alzheimer's disease. Alzheimer's disease is characterized by genetic instability. Genetic mutations, genetic risk factors and aneuploidy are causative factors and landmarks of the disease. Protein beta-amyloid originates from the post-transcriptional maturation of the amyloid precursor protein (APP). As the amyloid deposits in the brain, nerve cells start dying. The presenilin (PSEN) proteins are components of the gamma-secretase complex that plays a role in the maturation of APP into protein beta-amyloid. Neurofibrillary tangles are composed of intracellular deposits of hyperphosphorylated Tau proteins (Tau-P). The hyperphosphorylation of Tau proteins results in the aggregation and in the breakdown of microtubules. This leads to the formation of neurofibrillary tangles and cell death. Mutated forms of PSEN-1 are detected in interphase kinetochores and centrosomes of dividing cells, where they may be involved in the segragation and migration of chromosomes during cells division. The breakdown of microtubules causes the disruption in the mitotic spindle and promotes aneuploidy during cell division. Aneuploidy for genes involved in the pathology of AD, like *APP*, *PSEN-1*, *PSCN-2*, *TAU* and *ApoE*, would contribute to the pathogenesis of the disease, e.g. to the formation of amyloid plaques, neurofibrillary tangles and neurodegeneration, as a result of the over expression of those genes.

Protein beta-amyloid is a beta-peptide. It originates from the post-transcriptional maturation of the amyloid precursor protein (APP) [74]. Protein beta-amyloid is synthesized and secreted by nerve cells, as a soluble peptide. It aggregates to form deposits of amyloid fibrils or amyloid plaques after abnormal processing of APP under certain conditions, like in the presence of specific gene mutations for example. In physiological conditions, APP is cleaved primarily by the alpha- and gamma-secretases into a 40 amino acid beta-peptide [74]. Under pathological conditions, there is an increase in the cleavage of APP, by the beta- and gamma-secretases. This results in an increase in the synthesis of a 42 amino acid beta-amyloid peptide. This latter form of protein beta-amyloid aggregates into insoluble amyloid deposits or amyloid plaques, particularly in the brain (Figure 1).

According to the hypothesis knows as the amyloid hypothesis, deposits of protein beta-amyloid may be a causative factor of AD. As the amyloid deposits in the brain, nerve cells start dying, and the signs and symptoms of the disease appears. This hypothesis is the source of debates and controversies [75]. The main argument against the amyloid hypothesis is the lack of correlation between the density of amyloid plaques in the brain and the severity of the disease [76].

Neurofibrillary tangles are distributed throughout the brain of patients with AD. They are composed of intracellular deposits of hyperphosphorylated Tau proteins, in the brain of patients with AD [77]. Tau protein is microtubule-associated phosphoprotein [78]. Microtubules are involved in cell structure, intracellular transport and cell division. The hyperphosphorylation of Tau proteins results in their aggregation and in the breakdown of microtubules [79]. This leads to the formation of neurofibrillary tangles and cell death [80, 81] (Figure 1).

Genetic Mutations and Risks Factors in Alzheimer's Disease

Three genetic mutations causative for inherited forms of AD have been identified: mutations in the gene of APP, of presenilin-1 (PSEN-1) and of presenilin-2 (PSEN-2) [82]. APP is a 695-770 amino acid protein coding for the protein beta-amyloid. Mutations in *APP* cause excessive cleavage of APP by the beta- and gamma-secretases. This results in an excessive production of the 42 amino acid beta-amyloid peptide and the formation of amyloid deposits. The PSEN proteins are components of the gamma-secretase complex that plays a role in the maturation of APP into protein beta-amyloid [83]. Mutations in *PSEN-1* and *PSEN-2* lead to excessive cleavage of APP by gamma-secretase enzyme, resulting in an excessive production of the 42 amino acid beta-amyloid peptide and the formation of amyloid deposits [84] (Figure 1). Individuals carrying mutations in these genes, also known familial Alzheimer's disease (FAD) genes, will almost always develop AD or FAD, before age 65, or EOAD [85]. EOAD is primarily a genetic inherited disease. Cases of FAD can occur after age of 65 [86]. The causal mutations involved in these forms of LOAD remian unidentified.

Some of the genetic, acquired and environmental risk factors, causative for the sporadic forms of AD, have been identified like the presence of certain alleles such as the apolipoprotein E varepsilon 4 allele (*ApoE4*) in the genetic makeup of the individuals, hypertension, diabetis and oxidative stress [87-89]. ApoE is a plasma protein that is involved in the transport of cholesterol and lipids in the blood [90]. There are three major alleles of ApoE gene in humans: ApoE2, ApoE3 and ApoE4. Up to 50 percent of people who have AD have at least one *ApoE4* allele in their genetic make-up [91]. Individuals who have two *ApoE4* alleles have a higher risk of developing AD [92]. The presence *ApoE4* in the genes of the individuals accounts for most causes and risks to develop LOAD. Other genes have been been linked with the occurence of LOAD, among them variants for the genes coding for alpha2-macroglobulin, myeloperoxidase, cystatin C, the gene coding for neuronal sortilin-related receptor, the gene coding for FKBP52 and polymorphisms in the cholesteryl ester transfer protein gene [93-96]. These risk factors increase the probability of developing AD after age 65, or LOAD. However, sporadic cases of EOAD can occur, with no family history and no identified causal genetic mutations.

Aneuploidy in Region of Neurodegeneration

Lymphocyte preparations of patients with AD, EOAD and LOAD, reveal an increase in aneuploidy, particularly for chromosomes 13, 18 and 21 [97, 98]. Four to 10 percent of nerve cells in regions of neurodegeneration of the brain, like the hippocampus, of patients with AD are aneuploid and express proteins of the cell cycle, like cyclin B [99-101]. The nondisjunction of chromosomes during cell division in stem cells or somatic cells that retain their ability to divide is at the origin of aneuploidy in lymphocytes of patients with AD. In the adult brain, most nerve cells are post-mitotic. The characterization of markers of the cell cycle, like cyclin B, in nerve cells in regions of degeneration reveals that cell cycle re-entry and DNA duplication, without cell division, is at the origin of aneuploidy in those cells in the brain of AD patients [102, 103]. Aneuploid nerve cells originating from the re-expression of proteins of the cell cycle are fated to die. They may live in this state for months, undergoing a slow death process [104, 105]. Cell cycle re-entry and DNA duplication, without cell division, leading to aneuploidy would be an underlying mechanism of the neurodegenerative process in AD.

The genetic imbalance in aneuploid cells results in the over expression of genes by the cells. The genes for ApoE, APP, PSEN-1, PSEN-2 and TAU are located on chromosomes 19, 21, 1, 14 and 17, respectively [106-109]. Cells of AD patients elicit an elevation of aneuploidy for chromosomes 13, 18 and 21, particularly [97, 98]. Aneuploidy for genes involved in the pathology of AD would contribute to the pathogenesis of the disease, as a result of the over expression of those genes. Aneuploidy for chromosome 19 would result in the over expression of ApoE and in an increase risk for individuals who have *ApoE4* in the genetic make-up of developing the sporadic form of AD. Aneuploidy for chromosome 21 would result in the overexpression of APP and promote the formation of amyloid plaques. Aneuploidy for chromosomes 1 or 14 would promote the formation of amyloid plaques in patients carrying FAD mutations on PSEN genes and contribute to the pathogenesis of EOAD. Aneuploidy for chromosomes 17 would result in the overexpression of Tau protein and promote the formation of neurofibrillary tangles.

Protein beta-amyloid induces cell cycle re-entry and neuronal death [110]. Hence, aneuploidy for chromosome 21 would not only promote the formation of amyloid plaques, it would also promote cell cycle re-entry and DNA duplication, without cell division, leading to aneuploidy and neuronal cell death in regions of neurodegeneration in the brain. Hence, aneuploidy is landmark of the pathology of AD. It underlies the process of neurodegeneration and contributes to the pathogenesis of AD, by over-expressing genes involved in the disease and triggering a cascade of events amplifying the development of the disease.

Adult Neurogenesis and the Pathogenesis of Alzheimer's Disease

Neurogenesis is enhanced in the brain of patients with AD [7]. This reveals adult neurogenesis and newly generated neuronal cells of the adult brain play a role in the pathogenesis and pathology of AD, the contribution of which remains to be elucidated and determined.

Neurogenesis in Alzheimer's Disease

The expression of markers of immature neuronal cells, particularly doublecortin, is enhanced in the hippocampus of the brain of patients with AD, mostly patients with LOAD [7]. In animal models, adult neurogenesis is enhanced in the hippocampus of transgenic mice that express the Swedish and Indiana APP mutations. It is decreased in the hippocampus of mice deficient for APP or PSEN-1, of transgenic mice over expressing variants of APP or PSEN-1 and of PDAPP transgenic mice, a mouse model with age-dependent accumulation of protein beta-amyloid [111-115]. BrdU-labeling and/or immunohistochemistry for makers of the cell cycle were conducted to study and quantify neurogenesis in the adult hippocampus of AD patients and of animal models of AD. As such, due to the limitations and pitfalls over the use of BrdU-labeling and immunohistochemistry for makers of the cell cycle for studying cell proliferation and neurogenesis, these studies remain to further evaluated and confirmed [59, 60, 64]. In addition, the various animal models of AD used in those studies are not representative of complex diseases like AD, EOAD and LOAD, but rather of the genes deficient or mutated in AD [116]. Genetic modifications in transgenic mice may also have adverse effects during development, altering adult phenotypes, particularly adult neurogenesis.

Hence, these studies show that neurogenesis is enhanced in the hippocampus of patients with AD, but report conflicting data in animal models of AD. Studies of neurogenesis, in the adult hippocampus of AD patients and of animal models of AD, need to be confirmed and validated. Enhanced neurogenesis in the brain of patients with AD may contribute to regenerative attempts, to compensate for the neuronal loss.

In the SVZ, studies in patients with AD report a reduction in the number of neural progenitor cells in the SVZ, as revealed by immunohistology for nestin and Musashi1 [117]. Protein beta-amyloid stimulates neurogenesis in the SVZ of young APP/PS1 transgenic mice, but not of 12-month-old APP/PS1 transgenic models of AD [118]. The reduction in the number of neural progenitor cells in the SVZ of AD brain and the lack of stimulation of neural progenitor and stem cells of the adult SVZ by protein beta-amyloid suggest depletion in the pool of stem cells in the adult SVZ in AD. It may underlie the compromised olfaction also associated with the disease.

Aneuploid Newly Generated Neuronal Cells in the Adult Brain with Alzheimer's Disease

The hyperphosphorylation of Tau by kinases leads to the breakdown of microtubles and to the formation of neurofibrillary tangles [79]. The breakdown of microtubules causes the disruption in the mitotic spindle and promotes aneuploidy during cell division. Mutated forms of PSEN-1 are detected in interphase kinetochores and centrosomes of dividing cells, where they may be involved in the segragation and migration of chromosomes during cells division [119, 120]. Oxidative stress, an environmental risk factor for LOAD, promotes aneuploidy, particularly for chromosome 17 that carries the *TAU* gene [121]. Cells that are the most likely to develop aneuploidy are dividing cells. Hence, somatic cells that retain their ability to divide in AD are at high risk of aneuploidy. The process of adult neurogenesis holds the potential to generate populations of cells that are aneuploid, particularly in the neurogenic regions. The neurogenic regions are therefore sites of the adult brain with AD that are at particularly high risk of aneuploidy (Figure 1). The nondisjunction of chromosomes during the process of cell division of neural progenitor and stem cells of the adult brain could lead to newly generated neuronal cells that are aneuploid and/or to newly generated neuronal precursor cells that are aneuploid and would not proceed with their developmental program [8, 122]. These aneuploid cells may have their lifespan shortened, further contributing to the neurodegenerative process in AD, or they may survive for extended period of time, potentially contributing to the formation of amyloid plaques, neurofibrillary tangles, neurodegeneration and aneuploidy, locally, in the neurogenic regions of the adult brain, particularly the hippocampus (Figure 1).

The generation of new neuronal cells represents a relatively low frequency event in the adult brain of mammals, estimated that 0.1 and 0.004 percent of the granule cell population is generated per day in the DG of adult mice and macaque monkeys, respectively [19-21]. Hence, the generation of newly generated neuronal cells that are aneuploids and/or of newly generated neuronal precursor cells that are aneuploid and would not proceed with their developmental program in the adult brain would concern a relatively low fraction of cells of the hippocampus. Nonetheless, their pathological activity may be critical to the pathogenesis of AD, since these aneuploid neuronal cells are generated particularly in the hippocampus, a region involved in learning and memory and particularly affected in patients with AD. In addition, reports show that neurogenesis is enhanced in the brain of patients with AD [7]. So, adult neurogenesis may be a preferential target for generating aneuploid neuronal cells in the adult brain.

In all, causative factors of AD, like Tau protein, mutated PSEN-1 proteins and oxidative stress, may not only contribute to the pathogenesis of AD by promoting the formation of amyloid plaques and neurofibrillary tangles, the process of neurodegeneration, but also by promoting the generation of neuronal cells that are aneuploids in the brain with AD, particularly in the hippocampus. Enhanced neurogenesis may further contribute to the risk of generating neuronal cells that are aneuploids in the brain of patients with AD [123]. This reveals that neurogenesis in the adult brain may have a dual activity. On the one hand, it may contribute to regenerative attempts. On the other hand, it may contribute to the generation of aneuploid neuronal cells and the pathogenesis of AD. Adult neurogenesis would not only be beneficial, but also detrimental for patients with AD. This has important implications for therapeutic strategies for AD.

Novel Drug Targets for Alzheimer's Disease

Newly Generated Neuronal Cells of the Adult Brain

Three types of drugs are used for the treatment of patients with AD: blockers of the formation of amyloid plaques, inhibitors of acetylcholine esterase and N-methyl-D-aspartate glutamate receptor antagonists. These drugs improve both cognitive and behavioral symptoms of AD [124-126]. The activity of drugs used in the treatment of AD has been assessed for their effects on adult neurogenesis in rodents. Galantamine, an acetylcholine esterase inhibitor, and memantine, an N-methyl-D-aspartate glutamate receptor antagonist, increase neurogenesis by 26 to 45 percent in the hippocampus of adult rodents [127]. This reveals that adult neurogenesis may be the target of drugs used for treating AD and contribute to their activities [128]. The mechanisms and functions underlying the activities of these drugs on newly generated neuronal cells of the adult brain remain to be elucidated. Drugs may act directly or indirectly on those cells. They may act via their pharmacological activities, on messenger signaling pathways, and/or via a neurogenic activity, by modulating neurogenesis and/or compensating for neuronal loss [129].

Aneuploid Newly Generated Neuronal Cells of the Adult Brain

The generation of aneuploid new neuronal cells in the adult brain has implications for therapeutic treatments of AD. Factors and conditions promoting adult neurogenesis and aneuploidy would promote the generation of aneuploid new neuronal cells in the neurogenic regions of the adult brain, particularly the hippocampus, and further contribute to the development of AD. Novel drug therapies to treat neurological diseases and disorders aim at targeting the newly generated neuronal cells of the adult brain and at stimulating adult neurogenesis, particularly of the hippocampus [130-132]. This to compensate or reverse deficits associated with the hippocampus, like in AD and depression, and to promote functional recovery [46]. Such therapies may be associated with the risk of generating of aneuploid neuronal cells in the adult brain of those patients, contributing to pathological developments and deficits.

In all, adult neurogenesis and newly generated neuronal cells of the adult brain are the target of drugs used for treating neurological diseases and disorders and contribute to their activities, particularly in AD (Table 1). Drugs targeting the newly generated neuronal cells of the adult brain and adult neurogenesis carry the risk of promoting the generation of aneuploid neuronal cells in the adult brain (Table 1). Therapeutic strategies will aim at discovering and developing novel drugs that specifically target the newly generated neuronal cells of the adult brain to compensate or reverse deficits, particularly associated with the hippocampus. Such strategy will involve limiting the potential deleterious effects of the generation of aneuploid neuronal cells in the adult brain, without disrupting the regenerative capacity of adult neurogenesis [133].

Summary and Perspectives

The confirmation that neurogenesis occurs in the adult brain and NSCs reside in the adult CNS has tremendous implications and applications for our understanding of the nervous system and for therapy. Adult NSCs not only offer new opportunities for cellular therapy, to repair and restore degenerated and injured nerve pathways. They also provide novel opportunities for pharmacology, to compensate or reverse deficits, associated with neurological diseases and disorders. Current protocols to establish adult derived-neural progenitor and stem cells yield to heterogeneous populations of cells and the developmental potential of stem cells in under control of the microenvironment. This limits the potential of adult NSCs for cellular therapy for the treatment of neurological diseases and injuries, and particularly for AD. Neurogenesis is enhanced in the brain of patients with AD. Neurogenesis holds the potential to generate aneuploid new neuronal cells in the adult brain, a pathological hallmark of AD. Hence, adult neurogenesis may have a dual activity. It may be involved in regenerative attempts in AD, but also in the pathogenesis of AD. Adult neurogenesis would not only be beneficial, but also detrimental for patients with AD. This shows that a deep understanding of the mechanisms underlying adult neurogenesis and its contribution to the physio- and pathology of the nervous system is mandated, to bring adult NSCs to therapy. Future directions will aims at generating homogenous population of adult derived-self-renewing multipotent NSCs and to unravel the mechanisms underlying the neurogenic niches. They will also aim at discovering and developing novel drugs that specifically target the newly generated neuronal cells of the adult brain, or neurogenic drugs, to compensate or reverse deficits, particularly associated with the hippocampus; drugs that stimulate neurogenesis, compensate for neuronal loss and elicit potential for regenerative medicine. Such strategy will involve limiting the potential deleterious effects of the generation of aneuploid neuronal cells in the adult brain, without disrupting the regenerative capacity of adult neurogenesis.

Acknowledgments

Reproduced from: Taupin P. Neurogenesis, NSCs, pathogenesis and therapies for Alzheimer's disease. Alzheimer's disease. Frontiers in Bioscience (2011) 3:178-190. Copyright 2011, with kind permission from Frontiers in Bioscience.

References

[1] Eriksson, P.S., Perfilieva, E., Bjork-Eriksson, T., Alborn, A.M., Nordborg, C., Peterson, D.A. & F.H. Gage: Neurogenesis in the adult human hippocampus. *Nat. Med.*, 4, 1313-1317 (1998).

[2] Curtis, M.A., Kam M., Nannmark, U., Anderson, M.F., Axell, M.Z., Wikkelso, C., Holtas, S., van Roon-Mom, W.M., Bjork-Eriksson, T., Nordborg, C., Frisen, J., Dragunow, M., Faull, R.L. & P.S. Eriksson: Human neuroblasts migrate to the olfactory bulb via a lateral ventricular extension. *Science*, 315, 1243-1249 (2007).

[3] Duan, X., Kang, E., Liu, C.Y., Ming, G.L. & H. Song: Development of neural stem cell in the adult brain. *Curr. Opin. Neurobiol.*, 18, 108-115 (2008).

[4] P. Taupin: Neurogenesis in the adult central nervous system. *C. R. Biol.*, 329, 465-475 (2006).

[5] F.H. Gage: Mammalian neural stem cells. *Science*, 287, 1433-1438 (2000).

[6] P.H. St George-Hyslop: Piecing together *Alzheimer's. Sci. Am.*, 283, 76-83 (2000).

[7] Jin, K., Peel, A.L., Mao, X.O., Xie, L., Cottrell, B.A., Henshall, D.C. & D.A. Greenberg: Increased hippocampal neurogenesis in Alzheimer's disease. *Proc. Natl. Acad. Sci. U. S. A.*, 101, 343-347 (2004).

[8] P. Taupin: Adult neurogenesis, neural stem cells and Alzheimer's disease: developments, limitations, problems and promises. *Curr. Alzheimer Res.*, 6, 461-470 (2009).

[9] Corotto, F.S., Henegar, J.A. & J.A. Maruniak: Neurogenesis persists in the subependymal layer of the adult mouse brain. *Neurosci. Lett.*, 149, 111-114 (1993).

[10] Lois, C. & A. Alvarez-Buylla: Long-distance neuronal migration in the adult mammalian brain. *Science*, 264, 1145-1148 (1994).

[11] Stanfield, B.B. & J.E. Trice: Evidence that granule cells generated in the dentate gyrus of adult rats extend axonal projections. *Exp. Brain Res.*, 72, 399-406 (1988).

[12] Cameron, H.A., Woolley, C.S., McEwen, B.S. & E. Gould: Differentiation of newly born neurons and glia in the dentate gyrus of the adult rat. *Neurosci.*, 56, 337-344 (1993).

[13] Markakis, E.A. & F.H. Gage: Adult-generated neurons in the dentate gyrus send axonal projections to field CA3 and are surrounded by synaptic vesicles. *J. Comp. Neurol.*, 406, 449-460 (1999).

[14] Van Praag, H., Schinder, A.F., Christie, B.R., Toni, N., Palmer, T.D. & F.H. Gage: Functional neurogenesis in the adult hippocampus. Nature, 415, 1030-1034 (2002).

[15] Toni, N., Teng, EM.., Bushong, E.A., Aimone, J.B., Zhao, C., Consiglio, A., van Praag, H., Martone, M.E., Ellisman, M.H. & F.H. Gage: Synapse formation on neurons born in the adult hippocampus. *Nat. Neurosci.*, 10, 727-734 (2007).

[16] P. Taupin: Characterization and isolation of synapses of newly generated neuronal cells of the adult hippocampus at early stages of neurogenesis. *J. Neurodegener. Regene.*, 2, 9-17 (2009).

[17] Goldman, S.A. & M.B. Luskin: Strategies utilized by migrating neurons of the postnatal vertebrate forebrain, *Trends Neurosci.*, 21, 107-114 (1998).

[18] Temple, S. & A. Alvarez-Buylla: Stem cells in the adult mammalian central nervous system. *Curr. Opin. Neurobiol.*, 9, 135-141 (1999).

[19] Kempermann, G., Kuhn, H.G. & F.H. Gage: More hippocampal neurons in adult mice living in an enriched environment. *Nature*, 386, 493-495 (1997).

[20] Cameron, H.A. & R.D. McKay: Adult neurogenesis produces a large pool of new granule cells in the dentate gyrus. *J. Comp. Neurol.*, 435, 406-417 (2001).

[21] Kornack, D.R. & P. Rakic: Continuation of neurogenesis in the hippocampus of the adult macaque monkey. *Proc. Natl. Acad. Sci. U. S. A.*, 96, 5768-5773 (1999).

[22] Gould, E., Reeves, A.J., Graziano, M.S. & C.G. Gross: Neurogenesis in the neocortex of adult primates. *Science*, 286, 548-552 (1999).

[23] Rietze, R., Poulin, P. & S. Weiss: Mitotically active cells that generate neurons and astrocytes are present in multiple regions of the adult mouse hippocampus. *J. Comp. Neurol.*, 424, 397-408 (2000).

[24] Bedard, A., Gravel, C. & A. Parent: Chemical characterization of newly generated neurons in the striatum of adult primates. *Exp. Brain Res.*, 170, 501-512 (2006).

[25] Reynolds, B.A. & S. Weiss: Generation of neurons and astrocytes from isolated cells of the adult mammalian central nervous system. *Science*, 255, 1707-1710 (1992).

[26] Gage, F.H., Coates, P.W., Palmer, T.D., Kuhn, H.G., Fisher, L.J., Suhonen, J.O., Peterson, D.A., Suhr, S.T. & J. Ray: Survival and differentiation of adult neuronal progenitor cells transplanted to the adult brain. *Proc. Natl. Acad. Sci. U. S. A.*, 92, 11879-11883 (1995).

[27] Taupin, P. & F.H. Gage: Adult neurogenesis and neural stem cells of the central nervous system in mammals, *J. Neurosci. Res.*, 69, 745-749 (2002).

[28] Roy, N.S., Wang, S., Jiang, L., Kang, J., Benraiss, A., Harrison-Restelli, C., Fraser, R.A., Couldwell, W.T., Kawaguchi, A., Okano, H., Nedergaard, N. & S.A. Goldman: *In vitro* neurogenesis by progenitor cells isolated from the adult human hippocampus. *Nat. Med.*, 6, 271-277 (2000).

[29] Palmer, T.D., Schwartz, P.H. Taupin, P., Kaspar, B., Stein, S.A. & F.H. Gage: Cell culture. Progenitor cells from human brain after death. *Nature*, 411, 42-43 (2001).

[30] Potten, C.S. & M. Loeffler: Stem cells: attributes, cycles, spirals, pitfalls and uncertainties. Lessons for and from the crypt. *Development*, 110, 1001-1020 (1990).

[31] Chin, V.I., Taupin, P., Sanga, S., Scheel, J., Gage, F.H. & S.N. Bhatia: Microfabricated platform for studying stem cell fates. *Biotechnol. Bioeng.*, 88, 399-415 (2004).

[32] Lendahl, U., Zimmerman, L.B. & R.D. McKay: CNS stem cells express a new class of intermediate filament protein. *Cell*, 60, 585-595 (1990).

[33] Clarke, S.R., Shetty, A.K., Bradley, J.L. & D.A. Turner: Reactive astrocytes express the embryonic intermediate neurofilament nestin. *Neuroreport*, 5, 1885-1888 (1994).

[34] Sakakibara, S., Imai, T., Hamaguchi, K., Okabe, M., Aruga, J., Nakajima, K., Yasutomi, D., Nagata, T., Kurihara, Y., Uesugi, S., Miyata, T., Ogawa, M., Mikoshiba, K. & H. Okano: Mouse-Musashi-1, a neural RNA-binding protein highly enriched in the mammalian CNS stem cells. *Dev. Biol.*, 176, 230-242 (1996).

[35] Kaneko, Y., Sakakibara, S., Imai, T., Suzuki, A., Nakamura, Y., Sawamoto, K., Ogawa, Y., Toyama, Y., Miyata, T. & H. Okano: Musashi1: an evolutionally conserved

marker for CNS progenitor cells including neural stem cells. *Dev. Neurosci.*, 22, 139-153 (2000).

[36] Komitova, M. & P.S. Eriksson: Sox-2 is expressed by neural progenitors and astroglia in the adult rat brain. *Neurosci. Lett.*, 369, 24-27 (2004).

[37] Okuda, T., Tagawa, K., Qi, M.L. Hoshio, M., Ueda, H., Kawano, H., Kanazawa, I., Muramatsu, M. & H. Okazawa: Oct-3/4 repression accelerates differentiation of neural progenitor cells *in vitro* and *in vivo*. *Brain Res. Mol. Brain Res.*, 132, 18-30 (2004).

[38] P. Taupin: Adult neurogenesis in the mammalian central nervous system: functionality and potential clinical interest. *Med. Sci. Monit.*, 11, RA247-252 (2005).

[39] Gould, E., Beylin, A., Tanapat, P., Reeves, A. & T.J. Shors: Learning enhances adult neurogenesis in the hippocampal formation. *Nat. Neurosci.*, 2, 260-265 (1999).

[40] van Praag, H., Kempermann, G. & F.H. Gage: Running increases cell proliferation and neurogenesis in the adult mouse dentate gyrus. *Nat. Neurosci.*, 2, 266-270 (1999).

[41] Shors, T.J., Miesegaes, G., Beylin, A., Zhao, M., Rydel, T. & E. Gould: Neurogenesis in the adult is involved in the formation of trace memories. *Nature*, 410, 372-376 (2001) Erratum in: *Nature*, 414, 938 (2001).

[42] Parent, J.M., Yu, T.W., Leibowitz, R.T., Geschwind, D.H., Sloviter, R.S. & D.H. Lowenstein: Dentate granule cell neurogenesis is increased by seizures and contributes to aberrant network reorganization in the adult rat hippocampus. *J. Neurosci.*, 17, 3727-3738 (1997).

[43] Liu, J., Solway, K., Messing, R.O. & F.R. Sharp: Increased neurogenesis in the dentate gyrus after transient global ischemia in gerbils. *J. Neurosci.*, 18, 7768-7778 (1998).

[44] Dash, P.K., Mach, S.A. & A.N. Moore: Enhanced neurogenesis in the rodent hippocampus following traumatic brain injury. *J. Neurosci. Res.*, 63, 313-319 (2001).

[45] Curtis, M.A., Penney, E.B., Pearson, A.G., van Roon-Mom, W.M., Butterworth, N.J., Dragunow, M., Connor, B. & R.L. Faull: Increased cell proliferation and neurogenesis in the adult human Huntington's disease brain. *Proc. Natl. Acad. Sci. U. S. A.*, 100, 9023-9027 (2003).

[46] P. Taupin: Adult neurogenesis pharmacology in neurological diseases and disorders. *Exp. Rev. Neurother.*, 8, 311-320 (2008).

[47] P. Taupin: Adult neurogenesis and neuroplasticity. *Restor. Neurol. Neurosci.*, 24, 9-15 (2006).

[48] Ma, D.K., Bonaguidi, M.A., Ming, G.L. & H. Song: Adult neural stem cells in the mammalian central nervous system. *Cell. Res.*, 19, 672-682 (2009).

[49] Miller, M.W. & R.S. Nowakowski: Use of bromodeoxyuridine-immunohistochemistry to examine the proliferation, migration and time of origin of cells in the central nervous system. *Brain Res.*, 457, 44-52 (1998).

[50] Carpentier, P., Delamanche, I.S., Le Bert, M., Blanchet, G., & C. Bouchaud: Seizure-related opening of the blood-brain barrier induced by soman: possible correlation with the acute neuropathology observed in poisoned rats. *Neurotoxicology*, 11, 493-508 (1990).

[51] Pont, F., Collet, A. & G. Lallement: Early and transient increase of rat hippocampal blood-brain barrier permeability to amino acids during kainic acid-induced seizures. *Neurosci. Lett.*, 184, 52-54 (1995).

[52] Ide, K. & N.H. Secher: Cerebral blood flow and metabolism during exercise. *Prog. Neurobiol.*, 61, 397-414 (2000).

[53] Nowakowski, R.S. & N.L. Hayes: Stem cells: the promises and pitfalls. *Neuropsychopharmacology*, 25, 799-804 (2001).

[54] Gould, E. & C.G. Gross: Neurogenesis in adult mammals: some progress and problems. *J. Neurosci.*, 22, 619-623 (2002).

[55] P. Taupin: BrdU Immunohistochemistry for Studying Adult Neurogenesis: paradigms, pitfalls, limitations, and validation. *Brain Res. Rev.*, 53, 198-214 (2007).

[56] Arvidsson, A., Collin, T., Kirik, D., Kokaia, Z. & O. Lindvall: Neuronal replacement from endogenous precursors in the adult brain after stroke. *Nat. Med.*, 8, 963-970 (2002).

[57] Jin, K., Sun, Y., Xie, L., Peel, A., Mao, X.O. Batteur, S. & D.A. Greenberg: Directed migration of neuronal precursors into the ischemic cerebral cortex and striatum. *Mol. Cell. Neurosci.*, 24, 171-189 (2003).

[58] Brown, A.B., Yang, W., Schmidt, N.O., Carroll, R., Leishear, K.K., Rainov, N.G., Black, P.M., Breakefield, X.O. & K.S. Aboody: Intravascular delivery of neural stem cell lines to target intracranial and extracranial tumors of neural and non-neural origin. *Hum. Gene Ther.*, 14, 1777-1785 (2003).

[59] Pluchino, S., Quattrini, A., Brambilla, E., Gritti, A., Salani, G., Dina, G., Galli, R., Del Carro, U., Amadio, S., Bergami, A., Furlan, R., Comi, G., Vescovi, A.L. & G. Martino: Injection of adult neurospheres induces recovery in a chronic model of multiple sclerosis. *Nature*, 422, 688-694 (2003).

[60] P. Taupin: Adult neural stem cells, neurogenic niches and cellular therapy. *Stem Cell Rev.*, 2, 213-220 (2006).

[61] Mitsiadis, T.A., Barrandon, O., Rochat, A., Barrandon, Y. & C. De Bari: Stem cell niches in mammals. *Exp. Cell. Res.*, 313, 3377-3385 (2007).

[62] Palmer, T.D., Willhoite, A.R. & F.H. Gage: Vascular niche for adult hippocampal neurogenesis. *J. Comp. Neurol.*, 425, 479-494 (2000).

[63] Song, H., Stevens, C.F. & F.H. Gage: Astroglia induce neurogenesis from adult neural stem cells. *Nature*, 417, 39-44 (2002).

[64] P. Taupin: Editorial. Adult neural stem cells from promise to treatment: The road ahead. *J. Neurodegener. Regene.*, 1, 7-8 (2008).

[65] A. Alzheimer: Uber einen eigenartigen schweren erkrankungsprozeb der hirnrinde. *Neurologisches Cenrealblatt*, 23, 1129-1136 (1906).

[66] Lafreniere, D. & N. Mann: Anosmia: loss of smell in the elderly. *Otolaryngol Clin North Am*, 42, 123-131 (2009) Erratum in: *Otolaryngol Clin North Am*, 43, 691 (2010).

[67] Fusetti, M., Fioretti, AB., Silvagni, F., Simaskou, M., Sucapane, P., Necozione, S. & A. Eibenstein. Smell and preclinical Alzheimer disease: study of 29 patients with amnesic mild cognitive impairment. *J Otolaryngol Head Neck Surg*, 39, 175-181 (2010).

[68] Burns, A., Byrne, E.J. & K. Maurer: Alzheimer's disease. *Lancet*, 360, 163-165 (2002).

[69] Querfurth, H.W. & F.M. LaFerla FM: Alzheimer's disease. *N Engl. J Med.*, 362:329-44 (2010).

[70] R.J. Lederman: What tests are necessary to diagnose Alzheimer disease? *Cleve. Clin. J. Med.*, 67, 615-618 (2000).

[71] Dubois, B., Feldman, H.H., Jacova, C., DeKosky, S.T., Barberger-Gateau, P., Cummings, J., Delacourte, A., Galasko, D., Gauthier, S., Jicha, G., Meguro, K., O'Brien, J., Pasquier, F., Robert, P., Rossor, M., Salloway, S., Stern, Y., Visser, P.J. &

P. Schelten: Research criteria for the diagnosis of Alzheimer's disease: revising the NINCDS–ADRDA criteria. *The Lancet Neurology*, 6, 734-746 (2007).

[72] Brun, A. & L. Gustafson: Distribution of cerebral degeneration in Alzheimer's disease. A clinico-pathological study. *Arch. Psychiatr. Nervenkr.*, 223, 15-33 (1976).

[73] Anderson, D.H., Talaga, K.C., Rivest, A.J., Barron, E., Hageman, G.S. & L.V. Johnson: Characterization of beta amyloid assemblies in drusen: the deposits associated with aging and age-related macular degeneration. *Exp. Eye. Res.*, 78, 243-256 (2004).

[74] Kang, J., Lemaire, H.G., Unterbeck, A., Salbaum, J.M., Masters, C.L., Grzeschik. K.H., Multhaup. G., Beyreuther. K. & B. Müller-Hill: The precursor of Alzheimer's disease amyloid A4 protein resembles a cell-surface receptor. *Nature*, 325, 733-736 (1987).

[75] J. Hardy: The amyloid hypothesis for Alzheimer's disease: a critical reappraisal. *J. Neurochem.*, 110, 1129-1134 (2009).

[76] R.D. Terry: The pathogenesis of Alzheimer disease: an alternative to the amyloid hypothesis. *J. Neuropathol. Exp. Neurol.*, 55, 1023-1025 (1996).

[77] Fukutani, Y., Kobayashi, K., Nakamura, I., Watanabe, K., Isaki, K & N.J. Cairns: Neurons, intracellular and extra cellular neurofibrillary tangles in subdivisions of the hippocampal cortex in normal ageing and Alzheimer's disease. *Neurosci. Lett.*, 200, 57-60 (1995).

[78] Kim, H., Jensen, C.G. & L.I. Rebhun: The binding of MAP-2 and tau on brain microtubules *in vitro*: implications for microtubule structure. *Ann. N. Y. Acad. Sci.*, 466, 218-239 (1986).

[79] Kobayashi, K., Nakano, H., Hayashi, M., Shimazaki, M., Fukutani, Y., Sasaki, K., Sugimori, K. & Y. Koshino: Association of phosphorylation site of tau protein with neuronal apoptosis in Alzheimer's disease. *J. Neurol. Sci.*, 208, 17-24 (2003).

[80] Iqbal, K., Liu, F., Gong, C.X., Alonso Adel, C. & I. Grundke-Iqbal: Mechanisms of tau-induced neurodegeneration. *Acta. Neuropathol.*, 118, 53-69 (2009).

[81] Clavaguera, F., Bolmont, T., Crowther, R.A., Abramowski, D., Frank, S., Probst, A., Fraser, G., Stalder, A.K., Beibel, M., Staufenbiel, M., Jucker, M., Goedert, M. & M. Tolnay: Transmission and spreading of tauopathy in transgenic mouse brain. *Nat. Cell. Biol.*, 11, 909-913 (2009).

[82] Schellenberg, G.D., D'Souza, I. & P. Poorkaj: The genetics of Alzheimer's disease. *Curr. Psychiatry Rep.*, 2, 158-164 (2000).

[83] Nishimura, M., Yu, G. & P.H. St George-Hyslop: Biology of presenilins as causative molecules for Alzheimer disease. *Clin. Genet.*, 55, 219-225 (1999).

[84] Newman, M., Musgrave, F.I. & M. Lardelli: Alzheimer disease: amyloidogenesis, the presenilins and animal models. *Biochim. Biophys. Acta.*, 1772, 285-297 (2007).

[85] St George-Hyslop, P.H. & A. Petit: Molecular biology and genetics of Alzheimer's disease. *C. R. Biol.*, 328, 119-130 (2005).

[86] Wragg, M., Hutton, M. & C. Talbot: Genetic association between intronic polymorphism in presenilin-1 gene and late-onset *al*zheimer's disease. Alzheimer's Disease Collaborative Group. *Lancet*, 347, 509-512 (1996).

[87] Fassbender, K., Masters, C. & K. Beyreuther: Alzheimer's disease: an inflammatory disease? *Neurobiol. Aging*, 21, 433-436 (2000).

[88] Prasher, V.P. & M.S. Haque: Apolipoprotein E, Alzheimer's disease and Down's syndrome. *Br. J. Psychiatry*, 177, 469-470 (2000).

[89] Ferri, C.P., Prince, M., Brayne, C., Brodaty, H., Fratiglioni, L., Ganguli, M., Hall, K., Hasegawa, K., Filipcik, P., Cente, M., Ferencik, M., Hulin, I. & M. Novak: The role of oxidative stress in the pathogenesis of Alzheimer's disease. *Bratisl. Lek. Listy*, 107, 384-394 (2006).

[90] R.W. Mahley: Apolipoprotein E: cholesterol transport protein with expanding role in cell biology. *Science*, 240, 622-630 (1988).

[91] Raber, J., Huang, Y. & J.W. Ashford: ApoE genotype accounts for the vast majority of AD risk and AD pathology. *Neurobiol. Aging*, 25, 641-650 (2004).

[92] Strittmatter, W.J., Saunders, A.M., Schmechel, D., Pericak-Vance, M., Enghild, J., Salvesen, G.S. & A.D. Roses: Apolipoprotein E: high-avidity binding to beta-amyloid and increased frequency of type 4 allele in late-onset familial Alzheimer disease. *Proc. Natl. Acad. Sci. U. S. A.*, 90, 1977-1981 (1993).

[93] Finckh, U., von der Kammer, H., Velden, J., Michel, T., Andresen, B., Deng, A., Zhang, J., Müller-Thomsen, T., Zuchowski, K., Menzer, G., Mann, U., Papassotiropoulos, A., Heun, R., Zurdel, J., Holst, F., Benussi, L., Stoppe, G., Reiss, J., Miserez, A.R., Staehelin, H.B., Rebeck, G.W., Hyman, B.T., Binetti, G., Hock, C., Growdon, J.H. & R.M. Nitsch: Genetic association of a cystatin C gene polymorphism with late-onset alzheimer disease. *Arch. Neurol.*, 57, 1579-1583 (2000).

[94] Rogaeva, E., Meng, Y., Lee, J.H., Gu, Y., Kawarai, T., Zou, F., Katayama, T., Baldwin, C.T., Cheng, R., Hasegawa, H., Chen, F., Shibata, N., Lunetta, K.L., Pardossi-Piquard, R., Bohm, C., Wakutani, Y., Cupples, L.A., Cuenco, K.T., Green, R.C., Pinessi, L., Rainero, I., Sorbi, S., Bruni, A., Duara, R., Friedland, R.P., Inzelberg, R., Hampe, W., Bujo, H., Song, Y.Q., Andersen, O.M., Willnow, T.E., Graff-Radford, N., Petersen, R.C., Dickson, D., Der, S.D., Fraser, P.E., Schmitt-Ulms, G., Younkin, S., Mayeux, R., Farrer, L.A. & P. St George-Hyslop: The neuronal sortilin-related receptor SORL1 is genetically associated with Alzheimer disease. *Nat. Genet.*, 39, 168-177 (2007).

[95] Chambraud, B., Sardin, E., Giustiniani, J., Dounane, O., Schumacher, M., Goedert, M. & E.E. Baulieu: A role for FKBP52 in Tau protein function. *Proc. Natl. Acad. Sci. U. S. A.*, 107, 2658-2663 (2010).

[96] Sanders, A.E., Wang, C., Katz, M., Derby, C.A., Barzilai, N., Ozelius, L. & R.B. Lipton: Association of a functional polymorphism in the cholesteryl ester transfer protein (CETP) gene with memory decline and incidence of dementia. *J.A.M.A.*, 303, 150-158 (2010).

[97] Migliore, L., Testa, A., Scarpato, R., Pavese, N., Petrozzi, L. & U. Bonuccelli: Spontaneous and induced aneuploidy in peripheral blood lymphocytes of patients with Alzheimer's disease. *Hum. Genet.*, 101, 299-305 (1997).

[98] Migliore, L., Botto, N., Scarpato, R., Petrozzi, L., Cipriani, G. & U. Bonuccelli: Preferential occurrence of chromosome 21 malsegregation in peripheral blood lymphocytes of Alzheimer disease patients. *Cytogenet. Cell. Genet.*, 87, 41-46 (1999).

[99] Busser, J., Geldmacher, D.S. & K. Herrup: Ectopic cell cycle proteins predict the sites of neuronal cell death in Alzheimer's disease brain. *J. Neurosci.*, 18, 2801-2807 (1998).

[100] Yang, Y., Geldmacher, D.S. & K. Herrup: DNA replication precedes neuronal cell death in Alzheimer's disease. *J. Neurosci.*, 21, 2661-2668 (2001).

[101] Kingsbury, M.A., Yung, Y.C., Peterson, S.E., Westra, J.W. & J. Chun: Aneuploidy in the normal and diseased brain. *Cell. Mol. Life Sci.*, 63, 2626-2641 (2006).

[102] Vincent, I., Rosado, M. & P. Davies: Mitotic mechanisms in Alzheimer's disease? *J. Cell. Biol.*, 132, 413-425 (1996).

[103] Yang, Y., Mufson, E.J. & K.Herrup: Neuronal cell death is preceded by cell cycle events at all stages of Alzheimer's disease. *J. Neurosci.*, 23, 2557-2563 (2003).

[104] Herrup, K. & T. Arendt: Re-expression of cell cycle proteins induces neuronal cell death during Alzheimer's disease. *J. Alzheimers Dis.*, 4, 243-247 (2002).

[105] Yang, Y. & K. Herrup: Cell division in the CNS: protective response or lethal event in post-mitotic neurons? *Biochim. Biophys. Acta.*, 1772:457-66 (2007).

[106] Goldgaber, D., Lerman, M.I., McBride, O.W., Saffiotti, U. & D.C. Gajdusek: Characterization and chromosomal localization of a cDNA encoding brain amyloid of Alzheimer's disease. *Science*, 235, 877-880 (1987).

[107] Schellenberg, G.D., Bird, T.D., Wijsman, E.M., Orr, H.T., Anderson, L., Nemens, E., White, J.A., Bonnycastle, L., Weber, J.L., Alonso, M.E., Potter, H., Heston, L.L. & G.M. Martin: Genetic linkage evidence for a familial Alzheimer's disease locus on chromosome 14. *Science*, 258, 668-671 (1992).

[108] Iqbal, K., Grundke-Iqbal, I., Smith, A.J., George, L., Tung, Y.C. & T. Zaidi: Identification and localization of a tau peptide to paired helical filaments of Alzheimer disease. *Proc. Natl. Acad. Sci. U. S. A.*, 86, 5646-5650 (1989).

[109] Nishimura, M., Yu, G. & P.H. St George-Hyslop: Biology of presenilins as causative molecules for Alzheimer disease. *Clin. Genet.*, 55, 219-225 (1999).

[110] Chen, Y., McPhie, D.L., Hirschberg, J. & R.L. Neve: The amyloid precursor protein-binding protein APP-BP1 drives the cell cycle through the S-M checkpoint and causes apoptosis in neurons. *J. Biol. Chem.*, 275, 8929-8935 (2000).

[111] Wen, P.H., Shao, X., Shao, Z., Hof, P.R., Wisniewski, T., Kelley, K., Friedrich, V.L. Jr, Ho, L., Pasinetti, G.M., Shioi, J, Robakis, N.K. & G.A. Elder: Overexpression of wild type but not an FAD mutant presenilin-1 promotes neurogenesis in the hippocampus of adult mice. *Neurobiol. Dis.*, 10, 8-19 (2002).

[112] Jin, K., Galvan, V., Xie, L., Mao, X.O., Gorostiza, O.F., Bredesen, D.E. & D.A. Greenberg: Enhanced neurogenesis in Alzheimer's disease transgenic (PDGF-APPSw,Ind) mice. *Proc. Natl. Acad. Sci. U. S. A.*, 101, 13363-13367 (2004).

[113] Zhang, C., McNeil, E., Dressler, L. & R. Siman: Long-lasting impairment in hippocampal neurogenesis associated with amyloid deposition in a knock-in mouse model of familial Alzheimer's disease. *Exp. Neurol.*, 204, 77-87 (2007).

[114] Rodríguez, J.J., Jones, V.C., Tabuchi, M., Allan, S.M., Knight, E.M., LaFerla, F.M., Oddo, S. & A. Verkhratsky: Impaired adult neurogenesis in the dentate gyrus of a triple transgenic mouse model of Alzheimer's disease. *PLoS ONE*, 3, e2935 (2008).

[115] Yu, Y., He, J., Zhang, Y., Luo, H., Zhu, S., Yang, Y., Zhao, T., Wu, J., Huang, Y., Kong, J., Tan, Q. & X.M. Li: Increased hippocampal neurogenesis in the progressive stage of Alzheimer's disease phenotype in an APP/PS1 double transgenic mouse model. *Hippocampus*, 19, 1247-1253 (2009).

[116] German, D.C. & A.J. Eisch: Mouse models of Alzheimer's disease: insight into treatment. *Rev. Neurosci.*, 15, 353-369 (2004).

[117] Ziabreva, I., Perry, E., Perry, R., Minger, S.L., Ekonomou, A., Przyborski, S. & C. Ballard. Altered neurogenesis in Alzheimer's disease. *J Psychosom Res*, 61, 311-316 (2006).

[118] Sotthibundhu, A., Li, Q.X., Thangnipon, W. & E.J. Coulson. Abeta(1-42) stimulates adult SVZ neurogenesis through the p75 neurotrophin receptor. *Neurobiol Aging*, 30, 1975-1985 (2009).

[119] Li, J., Xu, M., Zhou, H., Ma, J. & H. Potter: Alzheimer presenilins in the nuclear membrane, interphase kinetochores, and centrosomes suggest a role in chromosome segregation. *Cell*, 90, 917-927 (1997).

[120] Boeras, D.I., Granic, A., Padmanabhan, J., Crespo, N.C., Rojiani, A.M. & H. Potter, H: Alzheimer's presenilin 1 causes chromosome missegregation and aneuploidy. *Neurobiol. Aging*, 29, 319-328 (2008).

[121] Ramírez, M.J., Puerto, S., Galofré, P., Parry, E.M., Parry, J.M., Creus, A., Marcos, R. & J. Surrallés: Multicolour FISH detection of radioactive iodine-induced 17cen-p53 chromosomal breakage in buccal cells from therapeutically exposed patients. *Carcinogenesis*, 21, 1581-1586 (2000).

[122] P. Taupin: Adult neurogenesis in the pathogenesis of Alzheimer's disease. *J. Neurodegener. Regene.*, 2, 6-8 (2009).

[123] P. Taupin: A dual activity of ROS and oxidative stress on adult neurogenesis and Alzheimer's disease. *Cent. Nerv. Syst. Agents Med. Chem.*, 10, 16-21 (2010).

[124] Arrieta, J.L. & F.R. Artalejo: Methodology, results and quality of clinical trials of tacrine in the treatment of Alzheimer's disease: a systematic review of the literature. *Age Ageing*, 27, 161-179 (1998).

[125] Wilkinson, D.G., Francis, P.T., Schwam, E. & J. Payne-Parrish: Cholinesterase inhibitors used in the treatment of Alzheimer's disease: the relationship between pharmacological effects and clinical efficacy. *Drugs Aging*, 21, 453-478 (2004).

[126] Creeley, C., Wozniak, D.F., Labruyere, J., Taylor, G.T. & J.W. Olney: Low doses of memantine disrupt memory in adult rats. *J. Neurosci.*, 26, 3923-3932 (2006).

[127] Jin, K., Xie, L., Mao, X.O. & D.A. Greenberg: Alzheimer's disease drugs promote neurogenesis. *Brain Res.*, 1085, 183-188 (2006).

[128] P. Taupin: Neurogenic factors are target in depression. *Drug. Discov. Today. Ther. Strateg.*, 5, 157-160 (2008).

[129] P. Taupin: Adult neurogenesis and drug therapy. *Cent. Nerv. Syst. Agents Med. Chem.*, 8, 198-202 (2008).

[130] P. Taupin: Nootropic agents stimulate neurogenesis. *Expert Opin. Ther. Pat.*, 19, 727-730 (2009).

[131] P. Taupin: Apigenin and related compounds stimulate adult neurogenesis. *Expert Opin. Ther. Pat.*, 19, 523-527 (2009).

[132] P. Taupin: Fourteen compounds and their derivatives for the treatment of diseases and injuries characterized by reduced neurogenesis and neurodegeneration. *Expert Opin. Ther. Pat.*, 19, 541-547 (2009).

[133] P. Taupin: Aneuploidy and adult neurogenesis in Alzheimer's disease: therapeutic strategies. *Drug Discov. Today*, In Press..

Chapter IV

Adult Neurogenesis and Drug Therapy[*]

Abstract

Current drug therapy strategies for the nervous system are based on the assumption that the adult central nervous system (CNS) lacks the capacity to make new nerve cells and regenerate after injury. Contrary to a long-held dogma, adult neurogenesis occurs in the adult brain and neural stem cells (NSCs) reside in the adult CNS. Neurogenesis in the adult brain is modulated in a broad range of environmental conditions, and physio- and pathological processes, as well as by trophic factors and drugs. This suggests that newborn neuronal cells of the adult brain may be involved in the functioning of the nervous system and may mediate a broad range of physio- and pathological processes, as well as the activities endogenous and exogenous factors and molecules. Hence, the confirmation that adult neurogenesis occurs in the adult brain and NSCs reside in the adult CNS force us to rethink how drugs are functioning and whether their activity may be mediated through adult neurogenesis. This will lead to the development and design of new strategies to treat neurological diseases and injuries, particularly drug therapy.

Introduction

The conventional belief was that we are born with a certain number of nerve cells and that the adult brain cannot generate new neurons and lacks the capacity for regeneration [1]. Hence, drug therapy to treat neurological diseases and injuries until now were focused on two main strategies, the control of neurotransmitter release and stimulation of nerve cells survival or capacity to make extra-numerous synapses, to compensate for neurotransmitters imbalance and neuronal loss.

---

*Copyright notice. Reproduced with permission from Bentham Science Publishers, Ltd.: Taupin P. Adult neurogenesis and drug therapy. Central Nervous System Agents in Medicinal Chemistry (2008) 8(3):198-202. Copyright 2008, Bentham Science Publishers, Ltd.

The first report that adult neurogenesis occurs in the adult mammalian brain came from studies conducted by Altman and Das in the early 60s. In their seminal studies, Altman and Das reported that new neuronal cells are generated in the adult dentate gyrus (DG) of the hippocampus, and that cell proliferation in the subventricular zone (SVZ), via migration, feeds persisting neurogenesis in the adult olfactory bulb in rodents [2, 3]. With the development of more sophisticated techniques to study neurogenesis [4], like bromodeoxyuridine (BrdU), retroviral labelings and confocal microscopy, studies in the 80s and 90s contributed to confirm that neurogenesis occurs in the adult brain of mammals, including humans [5]. The confirmation that neurogenesis occurs in the adult brain has tremendous implications for our understanding of the functioning and physio- and pathology of the nervous system, as well as for cellular therapy and pharmacology.

Neurogenesis in the Adult Mammalian Brain

In the adult mammalian brain, neurogenesis occurs primarily in two regions, the SVZ and DG of the hippocampus, in various species [5], including humans [6, 7]. It is postulated that newborn neuronal cells originate from stem cells in the adult brain. NSCs are the self-renewing multipotent cells that generate the main phenotypes of the nervous system [8]. Self-renewing multipotent neural progenitor and stem cells can be isolated and characterized in vitro, from various regions of the adult CNS, including the spinal cord [9-13]. Despite NSCs remaining to be fully identified and characterized in vitro and in vivo [14-17], it is well accepted that neurogenesis occurs in the adult brain and NSCs reside the in the adult CNS. Neurogenesis involves a relatively low fraction of neuronal cells in the adult brain, particularly the DG. It is reported that as many as 9,000 new neuronal cells are generated per day in the rodent DG, contributing to about 3.3% per month or about 0.1% per day of the granule cell population [18, 19]. Neurogenesis may also occur in other areas of the adult brain, like the CA1 area, neocortex, substantia nigra, 3rd ventricle, caudate nucleus, in some species [20-24]. However some of these data have been the sources of debates and controversies and remain to be further confirmed [25, 26]. The characterization that adult neurogenesis occurs in the adult brain and NSCs reside in the adult CNS suggests that the adult brain may be amenable to repair.

Adult neurogenesis is modulated by various conditions, like environment, various physio- and pathological processes, like aging, diseases, disorders and injuries, trophic factors, hormones and drug treatments [27]. The characterization that adult neurogenesis is modulated by a broad range of conditions, environment, physio- and pathological processes, endogenous and exogenous factors, suggests that newborn neuronal cells may contribute to these processes and the activities of endogenous and exogenous factors.

Neurogenesis and Neurological Diseases, Disorders and Injuries

Neurogenesis in Neurodegenerative Diseases and Disorders

Neurogenesis has been reported to be enhanced in the hippocampus of patients with neurological disease, like Alzheimer's disease (AD) and epilepsy.

Studies from autopsies reveal that the expression of markers of immature neuronal cells, like doublecortin, is increased in the DG, of the brains of patients with AD [28]. These results reveal that neurogenesis is enhanced in the brains of patients with AD. In animal models of AD, neurogenesis is enhanced in the DG of transgenic mice that express the Swedish and Indiana amyloid protein precursor (APP) mutations, [29], but it is decreased in the DG and SVZ of other models, like knock-out mice or mice deficient for presenilin 1 (PS1) and APP [30, 31]. The discrepancies of the data observed on adult neurogenesis in autopsies and animal models of AD may originate from the validity of animal models of AD, as representative models of the disease [32].

Neurogenesis is enhanced in the DG and SVZ, in animal models of epilepsy [33]. After pilocarpine treatment in rodents, ectopic granule-like cells in the hilus are labeled for marker of dividing cells, like BrdU. In these rodents, mossy fiber (MF)-like processes, in the stratum oriens of CA3 and inner molecular layer of the DG, are immunostained for markers of newly generated neuronal cells, like TOAD-64 [60]. This shows that ectopic granule-like cells in the hilus originate from newborn neuronal cells and MF remodeling derives from newborn granule cells rather than from preexisting mature dentate granule cells. X-ray irradiation of adult rat brains, after pilocarpine treatment, decreases neurogenesis, but does not prevent the induction of recurrent seizures, nor prevent seizure-induced ectopic granule-like cells and MF sprouting [34]. Hence, neurogenesis is enhanced in the DG and SVZ in animal models of epilepsy, and seizure-induced ectopic granule-like cells and MF sprouting arise not only from newborn neuronal cells, but also from mature dentate granule cells. These data provide a strong argument against a critical role of adult neurogenesis in epileptogenesis.

Immunohistochemistry and confocal microscopy analysis of autopsies for markers of the cell cycle and neuronal differentiation, like proliferating cell nuclear antigen and β-tubulin, reveal that cell proliferation and neurogenesis are increased in the SVZ of brains of patients with Huntington's disease (HD) [35]. In adult R6/1 transgenic mouse model of HD, neurogenesis is decreased in the DG [36]. After quinolinic acid striatal lesioning of adult brain, an experimental model of HD, neurogenesis is enhanced in the SVZ, leading to the migration of neuroblasts and formation of new neuronal cells in damaged areas of the striatum [37]. These data provide evidences that adult neurogenesis is enhanced in the SVZ of brains with HD. It shows that neural progenitor cells from the SVZ migrate toward the site of degeneration in HD. Data from R6/1 transgenic mouse model are difficult to interpret in the context of adult neurogenesis in HD, as mutated forms of huntingtin affect brain development [38]. This could underlie the decrease of adult neurogenesis reported in transgenic mice R6/1.

A post-mortem study reveals that adult neurogenesis is not altered in the hippocampus of patients suffering from depression [39]. Parkinson's disease (PD) is a chronic and progressive neurodegenerative disease, primarily associated with the loss of a specific type of dopamine neurons in the substantia nigra (SN) [40]. The rate of neurogenesis is stimulated in the SN, following lesion induced by a systemic dose of MPTP (1-methyl-4-phenyl-1,2,3,6-tetrahydropyridine) [22]. Another study reports no evidence of new dopaminergic neurons in the SN of 6-hydroxydopamine-lesioned hemi-Parkinsonian rodents [41]. Autopsy studies revealed that neurogenesis is decreased in the DG of patients suffering from schizophrenia [39]. The number of BrdU-positive cells decreased by 23% in the SGZ of the DG, 24 h after repeated injections of phencyclidine in rats, an experimental model of schizophrenia [42]. The level of newly generated cells returns to control level, one week after injection in the SGZ. These results show that neurogenesis is decreased in the DG of brains with schizophrenia.

In all, these results show that adult neurogenesis is modulated in a broad range of neurological diseases and disorders. In epilepsy, data presented provide a strong argument against a critical role of adult neurogenesis in epileptogenesis. However, although increased hippocampal neurogenesis may not be critical to epileptogenesis or to another disease, it could be a contributing factor to the disease when present. Hence, although these studies suggest that adult neurogenesis may contribute to the etiology of these diseases, its contribution to neurological diseases and disorders remains mostly unknown, and to be further evaluated and determined.

Table 1. Regulation of neurogenesis in the adult brain by trophic factors/cytokines and other molecules

Molecule	Area	Regulation	Reference #
EGF	SVZ	activation	49, 50
FGF-2 + CCg	DG	activation	50, 51
BDNF	SVZ	activation	52-54
IGF-I	DG	activation	55
TGF-α	SVZ	activation	56
Shh	DG	activation	57
VEGF	SVZ	activation	58
BDNF + noggin	SVZ/neostriatum	activation	59
CNTF	SVZ/DG	activation	60
PACAP	SVZ/DG	activation	62
NPY	DG	activation	63
Adrenal hormones	DG	inhibition	64, 65
NMDA receptor antagonist	DG	activation	66

Trophic factors, cytokines, and other factors, pituitary adenylate cyclase-activating polypeptide (PACAP), neuropeptide Y (NPY), nitric oxide (NO), N-methyl-D-aspartate (NMDA) receptor antagonists, have been administered in vivo, and tested for their neurogenic activities in the neurogenic areas of the adult brain; the dentate gyrus (DG) and subventricular zone (SVZ). The combination of BNDF and noggin mobilizes endogenous SVZ progenitor cells to the neostriatum, a non-neurogenic area of the adult brain, further emphasizing the potential of neural stem cells for repairing the CNS. EGF, epidermal growth factor; FGF-2, basic fibroblast growth factor, BDNF, brain derived neurotrophic factor, IGF-I, insulin growth factor-I; TGF-α, transforming growth factor-α; Shh, sonic hedgehog; VEGF, vascular endothelial growth factor; CNTF, ciliary neurotrophic factor.

Neurogenesis and Injuries

Neurogenesis is stimulated in the DG and SVZ, in the diseased brain and after CNS injuries, like strokes and traumatic brain injuries [43-45]. New neuronal cells are also generated at the sites of degeneration where they replace some of the degenerated nerve cells, after experimental strokes [43, 45]. Cell tracking studies revealed that new neuronal cells at the sites of degeneration originate from the SVZ. They migrate to the sites of degeneration, partially through the rostro-migratory stream [43, 45].

In all, newly generated neuronal cells are involved in the physiopathology of the adult CNS, but the function and relative contribution of newly generated neuronal cells to these processes versus the neuronal cells of the preexisting network remain to be determined. It is estimated that 0.2% of the degenerated nerve cells are replaced in the striatum after middle cerebral artery occlusion, a model of focal ischemia [45]. This low percentage of newly generated neuronal cells at the sites of injury may account for the lack of functional recovery in the injured CNS. The modulation of neurogenesis by environmental stimuli, and in physiopathological conditions may therefore contribute to CNS plasticity. The generation of newly generated neuronal cells, at the sites of injury in the diseased brain and after CNS injuries, may represent a regenerative attempt by the CNS [46, 47].

Discussion

The confirmation that neurogenesis occurs in the adult brain, and that NSCs reside in the adult CNS suggests that the adult CNS may be amenable to repair. Cell therapeutic intervention may involve the stimulation and transplantation of neural progenitor and stem cells of the adult CNS. Particularly, the ability of the CNS to regulate the generation of new neuronal cells may be use to promote brain repair in the diseased brain, and after CNS injury [48].

Stimulation of Neurogenesis

Trophic factors and cytokines have been reported to stimulate neurogenesis in vivo (Table 1). Epidermal growth factor administered by chronic infusions into the lateral ventricle of adult rats stimulates the proliferation of neural progenitor cells in the SVZ [49, 50]. The activity of basic fibroblast growth factor on adult hippocampal neurogenesis has been studied after chronic infusions into the lateral ventricle [48, 49] and subcutaneous injections [51]. In vivo, intracerebroventricular delivery of brain derived neurotrophic factor, by infusion or adenovirally administered, in adult rats increases the number of newly generated neuronal cells in the adult olfactory bulb. It also leads to new neurons in the parenchyma of the striatum, septum, thalamus, and hypothalamus [52-54]. The insulin-like growth factor-I stimulates neurogenesis in the adult rat DG [55]. Among other factors that have been reported to stimulate adult neurogenesis in vitro and in vivo are transforming growth factor-alpha [56], sonic hedgehog [57], vascular endothelial growth factor [58], noggin [59], ciliary neurotrophic factor [60], and neuropeptides like pituitary adenylate cyclase-activating polypeptide and neuropeptide Y [61-63]. Adrenal hormones and N-methyl-D-aspartate (NMDA) receptors also play an important role in the regulation of neurogenesis in the adult DG. Adrenal hormones suppress cell division in the adult rat DG, and treatment with NMDA receptor antagonists increase the birth of neurons and the overall density of neurons in the DG granule cell layer [64-68].

Since neural progenitor and stem cells reside throughout the adult CNS, the stimulation of endogenous neural progenitor and stem cells locally would represent a strategy to promote regeneration in the diseased brain and after CNS injury. Alternatively, since new neuronal cells that originate from the SVZ, are generated at the sites of degeneration in the diseased brain and after CNS injuries, strategies that promote regeneration and repair may focus on stimulating SVZ neurogenesis.

Drug Therapy

Neurogenesis is modulated in a broad range of neurological diseases and disorders, like AD. Studies reveal that drugs used to treat AD and depression, modulate neurogenesis. Two classes of drugs are currently used to treat patients with AD: acetylcholinesterase (AChE) inhibitors, like tacrine, donepezil, galantamine and rivastigmine, and NMDA glutamate receptor antagonists, like memantine [69-71]. Galantamine and memantine increase neurogenesis in the DG and SVZ of adult rodents, by 26-45% [72]. Various classes of drugs are currently prescribed for the treatment of depression [73, 74], among them, selective serotonin reuptake inhibitors (SSRIs) -like fluoxetine-, monoamine oxidase inhibitors -like tranylcypromine-, selective norepinephrine reuptake inhibitors -like reboxetine-, tricyclic antidepressants -like imipramine and desipramine- and phosphodiesterase-IV inhibitors -like rolipram-. Chronic administration of antidepressants, like fluoxetine, increases neurogenesis in the DG, but not the SVZ of adult rats and nonhuman primates [75-77]. Agomelatine, a melatonergic agonist and serotoninergic antagonist defining a new class of antidepressant [77], increases adult hippocampal neurogenesis in rodents [78].

This suggests that the activity of these drugs may be mediated through adult neurogenesis. In all, adult neurogenesis is enhanced in the brain of patients with AD and drugs used to treat AD, AChE and NMDA antagonists, modulate adult neurogenesis. Adult neurogenesis may also contribute to the activities of drugs used to treat depression. In support to this contention, X-irradiation of the hippocampal region, but not other brain regions, like the SVZ or the cerebellar region, prevents the behavioral effect of the antidepressants, like fluoxetine, in adult mice [79]. Hence, adult neurogenesis may mediate the activities of antidepressants, particularly SSRIs.

In all, drugs used to treat depression, particularly SSRIs, modulate adult neurogenesis that may mediate their behavioral activities. However, most studies performed in animal models use BrdU labeling as paradigm for studying neurogenesis. BrdU is a thymidine analog that incorporates DNA of dividing cells during the S-phase of the cell cycle, and is used for birthdating and monitoring cell proliferation [80]. As a thymidine analog, BrdU is not a marker for cell proliferation, but a marker for DNA synthesis. Some of the data observed by mean of immunohistochemistry for cell cycle markers and BrdU labeling may then not represent adult neurogenesis, but rather labeled nerve cells that may have entered the cell cycle and underwent DNA replication or duplication, but did not complete the cell cycle [81].

Furthermore, recent studies reveal that the blood-brain barrier may be affected in the patients with AD [82] and after drug treatments. In these conditions, an increase in BrdU labeling in the brain could originate from an increase in BrdU uptake rather than an increase in cell proliferation and neurogenesis [81]. In light of these data, adult neurogenesis must be re-evaluated and -examined, particularly in neurological diseases and disorders and after drug treatments.

Conclusion

Adult neurogenesis may contribute to the etiology and pathogenesis of neurological diseases and disorders and may mediate the activity of drugs used to treat neurological diseases and disorders, particularly AD and depression. However, the contribution and significance of adult neurogenesis to these processes remain to be further confirmed and elucidated. The mechanisms underlying the involvement of adult neurogenesis in the activities of drugs, used to treat AD and antidepressants remain also to be determined. Whether the drugs act directly or indirectly in newborn neuronal cells remain to be determined, and whether the drugs act via their pharmacological activities, on messenger signaling pathways, and/or via a neurogenic activity, by modulating neurogenesis, remain to be established. The involvement of adult neurogenesis in the activities of antidepressants has been challenged by other studies, reporting that antidepressant treatments do not result in an increase of neurogenesis in the adult DG of human, from autopsy studies [40]. Hence, the role and significance of the increased neurogenesis in the activity of drugs remain to be understood and further evaluated. Hence, the confirmation that neurogenesis occurs in the adult brain and NSCs reside in the adult CNS is not only important for our understanding of the functioning and physio- and pathology of the nervous system, but also for therapy and pharmacology [83]. The elucidation of the contribution of adult neurogenesis to neurological diseases and disorder may contribute to a better understanding of the etiology and mechanisms of neurological diseases and disorders, particularly AD and depression, as well as new drug design and strategies to treat these diseases and disorders. Future studies will aim at unraveling the mechanisms of action of drugs on neurogenesis.

References

[1]   Ramon y Cajal, S. Degeneration and Regeneration of the Nervous System, Hafner: New York, 1928.
[2]   Altman, J. (1969). *J. Comp. Neurol.*, 1969, 137, 433.
[3]   Rakic, P. *Science,* 1985, 227, 1054.
[4]   Taupin, P. *Regen. Med.*, 2007, 2, 51.
[5]   Taupin, P.; Gage, F.H. *J. Neurosci. Res.,* 2002, 69, 745.
[6]   Eriksson, P.S.; Perfilieva, E.; Bjork-Eriksson, T.; Alborn, A.M.; Nordborg, C.; Peterson, D.A.; Gage, F.H. *Nat. Med.,* 1998, 4, 1313.

[7]   Curtis, M.A.; Kam, M.; Nannmark, U.; Anderson, M.F.; Axell, M.Z.; Wikkelso, C.; Holtas, S.; van Roon-Mom, W,M.; Bjork-Eriksson, T.; Nordborg, C.; Frisen, J.; Dragunow, M.; Faull, R.L.; Eriksson, P.S. *Science,* 2007, 315, 1243.

[8]   Gage, F.H. *Science,* 2000, 287, 1433.

[9]   Reynolds, B.A.; Weiss, S. *Science,* 1992, 255, 1707.

[10] Gage, F.H.; Coates, P.W.; Palmer, T.D.; Kuhn, H.G.; Fisher, L.J.; Suhonen, J.O.; Peterson, D.A.; Suhr, S.T.; Ray, *J. Proc. Natl. Acad. Sci. USA,* 1995, 92, 11879.

[11] Gritti, A.; Parati, E.A.; Cova, L.; Frolichsthal, P.; Galli, R.; Wanke, E.; Faravelli, L.; Morassutti, D.J.; Roisen, F.; Nickel, D.D.; Vescovi, A.L. *J. Neurosci.,* 1996, 16, 1091.

[12] Weiss, S.; Dunne, C.; Hewson, J.; Wohl, C.; Wheatley, M.; Peterson, A.C.; Reynolds, B.A. *J. Neurosci.,* 1996, 16, 7599.

[13] Palmer, T.D.; Takahashi, J.; Gage, F.H. *Mol. Cell Neurosci.,* 1997, 8, 389.

[14] Kornblum, H.I.; Geschwind, D.H. *Nat. Rev. Neurosci.,* 2001, 2, 843.

[15] Seaberg, R.M.; van der Kooy, D. *J. Neurosci.,* 2002, 22, 1784.

[16] Suslov, O.N.; Kukekov, V.G.; Ignatova, T.N.; Steindler, D.A. *Proc. Natl. Acad. Sci. USA,* 2002, 99, 14506.

[17] Bull, N.D.; Bartlett, P.F. *J. Neurosci.,* 2005, 25, 10815.

[18] Kempermann, G.; Kuhn, H.G.; Gage, F.H. *Nature,* 1997,386, 493.

[19] Cameron, H.A.; McKay, R.D. *J. Comp. Neurol.,* 2001, 435, 406.

[20] Gould, E.; Reeves, A.J.; Graziano, M.S.; Gross, C.G. *Science*, 1999, 286, 548.

[21] Rietze, R.; Poulin, P.; Weiss, S. J. *Comp. Neurol.,* 2000, 424, 397.

[22] Zhao, M.; Momma, S.; Delfani, K.; Carlen, M.; Cassidy, R.M.; Johansson, C.B.; Brismar, H.; Shupliakov, O.; Frisen, J.; Janson, A.M. *Proc. Natl. Acad. Sci. USA,* 2003, 100, 7925.

[23] Xu, Y.; Tamamaki, N.; Noda, T.; Kimura, K.; Itokazu, Y.; Matsumoto, N.; Dezawa, M.; Ide, C. *Exp. Neurol.,* 2005, 192, 251.

[24] Luzzati, F.; De Marchis, S.; Fasolo, A.; Peretto, P. J. Neurosci., Behav., 2002, 1, 142.

[25] Kornack D.R.; Rakic P. *Science, 2001*, 294, 2127.

[26] Frielingsdorf, H.; Schwarz, K.; Brundin, P.; Mohapel, P. *Proc. Natl. Acad. Sci. USA,* 2004, 101, 10177.

[27] Taupin, P. *Med. Sci. Monit.,* 2005, 11, RA247.

[28] Jin, K.; Peel, A.L.; Mao, X.O.; Xie, L.; Cottrell, B.A.; Henshall, D.C.; Greenberg, D.A. *Proc. Natl. Acad. Sci. USA,* 2004, 101, 343.

[29] Jin, K.; Galvan, V.; Xie, L.; Mao, X.O.; Gorostiza, O.F.; Bredesen, D.E.; Greenberg, D.A. *Proc. Natl. Acad. Sci. USA,* 2004, 101, 13363.

[30] Feng, R.; Rampon, C.; Tang, Y.P.; Shrom, D.; Jin, J.; Kyin, M.; Sopher, B.; Miller, M.W.; Ware, C.B.; Martin, G.M.; Kim, S.H.; Langdon, R.B.; Sisodia, S.S.; Tsien, J.Z. Neuron, 2001, 32, 911. Erratum in: *Neuron,* 2002, 33, 313.

[31] Wen, P.H.; Shao, X.; Shao, Z.; Hof, P.R.; Wisniewski, T.; Kelley, K.; Friedrich, V.L. Jr; Ho, L.; Pasinetti, G.M.; Shioi, J.; Robakis, N.K.; Elder, G.A. *Neurobiol. Dis.,* 2002, 10, 8.

[32] Dodart, J.C.; Mathis, C.; Bales, K.R.; Paul, S.M. *Genes Brain Behav.,* 2002, 1, 142.

[33] Parent, J.M.; Yu, T.W.; Leibowitz, R.T.; Geschwind, D.H.; Sloviter, R.S.; Lowenstein, D.H. *J. Neurosci.,* 1997, 17, 3727.

[34] Parent, J.M.; Tada, E.; Fike, J.R.; Lowenstein, D.H. *J. Neurosci.,* 1999, 19, 4508.

[35] Curtis, M.A.; Penney, E.B.; Pearson, A.G.; van Roon-Mom, W.M.; Butterworth, N.J.; Dragunow, M.; Connor, B.; Faull, R.L. *Proc. Natl. Acad. Sci. USA*, 2003, 100, 9023.

[36] Lazic, S.E.; Grote, H.; Armstrong, R.J.; Blakemore, C.; Hannan, A.J.; van Dellen, A.; Barker, R.A. *Neuroreport*, 2004, 15, 811.

[37] Tattersfield, A.S.; Croon, R.J.; Liu, Y.W.; Kells, A.P.; Faull, R.L.; Connor, B. *Neuroscience*, 2004, 127, 319.

[38] White, J.K.; Auerbach, W.; Duyao, M.P.; Vonsattel, J.P.; Gusella, J.F.; Joyner, A.L.; MacDonald, M.E. *Nat. Genet.*, 1997, 17, 404.

[39] Reif, A.; Fritzen, S.; Finger, M.; Strobel, A.; Lauer, M.; Schmitt, A.; Lesch, K.P. *Mol. Psychiatry*, 2006, 11, 514.

[40] Fernandez-Espejo, E. *Mol. Neurobiol.*, 2004, 29, 15.

[41] Frielingsdorf, H.; Schwarz, K.; Brundin, P.; Mohapel, P. *Proc. Natl. Acad. Sci. USA*, 2004, 101, 10177.

[42] Liu, J.; Suzuki, T.; Seki, T.; Namba, T.; Tanimura, A.; Arai, H. Synapse, 2006, 60, 56.

[43] Liu, J.; Solway, K.; Messing, R.O.; Sharp, F.R. *J. Neurosci.*, 1998, 18, 7768.

[44] Dash, P.K.; Mach, S.A.; Moore, A.N. *J. Neurosci. Res.*, 2001, 63, 313.

[45] Jin, K.; Peel, A.L.; Mao, X.O.; Xie, L.; Cottrell, B.A.; Henshall, D.C.; Greenberg, D.A. *Proc. Natl. Acad. Sci. USA*, 2004, 101, 343.

[46] Taupin, P. *Restor. Neurol. Neurosci.*, 2006, 24, 9.

[47] Taupin, P. *Curr. Neurovasc. Res.*, 2006, 3, 67.

[48] Taupin, P. *Curr. Opin. Mol. Ther.*, 2006, 8, 225.

[49] Craig, C.G.; Tropepe, V.; Morshead, C.M.; Reynolds, B.A.; Weiss, S.; van der Kooy, D. *J. Neurosci.*, 1996, 16, 2649.

[50] Kuhn, H.G.; Winkler, J.; Kempermann, G.; Thal, L.J.; Gage, F.H. *J. Neurosci.*, 1997, 17, 5820.

[51] Wagner, J.P.; Black, I.B.; DiCicco-Bloom, E. *J. Neurosci.*, 1999, 19, 6006.

[52] Zigova, T.; Pencea, V.; Wiegand, S.J.; Luskin, M.B. *Mol. Cell. Neurosci.*, 1998, 11, 234.

[53] Pencea, V.; Bingaman, K.D.; Wiegand, S.J.; Luskin, M.B. *J. Neurosci.*, 2001, 21, 6706.

[54] Benraiss, A.; Chmielnicki, E.; Lerner, K.; Roh, D.; Goldman, S.A. *J. Neurosci.*, 2001, 21, 6718.

[55] Aberg, M.A.; Aberg, N.D.; Hedbacker, H.; Oscarsson, J.; Eriksson, P.S. *J. Neurosci.*, 2000, 20, 2896.

[56] Tropepe, V.; Craig, C.G.; Morshead, C.M.; van der Kooy, D. *J. Neurosci.*, 197, 17, 7850.

[57] Lai, K.; Kaspar, B.K.; Gage, F.H.; Schaffer, D.V. Nat. Neurosci., 2003, 6, 21. Erratum in: *Nat. Neurosci.*, 2003, 6, 645.

[58] Schanzer, A.; Wachs, F.P.; Wilhelm, D.; Acker, T.; Cooper-Kuhn, C.; Beck, H.; Winkler, J.; Aigner, L.; Plate, K.H.; Kuhn, H.G. *Brain Pathol.* 2004, 14, 237.

[59] Chmielnicki, E.; Benraiss, A.; Economides, A.N.; Goldman, S.A. *J. Neurosci.*, 2004, 24, 2133.

[60] Emsley, J.G.; Hagg, T. *Exp. Neurol.*, 2003, 183, 298.

[61] Hansel, D.E.; Eipper, B.A.; Ronnett, G.V. *J. Neurosci. Res.*, 2001, 66, 1.

[62] Mercer, A.; Ronnholm, H.; Holmberg, J.; Lundh, H.; Heidrich, J.; Zachrisson, O.; Ossoinak, A.; Frisen, J.; Patrone, C. *J. Neurosci. Res.*, 2004, 76, 205.

[63] Howell, O.W.; Doyle, K.; Goodman, J.H.; Scharfman, H.E.; Herzog, H.; Pringle, A.; Beck-Sickinger, A.G.; Gray, W.P. *J. Neuro-chem.*, 2005, 93, 560.

[64] Gould, E.; Cameron, H.A.; Daniels, D.C.; Woolley, C.S.; McEwen, B.S. *J. Neurosci.*, 1992, 12, 3642.

[65] Cameron, H.A.; Gould, E. *Neuroscience*, 1994, 61, 203.

[66] Cameron, H.A.; McEwen, B.S.; Gould, E. *J. Neurosci.*, 1995, 15, 4687.

[67] Cameron, H.A.; Gould, E. *J Comp Neurol.*, 1996, 369, 56.

[68] Cameron, H.A.; McKay, R.D. *Nat. Neurosci.*, 1999, 2, 894.

[69] Arrieta, J.L.; Artalejo, F.R. *Age Ageing*, 1998, 27, 161.

[70] Wilkinson, D.G.; Francis, P.T.; Schwam, E.; Payne-Parrish, J. *Drugs Aging*, 2004, 21, 453.

[71] McShane, R.; Areosa Sastre, A.; Minakaran, N. *Cochrane Database Syst. Rev.*, 2006. 2, CD003154.

[72] Jin, K.; Xie, L.; Mao, X.O.; Greenberg, D.A. *Brain Res.*, 2006, 1085, 183.

[73] Wong, M.L.; Licinio, J. *Nat. Rev. Neurosci.*, 2001, 2, 343.

[74] Brunello, N.; Mendlewicz, J.; Kasper, S.; Leonard, B.; Montgomery, S.; Nelson, J.; Paykel, E.; Versiani, M.; Racagni, G. *Eur. Neuropsychopharmacol.*, 2002, 12, 461.

[75] Malberg, J.E.; Eisch, A.J.; Nestler, E.J.; Duman, R.S. J. Neurosci., 2000, 20, 9104.

[76] Malberg, J.E. ; Duman, R.S. *Neuropsychopharmacology,* 2003, 28, 1562.

[77] Perera, T.D.; Coplan, J.D.; Lisanby, S.H.; Lipira, C.M.; Arif, M.; Carpio, C.; Spitzer, G.; Santarelli, L.; Scharf, B.; Hen, R.; Rosokli-ja, G.; Sackeim, H.A.; Dwork, A.J. *J. Neurosci.*, 2007, 27, 4894.

[78] Banasr, M.; Soumier, A.; Hery, M.; Mocaer, E.; Daszuta, A. *Biol. Psychiatry*, 2006, 59, 1087.

[79] Santarelli, L.; Saxe, M.; Gross, C.; Surget, A.; Battaglia, F.; Dulawa, S.; Weisstaub, N.; Lee, J.; Duman, R.; Arancio, O.; Belzung, C.; Hen, R. *Science*, 2003, 301, 805.

[80] Miller, M.W.; Nowakowski, R.S. *Brain Res.,* 1988, 457, 44.

[81] Taupin, P. *Brain Res. Rev.*, 2007, 53, 198.

[82] Desai, B.S.; Monahan, A.J.; Carvey, P.M.; Hendey, B. *Cell Transplant.*, 2007;16, 285.

[83] Taupin, P. *Exp. Rev. Neurother.*, 2008, 8, 311.

Chapter V

Neurogenic Factors Are Targets in Depression

Abstract

The confirmation that neurogenesis occurs in the adult brain and neural stem cells (NSCs) reside in the adult central nervous system (CNS) opens new avenues for our understanding of the physio- and pathology of the nervous system, as well as for therapy. Reports show that stress and antidepressants modulate neurogenesis in the adult hippocampus, and that the activity of antidepressants is mediated by adult neurogenesis. The mechanisms underlying the involvement of adult neurogenesis in depression and the activity of antidepressants might be mediated by trophic factors and cytokines. Hence, trophic factors, cytokines and their signaling pathways are potential targets in depression, and offer new opportunities to treat this disorder.

Introduction

Contrary to a long-held dogma, neurogenesis occurs in the adult mammalian brain, including in human [1,2]. It occurs primarily in two regions of the adult brain, the dentate gyrus (DG) of the hippocampus and the subventricular (SVZ) [3]. The confirmation that neurogenesis occurs in the adult mammalian brain, and the isolation and characterization of adult-derived neural progenitor and stem cells in vitro open new opportunities for cellular therapy; the stimulation of endogenous neural progenitor or stem cells, and the transplantation of neural progenitor and stem cells, to repair the degenerated or injured pathways [4]. Adult neurogenesis is modulated by a broad range of stimuli and conditions, including environmental enrichment, physiological processes, pathological conditions, trophic factors/cytokines and drugs [5,6]. Several studies have reported that stress and antidepressants modulate neurogenesis in the adult hippocampus. Hence, adult neurogenesis could be as important for cellular therapy, as for pharmacology, of the nervous system, particularly for depression.

Adult Neurogenesis and Depression

Stress is an environmental and causal factor in precipitating episodes of depression in human [7]. Neurogenesis is decreased in the hippocampus of adult monkeys and rats subjected to psychosocial and physical stress, like the establishment of dominant/subordinate relationship between two males unknown to each other, and acute or chronic restraint [8,9]. Chronic administration of antidepressants, like the selective serotonin reuptake inhibitor (SSRI) fluoxetine and the melatonergic agonist and serotoninergic antagonist agomelatine, increases neurogenesis in the DG, but not SVZ, of adult rats and nonhuman primates [10–13]. A postmortem study performed from the brains of patients with major depression reveals that neurogenesis is not altered in the hippocampus of those patients [14].

These results suggest that neurogenesis in the adult hippocampus plays an important role in biology of depression. Particularly, stress-induced decrease of neurogenesis in the adult DG would be an important causal factor in precipitating episodes of depression. It is proposed that the waning and waxing of neurogenesis in the adult hippocampus are important factors, in the precipitation of and recovery from episodes of clinical depression, respectively [15]. The mechanisms underlying the modulation of adult neurogenesis in depression remain to be fully determined. Glucocorticoids, stress-related hormones and serotonin (5-hydroxytryptamine or 5-HT), a neurotransmitter implicated in the modulation of mood and anxiety-related disorders, are among the factor and molecule candidates in modulating neurogenesis during episodes of depression [16]. Other factor candidates in modulating neurogenesis during episodes of depression are substances released by the immune cells, like cytokines. Recent studies have reported that inflammatory reactions could be causal factors of neurological diseases and disorders, particularly depression [17]. Interleukin-6 (IL-6) is released by the immune cells and involved in inflammatory reactions of the nervous system. A recent study reports that IL-6 decreases neurogenesis in the adult hippocampus in rodents [18]. Hence, IL-6 is a candidate for mediating neurogenesis in episode of depression.

Adult Neurogenesis and the Pharmacology of Depression

The modulation of adult neurogenesis by antidepressants, particularly SSRIs like fluoxetine, suggests that it might contribute or mediate their activity. X-irradiation of the hippocampal region inhibits neurogenesis in the DG and prevents the behavioral effect of antidepressants, like fluoxetine, in adult mice [19]. The behavioral effect of the antidepressants in this study was assessed by the novelty-suppressed feeding test, a test used to assess chronic antidepressant efficacy, in 129SvEvTac mice. In these mice the neurogenic activity of SSRIs is mediated by 5-HT, as fluoxetine does not elicit any neurogenic and behavioral effects in 5-HT1A receptor null mice [19]. These results provide evidences and support that adult neurogenesis might mediate the behavioral effects of antidepressants.

The mechanisms underlying the activity of antidepressants on adult neurogenesis remain to be fully determined. Studies show that it might be mediated by trophic factors, particularly that brain-derived neurotrophic factor (BDNF) [20]. BDNF has an antidepressant effects; the level of expression of BDNF is increased in the brains of patients subjected to antidepressant treatments and the administration of BDNF increases adult neurogenesis in the hippocampus [21–23]. The antidepressant activity of BDNF would be mediated through the TrkB neurotrophin receptor and the mitogen-activated protein kinase signaling pathway [24,25]. More recently, the expression of the angiogenic factor, vascular endothelial growth factor (VEGF), has been reported to be up-regulated in the brain of rodents administered with antidepressants [26]. This up-regulation mediates the increase in hippocampal neurogenesis induced by the antidepressants and is mediated by the VEGF-signaling pathway; Flk-1-signaling pathway. VEGF has previously been reported to stimulate adult neurogenesis in vivo [27]. These results show that neurogenic factors are potential therapeutic targets for the treatment of depression [28].

Discussion

In all, these data show that adult neurogenesis, the hippocampus and trophic factors are targets in depression. There are, however, controversies and debates over the involvement of adult neurogenesis and the hippocampus in the biology of depression and the activity of antidepressants.

Adult Neurogenesis and Depression

Several studies have reported that antidepressants, including SSRIs like fluoxetine, produce their activity independently of adult neurogenesis. In a postmortem study, performed from the brains of patients with major depression revealing that neurogenesis is not altered in the hippocampus of those patients, most of the patients were on antidepressant medication [14]. This argues against a role of antidepressants in adult neurogenesis. The anxiolytic/antidepressant SNAP 94847 (N-[3-(1-{[4-(3,4-difluorophenoxy)-phenyl]methyl} (4-piperidyl))-4-methylphenyl]-2-methylpropanamide), an antagonist of the melanin-concentrating hormone receptor, stimulates the proliferation of progenitor cells in the DG, but its activity is unaltered in mice in which neurogenesis was suppressed by X-irradiation [29]. More recently, it was reported that fluoxetine produces its antidepressant activity independently of neurogenesis in certain strains of mice, like BALB/cJ mice [30]. In these mice, the activity of SSRIs, like fluoxetine, was reported not to be mediated by 5-HT1A receptor [30]. This shows that antidepressants could elicit their activity independently of adult neurogenesis and/or that their activity might not be mediated through adult neurogenesis. Hence, antidepressants, particularly SSRIs, like fluoxetine, might produce their activities via distinct mechanisms, some independent of adult neurogenesis.

The Hippocampus and Depression

The modulation of adult neurogenesis by antidepressants and the mediation of the behavioral activity of antidepressants by adult neurogenesis link adult neurogenesis and the hippocampus to depression. Previous studies have reported conflicting data over the involvement of the hippocampus in clinical depression. On the one hand, clinical magnetic resonance imaging and postmortem studies in depressive patients reveal that chronic stress and depression result in atrophy of the hippocampus, an atrophy reversed by antidepressant treatment [31–33]. On the other hand, other studies show that hippocampal volume remains unchanged in depressive patients [34,35]. A link between adult neurogenesis, atrophy and loss of nerve cells in the hippocampus also remains to be demonstrated. Hence, the involvement of the hippocampus and adult neurogenesis remains to be further evaluated and characterized. The hippocampus could not be primarily involved in clinical depression, as other areas of the brain could play a critical role in depression [36]. As for adult neurogenesis, it could be more a contributing factor of plasticity of the central nervous system (CNS) and a consequence, rather than a causative factor, in neurological diseases and disorders [37–40].

Limitations of Paradigms and Models to Study Adult Neurogenesis and Depression

Most studies conducted in animal models, rodents and nonhuman primates, used the bromodeoxyuridine (BrdU) labeling paradigm to assess neurogenesis. BrdU is a thymidine analog that incorporates DNA of dividing cells during the S-phase of the cell cycle, and is used for birthdating and monitoring cell proliferation [41]. BrdU is a toxic and mutagenic substance; it alters the cell cycle, and has transcriptional and translational effects. As a thymidine analog, it is not a marker for cell proliferation, but a marker for DNA synthesis. As such its use is subject to limitations and pitfalls [42,43]. Particularly, the blood–brain barrier is affected by drug treatments [44]. An increase in BrdU labeling in the brain could then originate from an increase in BrdU uptake rather than an increase in cell proliferation and neurogenesis, as a result of antidepressant treatment. Neuroinflammation could be a causal factor of neurological diseases and disorders, particularly depression [17] and decreases neurogenesis in the adult brain [45,46]. Hence, neuroinflammation, either as a causative factor of depression or after X-irradiation of the adult brain or hippocampal region, might affect the experimental read-out of neurogenesis in vivo. In all, data on adult neurogenesis in depression and activity of antidepressants on adult neurogenesis are difficult to interpret in light of these data. In addition, recent reports have questioned the validity of antidepressants currently prescribed, for the treatment of depression [47,48].

Conclusion

In all, adult neurogenesis, the hippocampus and trophic factors are targets in depression. However, the contribution of adult neurogenesis and the hippocampus to the biology of depression and its pharmacology remains to be elucidated and determined. The confirmation that adult neurogenesis occurs in the adult brain and neural stem cells (NSCs) reside in the adult CNS in mammals has tremendous implications for our understanding of the functioning of the nervous system and for therapy. Evidence that adult neurogenesis is involved in depression and antidepressant activity might lead to a better understanding of the etiology of depression and its pharmacology. Future directions involve the design and development of new antidepressants targeting specifically newborn neuronal cells of the adult mammalian brain, and their validation. Specifically, neurogenic factors and their signaling pathways offer new targets to develop drugs and strategies for the treatment of depression.

Acknowledgments

Reproduced from: Taupin P. Neurogenic factors are target in depression. Drug Discovery Today: Therapeutic Strategies (2008) 5(3):157-160. Copyright (2008), with permission from Elsevier.

References

[1] Eriksson, P.S. et al. (1998) Neurogenesis in the adult human hippocampus. *Nat. Med.* 4, 1313–1317.

[2] Curtis, M.A. et al. (2007) Human neuroblasts migrate to the olfactory bulb via a lateral ventricular extension. *Science* 315, 1243–1249.

[3] Taupin, P. et al. (2002) Adult neurogenesis and neural stem cells of the central nervous system in mammals. *J. Neurosci. Res.* 69, 745–749.

[4] Taupin, P. (2006) The therapeutic potential of adult neural stem cells. *Curr. Opin. Mol. Ther.* 8, 225–231.

[5] van Praag, H. et al. (2000) Neural consequences of environmental enrichment. *Nat. Rev. Neurosci.* 1, 191–198.

[6] Taupin, P. (2005) Adult neurogenesis in the mammalian central nervous system: functionality and potential clinical interest. *Med. Sci. Monit.* 11, RA247–RA252.

[7] Miura, H. et al. (2008) A link between stress and depression: shifts in the balance between the kynurenine and serotonin pathways of tryptophan metabolism and the etiology and pathophysiology of depression. *Stress* 11, 198–209.

[8] Gould, E. et al. (1998) Proliferation of granule cell precursors in the dentate gyrus of adult monkeys is diminished by stress. *Proc. Natl. Acad. Sci. USA* 95, 3168–3171.

[9] Pham, K. et al. (2003) Repeated restraint stress suppresses neurogenesis and induces biphasic PSA-NCAM expression in the adult rat dentate gyrus. *Eur. J. Neurosci.* 17, 879–886.

[10] Malberg, J.E. et al. (2000) Chronic antidepressant treatment increases neurogenesis in adult rat hippocampus. *J. Neurosci.* 20, 9104–9110.

[11] Malberg, J.E. et al. (2003) Cell proliferation in adult hippocampus is decreased by inescapable stress: reversal by fluoxetine treatment. *Neuropsychopharmacology* 28, 1562–1571.

[12] Banasr, M. et al. (2006) Agomelatine, a new antidepressant, induces regional changes in hippocampal neurogenesis. *Biol. Psychiatry* 59, 1087–1096.

[13] Perera, T.D. et al. (2007) Antidepressant-induced neurogenesis in the hippocampus of adult nonhuman primates. *J. Neurosci.* 27, 4894–4901.

[14] Reif, A. et al. (2006) Neural stem cell proliferation is decreased in schizophrenia, but not in depression. *Mol. Psychiatry* 11, 514–522.

[15] Jacobs, B.L. et al. (2000) Adult brain neurogenesis and psychiatry: a novel theory of depression. *Mol. Psychiatry* 5, 262–269.

[16] Cameron, H.A. et al. (1994) Adult neurogenesis is regulated by adrenal steroids in the dentate gyrus. *Neuroscience* 61, 203–209.

[17] Minghetti, L. (2005) Role of inflammation in neurodegenerative diseases. *Curr. Opin. Neurol.* 18, 315–321.

[18] Vallieres, L. et al. (2002) Reduced hippocampal neurogenesis in adult transgenic mice with chronic astrocytic production of interleukin-6. *J. Neurosci.* 22, 486–492.

[19] Santarelli, L. et al. (2003) Requirement of hippocampal neurogenesis for the behavioral effects of antidepressants. *Science* 301, 805–809.

[20] Groves, J.O. (2007) Is it time to reassess the BDNF hypothesis of depression? *Mol. Psychiatry* 12, 1079–1088.

[21] Siuciak, J.A. et al. (1997) Antidepressant-like effect of brain-derived neurotrophic factor (BDNF). *Pharmacol. Biochem. Behav.* 56, 131–137.

[22] Chen, B. et al. (2001) Increased hippocampal BDNF immunoreactivity in subjects treated with antidepressant medication. *Biol. Psychiatry* 50, 260– 265.

[23] Scharfman, H. et al. (2005) Increased neurogenesis and the ectopic granule cells after intrahippocampal BDNF infusion in adult rats. *Exp. Neurol.* 192, 348–356.

[24] Saarelainen, T. et al. (2003) Activation of the TrkB neurotrophin receptor is induced by antidepressant drugs and is required for antidepressant-induced behavioral effects. *J. Neurosci.* 23, 349–357.

[25] Duman, C.H. et al. (2007) A role for MAP kinase signaling in behavioral models of depression and antidepressant treatment. *Biol. Psychiatry* 61, 661–670.

[26] Warner-Schmidt, J.L. et al. (2007) VEGF is an essential mediator of the neurogenic and behavioral actions of antidepressants. *Proc. Natl. Acad. Sci. USA* 104, 4647–4652.

[27] Schanzer, A. et al. (2004) Direct stimulation of adult neural stem cells in vitro and neurogenesis in vivo by vascular endothelial growth factor. *Brain Pathol.* 14, 237–248.

[28] Warner-Schmidt, J.L. et al. (2008) VEGF as a potential target for therapeutic intervention in depression. *Curr. Opin. Pharmacol.* 8, 14–19.

[29] David, D.J. et al. (2007) Efficacy of the MCHR1 antagonist N-[3-(1-{[4-(3,4-difluorophenoxy)phenyl]methyl}(4-piperidyl))-4-methylphenyl]-2-methylpropanamide (SNAP 94847) in mouse models of anxiety and depression following acute and chronic administration is independent of hippocampal neurogenesis. *J. Pharmacol. Exp. Ther.* 321, 237–248.

[30] Holick, K.A. et al. (2008) Behavioral effects of chronic fluoxetine in BALB/ cJ mice do not require adult hippocampal neurogenesis or the serotonin 1A receptor. *Neuropsychopharmacology* 33, 406–417.

[31] Czeh, B. et al. (2001) Stress-induced changes in cerebral metabolites, hippocampal volume, and cell proliferation are prevented by antidepressant treatment with tianeptine. *Proc. Natl. Acad. Sci. USA* 98, 12796–12801.

[32] Campbell, S. et al. (2004) Lower hippocampal volume in patients suffering from depression: a meta-analysis. *Am. J. Psychiatry* 161, 598–607.

[33] Colla, M. et al. (2007) Hippocampal volume reduction and HPA-system activity in major depression. *J. Psychiatr. Res.* 41, 553–560.

[34] Inagaki, M. et al. (2004) Hippocampal volume and first major depressive episode after cancer diagnosis in breast cancer survivors. *Am. J. Psychiatry* 161, 2263–2270.

[35] Bielau, H. et al. (2005) Volume deficits of subcortical nuclei in mood disorders. A postmortem study. *Eur. Arch. Psychiatry Clin. Neurosci.* 255, 401–412.

[36] Ebmeier, K.P. et al. (2006) Recent developments and current controversies in depression. *Lancet* 367, 153–167.

[37] Taupin, P. (2006) Adult neurogenesis and neuroplasticity. *Restor. Neurol. Neurosci.* 24, 9–15.

[38] Taupin, P. (2006) Neurogenesis and the effects of antidepressants. *Drug Target Insights* 1, 13–17.

[39] Taupin, P. (2008) Adult neurogenesis pharmacology in neurological diseases and disorders. *Exp. Rev. Neurother.* 8, 311–320.

[40] Thompson, A. et al. (2008) Changes in adult neurogenesis in neurodegenerative diseases: cause or consequence? *Genes Brain Behav.* 7, 28–42.

[41] Miller, M.W. et al. (1988) Use of bromodeoxyuridine-immunohistochemistry to examine the proliferation, migration and time of origin of cells in the central nervous system. *Brain Res.* 457, 44–52.

[42] Taupin, P. (2007) BrdU immunohistochemistry for studying adult neurogenesis: paradigms, pitfalls, limitations, and validation. *Brain Res. Rev.* 53, 198–214.

[43] Taupin, P. (2007) Protocols for studying adult neurogenesis: insights and recent developments. *Reg. Med.* 2, 51–62.

[44] Desai, B.S. et al. (2007) Blood–brain barrier pathology in Alzheimer's and Parkinson's disease: implications for drug therapy. *Cell Transplant.* 16, 285–299.

[45] Ekdahl, C.T. et al. (2003) Inflammation is detrimental for neurogenesis in adult brain. *Proc. Natl. Acad. Sci. USA* 100, 13632–13637.

[46] Monje, M.L. et al. (2003) Inflammatory blockade restores adult hippocampal neurogenesis. *Science* 302, 1760–1765.

[47] Kirsch, I. et al. (2008) Initial severity and antidepressant benefits: a meta-analysis of data submitted to the Food and Drug Administration. *PLoS Med.* 5, e45.

[48] Turner, E.H. et al. (2008) Selective publication of antidepressant trials and its influence on apparent efficacy. *N. Engl. J. Med.* 358, 252–260.

Chapter VI

Pharmacology of Adult Neurogenesis: Compensatory and Regenerative Processes

Neurogenesis occurs in the adult brain of mammals and is modulated by a broad range of stimuli and conditions. Drugs used in the treatment of Alzheimer's disease (AD) and depression stimulate neurogenesis in the adult hippocampus. Neurogenesis is enhanced in the brain of patients with neurological diseases and disorders and in the brain of animal models of neurological diseases and disorders. Despite controversies surrounding such studies and the need to confirm these data, adult neurogenesis and neural stem cells (NSCs) may be the target of drugs used in the treatment of neurological diseases and disorders, particularly AD and depression, and adult neurogenesis and the hippocampus may contribute to the pathology of neurological diseases and disorders. Enhanced neurogenesis in neurological diseases and disorders may represent regenerative attempts by the nervous system. Drug treatments may contribute to compensatory mechanisms in the adult hippocampus. It points to a broader involvement of the adult NSCs and the hippocampus in neurological diseases and drug therapy. Hence, adult NSCs represent not only a promising model for cellular therapy, but may also contribute to the physiopathology of the nervous system and its pharmacology, particularly for AD and depression, the understanding of which will lead to a better understanding of the nervous system, and the development of novel and more effective treatments and cures for neurological diseases and disorders.

Introduction

In the mammalian brain, neurogenesis occurs throughout adulthood primarily in two regions, the dentate gyrus (DG) of the hippocampus and the anterior part of the subventricular zone (SVZ) in various species, including humans (Eriksson et al. 1998; Curtis et al. 2007; Taupin 2008, "Adult neural"). In the DG, newly generated neuronal cells in the subgranular zone (SGZ) migrate to the granule cell layer, where they differentiate into granule-like cells and extend axonal projections to the CA3 region (Cameron et al. 1993; Toni et al. 2007;

Taupin 2009). In the SVZ, newly generated neuronal cells migrate to the olfactory bulb, through the rostro-migratory stream, where they differentiate into interneurons (Lois and Alvarez-Buylla 1994; Belluzzi et al. 2003; Curtis et al. 2007). About 0.1% of the granule cell population or 9,000 new neuronal cells are generated per day in the DG of young adult rodents and about 0.004% of the granule cell population is generated per day in the DG of adult macaque monkeys (Kornack and Rakic 1999; Cameron and McKay 2001). Though newly generated neuronal cells in the adult brain undergo programmed cell death rather than achieving maturity, the ones that survive survive for an extended period of time, at least two years in humans (Eriksson et al. 1998; Cameron and McKay 2001). It is postulated that newly generated neuronal cells in the adult brain originate from NSCs. NSCs are the self-renewing multipotent cells that generate the main phenotypes of the nervous system. Because of their potential to generate the main phenotypes of the nervous system, NSCs represent a promising model for cellular therapy for the treatment of a broad range of neurological diseases and injuries, particularly neurodegenerative diseases, cerebral strokes and spinal cord injuries. The stimulation of endogenous neural progenitor or stem cells and the transplantation of adult-derived neural progenitor and stem cells are proposed to restore and repair the degenerated or injured nerve pathways.

Neurogenesis in the adult hippocampus and SVZ is modulated by a broad range of stimuli and conditions, including environmental enrichment, physiological processes, pathological conditions, trophic factors/cytokines, and drugs (Taupin 2007). Neurogenesis in the adult hippocampus is modulated by drugs used in the treatments of AD and depression, and is modulated in the brain of patients with neurological diseases and disorders and in the brain of animal models of neurological diseases and disorders, like AD, epilepsy, and Huntington's disease (HD) (Parent et al. 1997; Malberg et al. 2000; Curtis et al. 2003; Jin, Galvan et al. 2004; Jin, Peel et al. 2004; Jin et al. 2006). Do adult neurogenesis and newly generated neuronal cells of the adult brain contribute to the pharmacology of drugs used in the treatments of neurological diseases and disorders? Do adult neurogenesis and the hippocampus contribute to the pathology of neurological diseases and disorders? In the following sections, we will review and discuss the potential involvement of adult neurogenesis and newly generated neuronal cells of the adult brain in the pharmacology of AD and depression, and in the pathology of neurological diseases and disorders.

Pharmacology of Adult Neurogenesis in Alzheimer's Disease

Alzheimer's Disease and Drug Therapy

Alzheimer's disease is a fatal neurodegenerative disease for which there is no cure. It is the most common dementia among elderly, affecting more than 26 million patients worldwide (Ferri et al. 2006). It starts with mild memory problems and ends with severe brain damages. AD is associated with loss of nerve cells, particularly in areas of the brain that are vital to memory and other mental abilities, like the hippocampus. The disease is characterized in the brain by amyloid or senile plaque deposits and neurofibrillary tangles (Caselli et al. 2006). There are two forms of the disease: the late-onset form (LOAD), diagnosed after age 65, and the early-onset form (EOAD), diagnosed at younger age. Most of the cases of LOAD are sporadic forms of the disease, whereas most cases of EOAD are inherited or familial forms of AD (FAD). Risks factors for LOAD include genetic, acquired, and environmental risk factors, like the presence of certain alleles in the genetic makeup of the individual (e.g., the apolipoprotein E varepsilon 4 allele), hypertension, diabetis, and oxidative stress (Raber, Huang, and Ashford 2004). Genetic mutations in the beta-amyloid precursor protein gene (APP), the presenilin-1 gene (PSEN1) and the presenilin-2 gene (PSEN2) have been identified as causative factors for FAD (Schellenberg 1995; St. George-Hyslop and Petit 2005). LOAD represents most cases of AD, with over 93% of all cases of the disease.

Actual treatments for AD consist in drug and occupational therapies (Scarpini, Scheltens, and Feldman 2003). Three types of drugs are currently used in the treatment of AD: blockers of the formation of amyloid plaques like alzhemed (Aisen 2005); inhibitors of acetylcholine esterase like galantamine, rivastigmine and tacrine (Wilkinson et al. 2004); and N-methyl-D-aspartate glutamate receptor antagonists like memantine (Creeley et al. 2006). Inhibitors of acetylcholine esterase improve cognitive functions by enhancing cholinergic neurotransmission that are important for learning and memory and that are affected in brain regions of patients with AD. N-methyl-D-aspartate glutamate receptor antagonists confer protection against excitotoxic neurodegeneration. These drugs produce improvements in cognitive and behavioral symptoms of AD. Other treatments that are considered and are being developed involve drugs for lowering cholesterol levels, anti-inflammatory drugs and protein beta-amyloid vaccination (Estrada and Soto 2007; Solomon 2007).

Adult Neurogenesis and Alzheimer's Disease Drugs

The drugs used in the treatment of AD have been assessed for their effects on adult neurogenesis in rodents. Galantamine and memantine increase neurogenesis in the DG and SVZ of adult rodents by 26–45%, as revealed by bromodeoxyuridine (BrdU) labeling (Jin et al. 2006) (see table 1). This suggests that adult neurogenesis may contribute to the activities of these drugs in the treatment of AD.

Pharmacology of Adult Neurogenesis in Depression

Depression and Antidepressants

Depression is a major public health issue. It affects an estimated 19 million Americans. Twenty-five percent of adults will have a major depressive episode sometime in their life (Kessler et al. 1994). It is proposed that an imbalance in the 5-hydroxytryptamine (serotonin or 5-HT) and noradrenaline pathways underlies the pathogenesis of depressive disorders (Hindmarch 2001; Owens 2004). Stress and neuroinflammation are causal factors precipitating episodes of depression in humans (Minghetti 2005; Miura et al. 2008).

Table 1. Adult neurogenesis in drug activities and neurological diseases and disorders

Alzheimer's disease drugs	- Galantamine and memantine increase neurogenesis in the DG of adult rodents by 26-45 %
Antidepressants	- Chronic administration of fluoxetine increases neurogenesis in the DG of adult rodents and non-human primates (a)
Alzheimer's disease	- Neurogenesis is enhanced in the hippocampus of AD patients (b)
	- Neurogenesis is decreased in the DG of adult mice deficient for APP and/or PSEN1
	- Neurogenesis is decreased in the DG of adult PDAPP transgenic mice
	- Neurogenesis is increased in the DG of adult transgenic mice that express the Swedish and Indiana APP mutations
Depression	- Post-mortem studies do not reveal any increase in neurogenesis in the hippocampus of patients with depression (c)
Epilepsy	- Neurogenesis is increased in the DG of animal models of epilepsy, like after pilocarpine treatment
Huntington's disease	- Neurogenesis is enhanced in the SVZ of HD patients
	- Neurogenesis is decreased in the DG of adult R6/1 transgenic mice
	- Neurogenesis is increased in the SVZ of adult rodents after quinolinic acid striatal lesioning

Notes: Study and quantification of adult neurogenesis was performed primarily by immunohistology for markers of the cell cycle and for the thymidine analog BrdU.

a. In other strains of mice, fluoxetine and other antidepressants were reported to produce their activities independently of adult neurogenesis.

b. Autopsies in this study were performed most likely on patients with the sporadic form of AD.

c. Autopsies in this study were performed on patients that were on antidepressant medication. Adult neurogenesis may mediate the activities of drugs used in the treatment of AD and depression. The modulation of neurogenesis in the adult hippocampus would represent a phenomenon of plasticity or compensatory mechanisms of recovery. Neurogenesis is enhanced in the brain of patients with and of animal models of neurological diseases and disorders, particularly AD, epilepsy and HD. Enhanced neurogenesis in the DG of the brain with neurological diseases and disorders, particularly neurodegenerative diseases, may contribute to regenerative attempts, to compensate for the neuronal losses. Due to the limitations and pitfalls over the methodologies and paradigms used to study and quantify neurogenesis, these data remain to be validated and confirmed.

Actual treatments for depression consist in drug therapy, and psychological support and therapy. Five types of drugs are used in the treatment of depression: selective serotonin reuptake inhibitors like fluoxetine, monoamine oxidase inhibitors like tranylcypromine, selective norepinephrine reuptake inhibitors like reboxetine, tricyclic antidepressants like imipramine and desipramine, and phosphodiesterase-IV inhibitors, like rolipram (Wong and Licinio 2001; Brunello et al. 2002). The efficiency and therapeutic benefits of some of the antidepressants currently prescribed for the treatment of depression have been questioned in recent publications (Kirsch et al. 2008), mandating the development of new drugs for treating depression.

Adult Neurogenesis and Antidepressants

The activity of antidepressants has been assessed for their effects on adult neurogenesis in rodents and nonhuman primates (see table 1). The chronic administration of fluoxetine and of agomelatine, the melatonergic agonist and serotoninergic antagonist, increases neurogenesis in the DG, but not SVZ of adult rats and nonhuman primates (Malberg et al. 2000; Banasr et al. 2006; Perera et al. 2007). The X-irradiation of the hippocampal region inhibits neurogenesis in the DG and prevents the behavioral effect of fluoxetine in adult mice *in vivo* (Santarelli et al. 2003). In this report, the activity of fluoxetine was reported to be mediated by 5-HT1A receptor in 129SvEvTac mice. In other strains of mice, BALB/cJ mice, fluoxetine activity was reported not to be mediated by 5-HT1A receptor and produces its antidepressant activity independently of neurogenesis (Holick et al. 2008). Autopsy studies report that neurogenesis is not altered in the hippocampus of adult patients who were on antidepressant medication (Reif et al. 2006). The anxiolytic/antidepressant N-[3-(1-{[4-(3,4-difluorophenoxy)-phenyl]methyl}(4-piperidyl))-4-methylphenyl]-2-methylpropanamide (SNAP 94847) stimulates the proliferation of progenitor cells in the DG, but its activity is unaltered in mice in which neurogenesis was suppressed by X-irradiation (David et al. 2007).

This shows that adult neurogenesis may mediate the activities of antidepressants, particularly selective serotonin reuptake inhibitors like fluoxetine, but that fluoxetine and other antidepressants may also produce their activity via distinct mechanisms, some independently of adult neurogenesis. The mechanisms underlying the activity of antidepressants on adult neurogenesis remain to be determined. It may be mediated by glucocorticoids, stress-related hormones, interleukin-6, a cytokine involved in neuroinflammation, and brain-derived neurotrophic factor, a trophic factor that has antidepressant effects (Siuciak et al. 1997; Cameron, Tanapat, and Gould 1998; Vallieres et al. 2002; Scharfman et al. 2005).

Discussion

The data reviewed show that adult neurogenesis and newly generated neuronal cells of the adult brain contribute to the pharmacology of drugs used in the treatments of AD and depression. There are, however, controversies and debates over the involvement of adult neurogenesis and newly generated neuronal cells in the activity of drugs used in the treatments of these diseases, particularly in the treatment of depression, and over the involvement of adult neurogenesis in neurological diseases and disorders.

Drug Therapy: Compensatory Processes

Neurogenesis occurs and is modulated in specialized microenvironments or "niches" (Taupin 2006, "Adult neural stem cells"; Mitsiadis et al. 2007). Neurogenesis in the adult hippocampus is modulated by drugs used in the treatment of AD and depression. This suggests that adult neurogenesis and newly generated neuronal cells of the adult hippocampus contribute to and may play an important role in the activities of these drugs. This is particularly striking for antidepressants, as the hippocampus is not the brain region primarily involved in depressive episodes (Campbell and Macqueen 2004).

Neurogenesis in the adult hippocampus plays a critical role in the activity of antidepressants like fluoxetine. Stress, a causal factor precipitating episodes of depression, decreases neurogenesis in the hippocampus in rodents and nonhuman primates (Gould et al. 1998; Pham et al. 2003), an effect that is reversed after administration of fluoxetine (Malberg and Duman 2003). This led to the theory that the waning and waxing of hippocampal neurogenesis in the adult brain are important causal factors in the precipitation and recovery from episodes of clinical depression (Jacobs, Praag, and Gage 2000). Hence, adult neurogenesis and newly generated neuronal cells of the adult hippocampus are targets of drugs used for the treatment of neurological diseases and disorders.

The modulation of neurogenesis in the adult hippocampus would represent a phenomenon of plasticity or compensatory mechanisms of recovery involving this area of the brain (Taupin 2006, "Adult neurogenesis"), the role and mechanisms of which remain to be determined. Drugs may act directly or indirectly on newly generated neuronal cells of the adult brain, and they may act via their pharmacological activities on messenger signaling pathways and/or via a neurogenic activity by modulating neurogenesis (Taupin 2008, "Adult neurogenesis").

Adult Neurogenesis in Neurological Diseases and Disorders: Regenerative Processes

Autopsy studies reveal that the expression of markers of immature neuronal cells, like doublecortin and polysialylated nerve cell adhesion molecule, is increased in the DG in the brain of patients with AD, with the sporadic form of the disease (Jin, Peel et al. 2004). Experimental studies in animal models show that neurogenesis is decreased in the DG of adult mice deficient for APP and/or PSEN1, decreased in the DG of adult PDAPP transgenic mice, and increased in the DG of adult transgenic mice that express the Swedish and Indiana APP mutations (Wen et al. 2002; Jin, Galvan et al. 2004; Donovan et al. 2006; Verret et al. 2007; Zhang et al. 2007; Rodríguez et al. 2008). These studies highlight discrepancies in the effect of AD on adult neurogenesis between patients and animal models of AD. They may originate from the validity of the animal models used in those studies, as representative of the diseases, and to study adult phenotypes (German and Eisch 2004). They may also originate from the validity of the protocols used, like immunohistochemistry for markers of the cell cycle and for the thymidine analog BrdU, as paradigms to study adult neurogenesis (Nowakowski and Hayes 2000; Taupin 2007). Despite data suggesting that neurogenesis is enhanced in the hippocampus of AD patients, these studies need to be further confirmed and validated.

In patients with depressive disorders, post-mortem studies do not reveal any increase in neurogenesis in the hippocampus (Reif et al. 2006). These data show that neurogenesis in the adult hippocampus may not be modulated by episodes of depression. However, the autopsies in these studies were performed on patients that were on antidepressant medication, known to affect neurogenesis in the adult hippocampus (Malberg et al. 2000). In addition, there are conflicting data on the effects of depression on the hippocampus. On the one hand, the hippocampus of patients with depression show signs of atrophy and neuronal loss (Sheline et al. 1996; Colla et al. 2007). On the other hand, hippocampal volume remains unchanged in depressive patients (Inagaki et al. 2004; Bielau et al. 2005). Therefore, it is unclear how neurogenesis in altered and what is the involvement of the hippocampus in patients with depression.

Epilepsy is a brain disorder in which populations of neurons signal abnormally. Neurogenesis is enhanced in the DG of animal models of epilepsy, like after pilocarpine treatment (Parent et al. 1997). Low-dose, whole-brain, X-ray irradiation in adult rats after pilocarpine treatment does not prevent the induction of recurrent seizures or prevent seizure-induced ectopic granule-like cells and MF sprouting (Parent et al. 1999). These data provide a strong argument against a critical role of adult neurogenesis in epileptogenesis.

HD is a familial disease, inherited through a mutation; a polyglutamine repeat/expansion that lengthens a glutamine segment in the huntingtin protein (Li and Li 2004). This causes degeneration of neuronal cells in certain areas of the brain, particularly the caudate nucleus and results in uncontrolled movements, loss of intellectual faculties and emotional disturbance in the patients (Sawa, Tomoda, and Bae 2003). Autopsy studies for markers of the cell cycle and of neuronal differentiation, like proliferating cell nuclear antigen and beta-tubulin, show that cell proliferation and neurogenesis are increased in the SVZ of brains of patients with HD (Curtis et al. 2003). Neurogenesis is decreased in the DG in adult R6/1 transgenic mouse model of HD (Lazic et al. 2004). It is increased in the SVZ after quinolinic acid striatal lesioning of the adult brain of rodents, leading to the migration of neuroblasts and the formation of new neuronal cells in damaged areas of the striatum, as observed in the brains of HD patients (Tattersfield et al. 2004). These data suggest that adult neurogenesis is enhanced in the hippocampus of patients with HD.

In all, neurogenesis is enhanced in the brain of patients with and of animal models of neurological diseases and disorders, particularly AD, epilepsy and HD (see table 1). Enhanced neurogenesis in the DG of the brain with neurological diseases and disorders, particularly neurodegenerative diseases, may contribute to regenerative attempts, to compensate for the neuronal losses. However, due to the limitations and pitfalls over the methodologies and paradigms used to study and quantify neurogenesis, these data remain to be further validated and confirmed (Taupin 2007). After excitotoxic and mechanical lesions in the dentate granule cell layer of adult rats, neurogenesis is enhanced in the DG (Gould and Tanapat 1997). The increased neurogenesis in many of these illnesses would result from damage or stimulation induction of neurogenesis. This indicates that enhanced neurogenesis may be a result, rather than a cause, of the illnesses (Taupin 2008, "Adult neurogenesis pharmacology").

Adult Neural Stem Cells and Regenerative Medicine

NSCs hold the promise to cure a broad range of neurological diseases and injuries. The confirmation that neurogenesis occurs in the adult brain and NSCs reside in the adult CNS of mammals including humans, reveals that the adult brain has the potential for self-repair. Two strategies are envisioned to bring adult NSCs to therapy; the stimulation or transplantation of neural progenitor and stem cells of the adult CNS. The isolation and characterization of adult-derived neural progenitor and stem cells from various regions of the adult CNS show that they may reside throughout the adult CNS. Studies have reported that new neuronal cells are generated at sites of degeneration in the diseased brain and after CNS injuries, like in HD and in experimental models of cerebral strokes. These cells originate from the SVZ; they migrate partially through the rostro-migratory stream to the sites of degeneration (Arvidsson et al. 2002; Curtis et al. 2003). Hence, therapeutic strategies aiming at stimulating endogenous neural progenitor or stem cells to treat neurological diseases or injures could involve either the stimulation, by trophic factor or cytokines, locally of neural progenitor or stem cells or the simulation of neural progenitor or stem cells of the SVZ. Alternatively, adult human-derived neural progenitor and stem cells provide a source a tissue for therapeutic strategies of transplantation, to restore and repair degenerated or injured nerve pathways (Roy et al. 2000; Palmer et al. 2001).

There are, however, limitations and constraints over the use of adult NSCs for cellular therapy, and particularly for the treatment of AD. First, stem cells, including NSCs, reside in specialized microenvironments or "niches" (Taupin 2006, "Adult neural stem cells"; Mitsiadis et al. 2007). These "niches" control the developmental potential of the stem cells that reside within. This has tremendous consequences, not only for regeneration of tissues by stimulating endogenous stem or progenitor cells, but also when transplanting such cells. The microenvironment may not be permissive, limiting the chance of success of such strategies. Second, current protocols for isolating and culturing NSCs *in vitro* lead to heterogeneous population of neural progenitor and stem cells, limiting their potential for transplantation therapies. Third, in the case of AD, neurodegeneration is widespread through the brain, targeting areas like the entorhinal cortex, hippocampus, and neocortex. As consequence, any strategies involving cellular therapy will need to restore and repair multiple neuronal pathways. This would involve the stimulation of endogenous neural progenitor or stem cells, or transplantation of adult-derived neural progenitor and stem cells, at multiple sites to maximize the recovery of deficits and impairments. This makes such strategies rather challenging. To limit the secondary effects associated with intracerebral transplantations, it is proposed to administer the transplanted cells intravenously. Following intravenous administration of adult-derived neural progenitor and stem cells, these cells migrate to sites of degeneration, diseases and injuries, providing a promising method to treat a broad range of neurological diseases and injuries (Brown et al. 2003; Pluchino et al. 2003). Intravenous administration of adult-derived neural progenitor and stem cells would represent a more practical route of administration for NSC-based transplantation strategy for treating AD.

In all, adult NSCs provide a promising strategy for the treatment of a broad range of neurological diseases and disorders, but there are limitations and constraints to overcome before such strategy is brought to therapy, particularly for AD.

Conclusion and Perspectives

Adult neurogenesis and newly generated neuronal cells contribute to the pathology of neurological diseases and disorders, and are targets of drugs used for the treatment of these diseases, particularly AD and depression. This reveals that adult neurogenesis and the hippocampus are involved in a broad range of physiopathological and pharmacological processes. There are, however, many controversies and debates that rise from the studies reported. Beside the validation and confirmation of the techniques and protocols used in these reports, the role of adult neurogenesis and the hippocampus in neurological diseases and disorders, and drug activities, remain to be elucidated. Adult NSCs represent a promising model for cellular therapy. These studies reveal that adult NSCs may be as important for our understanding of development and physiopathology of the nervous system, as for its pharmacology, thereby opening new opportunities for the treatment and cure neurological diseases and disorders. Future studies will aim at unraveling the contribution of adult neurogenesis and newly generated neuronal cells to the etiology, pathogenesis and pathology of neurological diseases and disorders, and to develop novel and more effective treatments for these diseases and disorders, particularly for AD, for which there is still no cure, and for depression, which mandates the development of new drugs.

Acknowledgments

Reproduced from: Taupin P. Alzheimer's disease: increased neurogenesis and possible disease mechanisms related to neurogenesis. Dementia: Volume III: Treatments and developments. Praeger Publishers (2011), pp 135-150, chpt. 7. Copyright 2011, with kind permission from Praeger Publishers.

References

Aisen, P. S. 2005. The development of anti-amyloid therapy for Alzheimer's disease: From secretase modulators to polymerisation inhibitors. *CNS Drugs* 19: 989–996.

Arvidsson, A., T. Collin, D. Kirik, Z. Kokaia, and O. Lindvall. 2002. Neuronal replacement from endogenous precursors in the adult brain after stroke. *Nat Med* 8: 963–970.

Banasr, M., A. Soumier, M. Hery, E. Mocaër, and A. Daszuta. 2006. Agomelatine, a new antidepressant, induces regional changes in hippocampal neurogenesis. *Biol Psychiatry* 59: 1087–1096.

Belluzzi, O., M. Benedusi, J. Ackman, and J. J. LoTurco. 2003. Electrophysiological differentiation of new neurons in the olfactory bulb. *J Neurosci* 23: 10411–10418.

Bielau, H., K. Trübner, D. Krell, M. W. Agelink, H. G. Bernstein, R. Stauch, C. Mawrin, et al. 2005. Volume deficits of subcortical nuclei in mood disorders A postmortem study. Eur Arch Psychiatry. *Clin Neurosci* 255: 401–412.

Brown, A. B., W. Yang, N. O. Schmidt, R. Carroll, K. K. Leishear, N. G. Rainov, P. M. Black, X. O. Breakefield, and K. S. Aboody. 2003. Intravascular delivery of neural stem cell lines to target intracranial and extracranial tumors of neural and non-neural origin. *Hum Gene Ther* 14: 1777–17785.

Brunello, N., J. Mendlewicz, S. Kasper, B. Leonard, S. Montgomery, J. Nelson, E. Paykel, M. Versiani, and G. Racagni. 2002. The role of noradrenaline and selective noradrenaline reuptake inhibition in depression. *Eur Neuropsychopharmacol* 12: 461–475.

Cameron, H. A., and R. D. McKay. 2001. Adult neurogenesis produces a large pool of new granule cells in the dentate gyrus. *J Comp Neurol* 435: 406–417.

Cameron, H. A., P. Tanapat, and E. Gould. 1998. Adrenal steroids and N-methyl-D-aspartate receptor activation regulate neurogenesis in the dentate gyrus of adult rats through a common pathway. *Neurosci* 82: 349–354.

Cameron, H. A., C. S. Woolley, B. S. McEwen, and E. Gould. 1993. Differentiation of newly born neurons and glia in the dentate gyrus of the adult rat. *Neurosci* 56: 337–344.

Campbell, S., and G. Macqueen. 2004. The role of the hippocampus in the pathophysiology of major depression. *J Psychiatry Neurosci* 29: 417–426.

Caselli, R. J., T. G. Beach, R. Yaari, and E. M. Reiman. 2006. Alzheimer's disease a century later. J *Clin Psychiatry* 67: 1784–1800.

Colla, M., G. Kronenberg, M. Deuschle, K. Meichel, T. Hagen, M. Bohrer, and I. Heuser. 2007. Hippocampal volume reduction and HPA-system activity in major depression. *J Psychiatr* Res 41: 553–560.

Creeley, C., D. F. Wozniak, J. Labruyere, G. T. Taylor, and J. W. Olney. 2006. Low doses of memantine disrupt memory in adult rats. *J Neurosci* 26: 3923–3932.

Curtis, M. A., M. Kam, U. Nannmark, M. F. Anderson, M. Z. Axell, C. Wikkelso, S. Holtas, et al. 2007. Human neuroblasts migrate to the olfactory bulb via a lateral ventricular extension. *Science* 315: 1243–1249.

Curtis, M. A., E. B. Penney, A. G. Pearson, W. M. van Roon-Mom, N. J. Butterworth, M. Dragunow, B. Connor, and R. L. Faull. 2003. Increased cell proliferation and neurogenesis in the adult human Huntington's disease brain. *Proc Natl Acad Sci USA* 100: 9023–9027.

David, D. J., K. C. Klemenhagen, K. A. Holick, M. D. Saxe, I. Mendez, L. Santarelli, D. A. Craig, et al. 2007. Efficacy of the MCHR1 antagonist N-[3-(1-{[4-(3,4-difl uorophenoxy)phenyl]methyl}(4-piperidyl))-4-methylphenyl]-2-methylpropanamide (SNAP 94847) in mouse models of anxiety and depression following acute and chronic administration is independent of hippocampal neurogenesis. *J Pharmacol Exp Ther* 321: 237–248.

Donovan, M. H., U. Yazdani, R. D. Norris, D. Games, D. C. German, and A. J. Eisch. 2006. Decreased adult hippocampal neurogenesis in the PDAPP mouse model of Alzheimer's disease. *J Comp Neurol* 495: 70–83.

Eriksson, P. S., E. Perfilieva, T. Bjork-Eriksson, A. M. Alborn, C. Nordborg, D. A. Peterson, and F. H. Gage. 1998. Neurogenesis in the adult human hippocampus. *Nat Med* 4: 1313–1317.

Estrada, L. D., and C. Soto. 2007. Disrupting beta-amyloid aggregation for Alzheimer disease treatment. *Curr Top Med Chem* 7: 115–126.

Ferri, C. P., M. Prince, C. Brayne, H. Brodaty, L. Fratiglioni, M. Ganguli, K. Hall, et al. 2006. The role of oxidative stress in the pathogenesis of Alzheimer's disease. *Bratisl Lek Listy* 107: 384–394.

German, D. C., and A. J. Eisch. 2004. Mouse models of Alzheimer's disease: Insight into treatment. *Rev Neurosci* 15: 353–369.

Gould, E., and P. Tanapat. 1997. Lesion-induced proliferation of neuronal progenitors in the dentate gyrus of the adult rat. *Neurosci* 80: 427–436.

Gould, E., P. Tanapat, B. S. McEwen, G. Flügge, and E. Fuchs. 1998. Proliferation of granule cell precursors in the dentate gyrus of adult monkeys is diminished by stress. *Proc Natl Acad Sci USA* 95: 3168–3171.

Hindmarch, I. 2001. Expanding the horizons of depression: Beyond the monoamine hypothesis. *Hum Psychopharmacol* 16: 203–218.

Holick, K. A., D. C. Lee, R. Hen, and S. C. Dulawa. 2008. Behavioral effects of chronic fluoxetine in BALB/cJ mice do not require adult hippocampal neurogenesis or the serotonin 1A receptor. *Neuropsychopharmacology* 33: 406–417.

Inagaki, M., Y. Matsuoka, Y. Sugahara, T. Nakano, T. Akechi, M. Fujimori, S. Imoto, K. Murakami, and Y. Uchitomi. 2004. Hippocampal volume and first major depressive episode after cancer diagnosis in breast cancer survivors. *Am J Psychiatry* 161: 2263–2270.

Jacobs, B. L., H. Praag, and F. H. Gage. 2000. Adult brain neurogenesis and psychiatry: A novel theory of depression. *Mol Psychiatry* 5: 262–269.

Jin, K., V. Galvan, L. Xie, X. O. Mao, O. F. Gorostiza, D. E. Bredesen, and D. A. Greenberg. 2004. Enhanced neurogenesis in Alzheimer's disease transgenic (PDGF-APPSw, Ind) mice. *Proc Natl Acad Sci USA* 101: 13363–13367.

Jin, K., A. L. Peel, X. O. Mao, L. Xie, B. A. Cottrell, D. C. Henshall, and D. A. Greenberg. 2004. Increased hippocampal neurogenesis in Alzheimer's disease. *Proc Natl Acad Sci USA* 101: 343–347.

Jin, K., L. Xie, X. O. Mao, and D. A. Greenberg. 2006. Alzheimer's disease drugs promote neurogenesis. *Brain Res* 1085: 183–188.

Kessler, R. C., K. A. McGonagle, S. Zhao, C. B. Nelson, M. Hughes, S. Eshleman, H. U. Wittchen, and K. S. Kendler. 1994. Lifetime and 12-month prevalence of DSM-III-R psychiatric disorders in the United States. Results from the National Comorbidity Survey. *Arch Gen Psychiatry* 51: 8–19.

Kirsch, I., B. J. Deacon, T. B. Huedo-Medina, A. Scoboria, T. J. Moore, and B. T. Johnson. 2008. Initial severity and antidepressant benefits: A meta-analysis of data submitted to the Food and Drug Administration. *PLoS Med* 5: e45.

Kornack, D. R., and P. Rakic. 1999. Continuation of neurogenesis in the hippocampus of the adult macaque monkey. *Proc Natl Acad Sci USA* 96: 5768–5773.

Lazic, S. E., H. Grote, R. J. Armstrong, C. Blakemore, A. J. Hannan, A. van Dellen, and R. A. Barker. 2004. Decreased hippocampal cell proliferation in R6/1 Huntington's mice. *Neuroreport* 15: 811–813.

Li, S. H., and X. J. Li. 2004. Huntingtin-protein interactions and the pathogenesis of Huntington's disease. *Trends Genet* 20: 146–154.

Lois, C., and A. Alvarez-Buylla. 1994. Long-distance neuronal migration in the adult mammalian brain. *Science* 264: 1145–1148.

Malberg, J. E., and R. S. Duman. 2003. Cell proliferation in adult hippocampus is decreased by inescapable stress: Reversal by fluoxetine treatment. *Neuropsychopharmacol* 28: 1562–1571.

Malberg, J. E., A. J. Eisch, E. J. Nestler, and R. S. Duman. 2000. Chronic antidepressant treatment increases neurogenesis in adult rat hippocampus. *J Neurosci* 20: 9104–9110.

Minghetti, L. 2005. Role of inflammation in neurodegenerative diseases. *Curr Opin Neurol* 18: 315–321.

Mitsiadis, T. A., O. Barrandon, A. Rochat, Y. Barrandon, and C. De Bari. 2007. Stem cell niches in mammals. *Exp Cell Res* 313: 3377–3385.

Miura, H., N. Ozaki, M. Sawada, K. Isobe, T. Ohta, and T. Nagatsu. 2008. A link between stress and depression: Shifts in the balance between the kynurenine and serotonin pathways of tryptophan metabolism and the etiology and pathophysiology of depression. *Stress* 11: 198–209.

Nowakowski, R. S., and N. L. Hayes. 2000. New neurons: Extraordinary evidence or extraordinary conclusion? *Science* 288: 771.

Owens, M. J. 2004. Selectivity of antidepressants: From the monoamine hypothesis of depression to the SSRI revolution and beyond. *J Clin Psychiatry* 65: 5–10.

Palmer, T. D., P. H. Schwartz, P. Taupin, B. Kaspar, S. A. Stein, and F. H. Gage. 2001. Cell culture. Progenitor cells from human brain after death. *Nature* 411: 42–43.

Parent, J. M., E. Tada, J. R. Fike, and D. H. Lowenstein. 1999. Inhibition of dentate granule cell neurogenesis with brain irradiation does not prevent seizure-induced mossy fiber synaptic reorganization in the rat. *J Neurosci* 19: 4508–4519.

Parent, J. M., T. W. Yu, R. T. Leibowitz, D. H. Geschwind, R. S. Sloviter, and D. H. Lowenstein. 1997. Dentate granule cell neurogenesis is increased by seizures and contributes to aberrant network reorganization in the adult rat hippocampus. *J Neurosci* 17: 3727–3738.

Perera, T. D., J. D. Coplan, S. H. Lisanby, C. M. Lipira, M. Arif, C. Carpio, G. Spitzer, et al. 2007. Antidepressant-induced neurogenesis in the hippocampus of adult nonhuman primates. *J Neurosci* 27: 4894–4901.

Pham, K., J. Nacher, P. R. Hof, and B. S. McEwen. 2003. Repeated restraint stress suppresses neurogenesis and induces biphasic PSA-NCAM expression in the adult rat dentate gyrus. *Eur J Neurosci* 17: 879–886.

Pluchino, S., A. Quattrini, E. Brambilla, A. Gritti, G. Salani, G. Dina, R. Galli, et al. 2003. Injection of adult neurospheres induces recovery in a chronic model of multiple sclerosis. *Nature* 422: 688–694.

Raber, J., Y. Huang, and J. W. Ashford. 2004. ApoE genotype accounts for the vast majority of AD risk and AD pathology. *Neurobiol Aging* 25: 641–650.

Reif, A., S. Fritzen, M. Finger, A. Strobel, M. Lauer, A. Schmitt, and K. P. Lesch. 2006. Neural stem cell proliferation is decreased in schizophrenia, but not in depression. *Mol Psychiatry* 11: 514–522.

Rodríguez, J. J., V. C. Jones, M. Tabuchi, S. M. Allan, E. M. Knight, F. M. LaFerla, S. Oddo, and A. Verkhratsky. 2008. *Impaired adult neurogenesis in the dentate gyrus of a triple transgenic mouse model of Alzheimer's disease.* PLoS ONE 3: e2935.

Roy, N. S., S. Wang, L. Jiang, J. Kang, A. Benraiss, C. Harrison-Restelli, R. A. Fraser, et al. 2000. In vitro neurogenesis by progenitor cells isolated from the adult human hippocampus. *Nat Med* 6: 271–277.

Santarelli, L., M. Saxe, C. Gross, A. Surget, F. Battaglia, S. Dulawa, N. Weisstaub, et al. 2003. Requirement of hippocampal neurogenesis for the behavioral effects of antidepressants. *Science* 301: 805–809.

Scarpini, E., P. Scheltens, and H. Feldman. 2003. Treatment of Alzheimer's disease: Current status and new perspectives. *Lancet Neurol* 2: 539–547.

Sawa, A., T. Tomoda, and B. I. Bae. 2003. Mechanisms of neuronal cell death in Huntington's disease. *Cytogenet Genome Res* 100: 287–295.

Scharfman, H., J. Goodman, A. Macleod, S. Phani, C. Antonelli, and S. Croll. 2005. Increased neurogenesis and the ectopic granule cells after intrahippocampal BDNF infusion in adult rats. *Exp Neurol* 192: 348–356.

Schellenberg, G. D. 1995. Genetic dissection of Alzheimer disease, a heterogeneous disorder. *Proc Natl Acad Sci USA* 92: 8552–8559.

Sheline, Y. I., P. W. Wang, M. H. Gado, J. G. Csernansky, and M. W. Vannier. 1996. Hippocampal atrophy in recurrent major depression. *Proc Natl Acad Sci USA* 93: 3908–3913.

Siuciak, J. A., D. R. Lewis, S. J. Wiegand, and R. M. Lindsay. 1997. Antidepressant-like effect of brain-derived neurotrophic factor (BDNF). *Pharmacol Biochem Behav* 56: 131–137.

Solomon, B. 2007. Intravenous immunoglobulin and Alzheimer's disease immunotherapy. *Curr Opin Mol Ther* 9: 79–85.

St. George-Hyslop, P. H., and A. Petit. 2005. Molecular biology and genetics of Alzheimer's disease. *C R Biol* 328: 119–130.

Tattersfield, A. S., R. J. Croon, Y. W. Liu, A. P. Kells, R. L. Faull, and B. Connor. 2004. Neurogenesis in the striatum of the quinolinic acid lesion model of Huntington's disease. *Neurosci* 127: 319–332.

Taupin, P. 2006. Adult neural stem cells, neurogenic niches and cellular therapy. *Stem Cell Reviews* 2: 213–219.

Taupin, P. 2006. Adult neurogenesis and neuroplasticity. *Restor Neurol Neurosci* 24: 9–15.

Taupin, P. 2007. Protocols for studying adult neurogenesis: Insights and recent developments. *Regenerative Medicine* 2: 51–62.

Taupin, P. 2008. Adult neural stem cells: Redefining the physio- and pathology of the CNS. *International Journal of Biomedical Science* 4: 100–106.

Taupin, P. 2008. Adult neurogenesis and drug therapy. *Central Nervous System Agents in Medicinal Chemistry* 8: 198–202.

Taupin, P. 2008. Adult neurogenesis pharmacology in neurological diseases and disorders. *Expert Review of Neurotherapeutics* 8: 311–320.

Taupin, P. 2009. Characterization and isolation of synapses of newly generated neuronal cells of the adult hippocampus at early stages of neurogenesis. *Journal of Neurodegeneration and Regeneration* 2: 9–17.

Toni, N., E. M. Teng, E. A. Bushong, J. B. Aimone, C. Zhao, A. Consiglio, H. van Praag, M. E. Martone, M. H. Ellisman, and F. H. Gage. 2007. Synapse formation on neurons born in the adult hippocampus. *Nat Neurosci* 10: 727–734.

Vallieres, L., I. L. Campbell, F. H. Gage, and P. E. Sawchenko. 2002. Reduced hippocampal neurogenesis in adult transgenic mice with chronic astrocytic production of interleukin-6. *J Neurosci* 22: 486–492.

Verret, L., J. L. Jankowsky, G. M. Xu, D. R. Borchelt, and C. Rampon. 2007. Alzheimer's-type amyloidosis in transgenic mice impairs survival of newborn neurons derived from adult hippocampal neurogenesis. *J Neurosci* 27: 6771–6780.

Wen, P. H., X. Shao, Z. Shao, P. R. Hof, T. Wisniewski, K. Kelley, V. L. Friedrich Jr., et al. 2002. Overexpression of wild type but not an FAD mutant presenilin-1 promotes neurogenesis in the hippocampus of adult mice. *Neurobiol Dis* 10: 8–19.

Wilkinson, D. G., P. T. Francis, E. Schwam, and J. Payne-Parrish. 2004. Cholinesterase inhibitors used in the treatment of Alzheimer's disease: The relationship between pharmacological effects and clinical efficacy. *Drugs Aging* 21: 453–478.

Wong, M. L., and J. Licinio. 2001. Research and treatment approaches to depression. *Nat Rev Neurosci* 2: 343–351.

Zhang, C., E. McNeil, L. Dressler, and R. Siman. 2007. Long-lasting impairment in hippocampal neurogenesis associated with amyloid deposition in a knock-in mouse model of familial Alzheimer's disease. *Exp Neurol* 204: 77–87.

Chapter VII

Adult Neurogenesis, Neuroinflammation, and Therapeutic Potential of Adult Neural Stem Cells

Abstract

Contrary to a long-held dogma, neurogenesis occurs throughout adulthood in mammals, including humans. Neurogenesis occurs primarily in two regions of the adult brain, the hippocampus and the subventricular zone (SVZ), along the ventricles. Neural progenitor and stem cells have been isolated from various regions of the adult central nervous system (CNS) and characterized in vitro, providing evidence that neural stem cells (NSCs) reside in the adult CNS and are potential sources of tissue for therapy. Adult neurogenesis is modulated in animal models and patients with neurological diseases and disorders, such as Alzheimer's disease, depression, and epilepsy. The contribution of adult neurogenesis to neurological diseases and disorders, and its significance, remain to be elucidated. The confirmation that neurogenesis occurs in the adult brain and that NSCs reside in the adult CNS is as important for our understanding of the development, physiology, and pathology of the nervous system as it is for therapy. Cellular therapy may involve the stimulation of endogenous neural progenitor or stem cells and the grafting of neural progenitor and stem cells to restore the degenerated or injured pathways. Mounting evidence suggests that neuroinflammation is involved in the pathogenesis of neurological diseases and disorders. Neural progenitor and stem cells express receptors involved in neuroinflammation, and neuroinflammation modulates neurogenesis in the adult brain. Hence, neuroinflammation may underlie the contribution of adult neurogenesis to the pathologies of the nervous system and the therapeutic potential of adult NSCs.

Introduction

Most nerve cells in the adult mammalian central nervous system (CNS) are post-mitotic and differentiated cells (Cajal 1928). They are born from primordial stem cells during development. It was believed that the adult brain was devoid of stem cells, and hence lacked the capacity to generate new nerve cells and regenerate after injury. Studies in the 1960s and mostly in the 1980s and 1990s have reported and confirmed that, contrary to this long-held dogma, neurogenesis occurs in the adult brain of mammals (Gross 2000; Kaplan 2001; Taupin, Gage 2002). The confirmation that neurogenesis occurs in the adult mammalian brain has tremendous consequences for our understanding of brain development and functioning, as well as for therapy.

Neurogenesis and Neural Stem Cells in the Adult CNS

Neurogenesis occurs primarily in two discrete regions of the adult brain, the dentate gyrus (DG) of the hippocampus and the anterior part of the subventricular zone (SVZ), in various species (Taupin, Gage 2002), including humans (Eriksson, Perfilieva, Bjork-Eriksson et al. 1998; Curtis, Kam, Nannmark et al. 2007). Newborn neuronal cells in the anterior part of the SVZ migrate to the olfactory bulb (OB) through the rostro-migratory stream (RMS) (Luskin 1993; Lois, Alvarez-Buylla 1994). They differentiate in the OB into functional interneurons (Belluzzi, Benedusi, Ackman et al. 2003). In humans, the RMS is organized differently than in other species, around a lateral ventricular extension reaching the OB (Curtis, Kam, Nannmark et al. 2007). In the DG, newborn neuronal cells in the subgranular zone (SGZ) migrate to the granule cell layer, where they differentiate into granule-like cells (Cameron, Woolley, McEwen et al. 1993). They establish functional connections with neighboring cells (van Praag, Schinder, Christie et al. 2002; Toni, Teng, Bushong et al. 2007) and extend axonal projections to the CA3 region of Ammon's horn (Stanfield, Trice 1988; Markakis, Gage 1999). Newborn granule-like cells in the DG survive for an extended period of time—at least 2 years in humans (Eriksson, Perfi lieva, Bjork-Eriksson et al. 1998). Neurogenesis may also occur in other areas of the adult brain, such as the neocortex (Gould, Reeves, Graziano et al. 1999), CA1 area (Rietze, Poulin, Weiss et al. 2000), and substantia nigra (SN) (Zhao, Momma, Delfani et al. 2003). However, some of these data have been the source of debates and controversies (Kornack, Rakic 2001; Frielingsdorf, Schwarz, Brundin et al. 2004), and remain to be further confirmed.

In rodents, 65.3% to 76.9% of bulbar neurons are replaced during a 6-week period (Kato, Yokouchi, Fukushima et al. 2001). In the DG, as many as 9000 new neuronal cells are generated per day in young adult rodents, contributing to about 3.3% per month or about 0.1% per day of the granule cell population (Kempermann, Kuhn, Gage et al. 1997; Cameron, McKay 2001). In the adult macaque monkey, at least 0.004% of the neuronal population in the granule cell layer consists of new neurons generated per day (Kornack, Rakic 1999). The rate of neurogenesis in the human DG was also reported to be low (Eriksson, Perfilieva, Bjork-Eriksson et al. 1998). The reasons for the apparent decline of adult neurogenesis in primates are unclear. The decline of adult neurogenesis during vertebrate evolution could be an adaptive strategy to maintain stable neuronal populations throughout life (Rakic 1985).

It is hypothesized that newborn neuronal cells in the adult brain originate from residual stem cells. Neural stem cells (NSCs) are the self-renewing multipotent cells that generate the main phenotypes of the nervous system (Gage 2000) (Figure 1). Neural progenitor cells are multipotent cells with limited proliferative capabilities. Self-renewing multipotent neural progenitor and stem cells have been isolated and characterized in vitro from various regions of the adult CNS, including the spinal cord (Reynolds, Weiss 1992; Gage, Coates, Palmer et al. 1995; Gritti, Parati, Cova et al. 1996; Palmer, Takahashi, Gage 1997; Shihabuddin, Horner, Ray et al. 2000). In the adult brain, populations of ependymocytes and astrocytes have been identified and proposed as candidates for stem cells in the DG and SVZ (Chiasson, Tropepe, Morshead et al. 1999; Doetsch, Caille, Lim et al. 1999; Johansson, Momma, Clarke et al. 1999; Seri, Garcia-Verdugo, McEwen et al. 2001). Despite being characterized in vitro and in situ, NSCs are still elusive cells in the adult CNS. They remain to be unequivocally identified and characterized (Kornblum, Geschwind 2001; Suslov, Kukekov, Ignatova et al. 2002; Fortunel, Out, Ng et al. 2003).

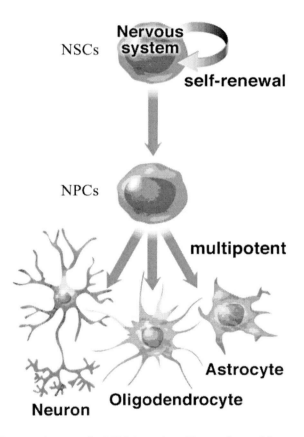

Figure 1 Neural stem cells. Neural stem cells (NSCs) are the self-renewing multipotent cells that generate the main phenotypes of the nervous system. Neural progenitor cells (NPCs) are multipotent cells, with limited proliferative capabilities. In the adult brain, populations of ependymocytes and astrocytes have been identified and proposed as candidates for stem cells. Self-renewing multipotent neural progenitor and stem cells have been isolated and characterized in vitro from various regions of the adult CNS. Adapted with permission from Taupin and Gage 2002.

In all, neurogenesis occurs in the adult brain and NSCs reside in the adult CNS, in mammals. It is a functional neurogenesis and NSCs remain to be unequivocally identified and characterized in the adult CNS. The confirmation that neurogenesis occurs in the adult brain and NSCs reside in the adult CNS has tremendous implications for our understanding of the development and functioning of the nervous system, particularly for our understanding of the etiology and pathogenesis of neurological diseases and disorders, as well as for therapy.

Adult Neurogenesis in Neurological Diseases and Disorders

Adult neurogenesis is modulated in a broad range of neurological diseases and disorders, such as Alzheimer's disease, depression, epilepsy, and Huntington's and Parkinson's diseases, and in animal models of these conditions (Table 1).

Alzheimer's Disease

Alzheimer's disease (AD) is a progressive neurodegenerative disease that starts with mild memory problems and ends with severe brain damage. It is associated with the loss of nerve cells in areas of the brain that are vital to memory and other mental abilities, such as the hippocampus. AD is characterized by amyloid plaque deposits and neurofibrillary tangles in the brain (Caselli, Beach, Yaari et al. 2006). There are two forms of the disease: the early-onset, or familial, form, and the late-onset, or sporadic, form of AD. The early-onset form of AD is a rare form of the disease. Approximately 10% of patients with AD have the familial form. It is the genetic form of the disease and is inherited. It appears at a young age. Mutations in three genes, presenilin 1, presenilin 2, and amyloid precursor protein (APP), have been identified as causes of the early-onset form of AD (St George-Hyslop, Petit 2005). The late-onset form is not inherited. It appears generally at an older age (above age 65). The origin of the late-onset form of AD remains unknown; risk factors include expression of different forms of the gene apolipoprotein (Raber, Huang, Ashford et al. 2004) and reduced expression of neuronal sortilin-related receptor gene (Rogaeva, Meng, Lee et al. 2007). The late-onset form of AD is the most common type of dementia among older people. AD is the fourth highest cause of death in the developed world. There is currently no cure for AD. Actual treatments consist of drug therapy, physical support, and assistance (Caselli, Beach, Yaari et al. 2006).

Neurogenesis is increased in the hippocampus of brains of patients with AD, as revealed after autopsies by an increase in the expression of markers for immature neuronal cells, such as doublecortin and polysialylated nerve cell adhesion molecule, in hippocampal regions (Jin, Peel, Mao et al. 2004). In animal models of AD, neurogenesis is increased in the DG of transgenic mice expressing the Swedish and Indiana APP mutations, mutant forms of human APP (Jin, Galvan, Xie et al. 2004), and decreased in the DG and SVZ of knockout mice for presenilin 1 and APP (Feng, Rampon, Tang et al. 2001; Wen, Shao, Shao et al. 2002).

Table 1. Modulation of adult neurogenesis in neurological diseases and disorders

Disease/Model	Regulation	References
Alzheimer's disease		
Autopsies	increase	Jin (2004a)
Transgenic mice Swedish and Indiana APP mutations	increase	Jin (2004b)
Knock-out/deficient mice for presenilin-1 (PS-1) and APP	decrease	Feng (2001) Wen (2002)
Depression		
Autopsies	not altered	Reif (2006)
Epilepsy		
Animal model - pilocarpine treatment	increase	Parent (1997)
Huntington's disease		
Autopsies	increase	Curtis (2003)
R6/1 transgenic mouse model of HD	decrease	Lazic (2005)
Quinolinic acid striatal lesion	increase	Tattersfield (2004)
Parkinson's disease		
MPTP lesion	increase	Zhao (2003)
6-hydroxydopamine lesion	not altered	Frielingsdorf (2004)

Hence, there are discrepancies in the data observed on adult neurogenesis in brain autopsies of patients with AD and animal models of AD. These Hence, there are discrepancies in the data observed on adult neurogenesis in brain autopsies of patients with AD and animal models of AD. These discrepancies may originate from the limitations of animal models, particularly transgenic mice, as representative models of complex diseases, particularly AD (Dodart, Mathis, Bales et al. 2002), and for studying adult phenotypes, such as adult neurogenesis. Further, high levels (4% to 10%) of tetraploid nerve cells have been reported in regions in which degeneration occurs in AD, such as in the hippocampus (Yang, Geldmacher, Herrup et al. 2001). It is proposed that cell cycle re-entry and DNA duplication, without cell proliferation, precede neuronal death in degenerating regions of the CNS (Herrup, Neve, Ackerman et al. 2004). Some of the data, observed by means of immunohistochemistry for cell cycle proteins and bromodeoxyridine (BrdU) labeling, may therefore represent not adult neurogenesis but rather labeled nerve cells that may have entered the cell cycle and undergone DNA replication without completing the cell cycle (Taupin 2007). In the end, though adult neurogenesis is increased in the adult brain with AD, these data remain to be further investigated and confirmed.

Adult neurogenesis is modulated in a broad range of neurological diseases and disorders, and in animal models, such as Alzheimer's disease, depression, epilepsy, and Huntington's and Parkinson's diseases. The contribution and significance of this modulation is yet to be elucidated. Newborn neuronal cells may be involved in regenerative attempts and plasticity of the nervous system.

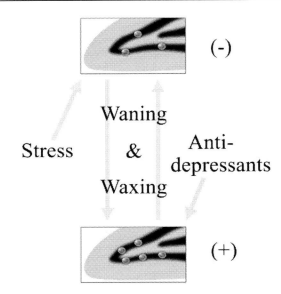

Figure 2 Adult neurogenesis, depression, and the effects of antidepressants. Stress is an important causal factor in precipitating episodes of depression and decreases hippocampal neurogenesis in adult monkeys. It is proposed that the waning and waxing of hippocampal neurogenesis are important causal factors in the precipitation and recovery from episodes of clinical depression. Chronic administration of antidepressants, such as fluoxetine, increases neurogenesis in the DG. Hence, adult neurogenesis may be important in the etiology of depression and for the mediation of drug activity to treat of depression. However, the importance of the hippocampus and adult neurogenesis in the depression remain to be established.

Depression

Depression is a major public health issue; 8% of adolescents and 25% of adults will have a major depressive episode sometime in their life (Kessler, McGonagle, Zhao et al. 1994). The hippocampus of patients with depression shows signs of atrophy and neuronal loss (Sheline, Wang, Gado et al. 1996; Colla, Kronenberg, Deuschle et al. 2007). Current treatments consist of drug therapy and psychological support (Wong, Licinio 2001). Among the drugs used to treat depression are selective serotonin reuptake inhibitors, such as fluoxetine.

Chronic administration of antidepressants such as fluoxetine increases neurogenesis in the DG but not in the SVZ in adult rats (Malberg, Eisch, Nestler et al. 2000; Malberg, Duman 2003). Stress is an important causal factor in precipitating episodes of depression, and it decreases hippocampal neurogenesis in adult monkeys (Gould, Tanapat, McEwen et al. 1998). It is proposed that the waning and waxing of hippocampal neurogenesis are important causal factors in the precipitation of and recovery from episodes of clinical depression (Jacobs, Praag, Gage 2000) (Figure 2).

Further support for the role of adult neurogenesis in depression has come from pharmacological studies (Santarelli, Saxe, Gross et al. 2003). These show that adult neurogenesis may be important in the etiology of depression and for the mediation of the activity of drugs such as selective serotonin reuptake inhibitors to treat depression. However, the importance of the hippocampus and adult neurogenesis in depression has been challenged by others (Campbell, Macqueen 2004; Reif, Fritzen, Finger 2006). In particular, some studies report that hippocampal volume and neurogenesis remain unchanged in depressive patients.

Hence, the links among the hippocampus, adult neurogenesis, and depression remain to be further established.

Epilepsy

Epilepsy is a brain disorder in which populations of neurons signal abnormally. In the individual, this translates into a variety of seizures with symptoms that range from mild changes in behavior to more severe symptoms, such as convulsions, muscle spasms, and loss of consciousness. The hippocampal formation is a critical area in the pathology of epilepsy. Patients suffering from temporal lobe epilepsy show a hippocampal formation with a dispersed granular cell layer and ectopic granule-like cells in the hilus (Houser 1990). Dentate granule cells give rise to abnormal axonal projections, or mossy fiber (MF) sprouting, in the supragranular inner molecular layer of the DG and basal dendrites of CA3 pyramidal cells in the stratum oriens (Sutula, Cascino, Cavazos et al. 1989; Represa, Tremblay, Ben-Ari 1990). Epilepsy is one of the most prevalent neurological disorders, affecting approximately 1% of Americans.

Neurogenesis is increased in the DG of animal models of epilepsy, such as after pilocarpine treatment (Parent, Yu, Leibowitz et al. 1997). In this model, ectopic granule-like cells in the hilus of the DG and the CA3 cell layer are labeled for BrdU. The authors present data suggesting that MF remodeling derives from newborn granule-like cells rather than from pre-existing mature dentate granule cells. These data indicate that neurogenesis is enhanced in the brain following limbic-induced seizures and that newborn cells in the DG contribute to hippocampal plasticity associated with seizures, such as the generation of ectopic granule-like cells and MF sprouting.

These data have been challenged by subsequent studies (Parent, Tada, Fike et al. 1999). Low-dose, whole-brain, X-ray irradiation in adult rats inhibits dentate granule cell neurogenesis (Tada, Parent, Lowenstein et al. 2000). Low-dose, whole-brain, X-ray irradiation in adult rats, after pilocarpine treatment, does not prevent the induction of recurrent seizures or the generation of seizure-induced ectopic granule-like cells and MF sprouting. These data show that seizure-induced ectopic granule-like cells and MF sprouting arise not only from newborn neuronal cells, as previously reported (Parent, Tada, Fike et al. 1999), but also from mature dentate granule cells. These data provide a strong argument against a critical role of adult neurogenesis in epileptogenesis. However, although increased hippocampal neurogenesis may not be critical to epileptogenesis, it could be a contributing factor to limbic seizures when present.

Huntington's Disease

Huntington's disease (HD) results from genetically programmed degeneration of neuronal cells in certain areas of the brain (Sawa, Tomoda, Bae et al. 2003). This degeneration causes uncontrolled movements, loss of intellectual faculties, and emotional disturbance. The caudate nucleus is the most severely and preferentially affected region of the brain in HD. HD is a familial disease, inherited through a mutation—a polyglutamine repeat/expansion that lengthens a glutamine segment in the huntingtin protein (Li, Li 2004).

Immunohistochemistry and confocal microscopy analysis at autopsies for markers of the cell cycle and neuronal differentiation, such as proliferating cell nuclear antigen and β-tubulin, show that cell proliferation and neurogenesis are increased in the SVZ of brains of patients with HD (Curtis, Penney, Pearson et al. 2003). In the adult R6/1 transgenic mouse model of HD, neurogenesis decreases in the DG (Lazic, Grote, Armstrong et al. 2004). Tattersfield et al. (2004) reported that after quinolinic acid striatal lesioning of adult brain, neurogenesis is increased in the SVZ, leading to the migration of neuroblasts and formation of new neurons in damaged areas of the striatum, as observed in brains of HD patients (Curtis, Penney, Pearson et al. 2003).

These data provide evidence that adult neurogenesis is increased in the SVZ of brains with HD. It also shows that neural progenitor cells from the SVZ migrate toward the site of degeneration in HD. Data from an R6/1 transgenic mouse model of HD are difficult to interpret in the context of adult neurogenesis in HD, as mutated forms of huntingtin affect brain development (White, Auerbach, Duyao et al. 1997). This could underlie the decrease of neurogenesis reported in adult R6/1 transgenic mice.

Parkinson's Disease

Parkinson's disease (PD) is a chronic and progressive neurodegenerative disease, primarily associated with the loss of a specific type of dopamine neuron in the SN (Fernandez-Espejo 2004). The four primary symptoms of PD are tremors, rigidity, bradykinesia, and postural instability. The disease is considerably more common in the above 50 age group. The cause of PD is mostly unknown. Certain mutations in genes such as α-synuclein and Parkin have been associated with a risk of developing PD, but PD is not usually inherited (Douglas, Lewthwaite, Nicholl 2007). A variety of medications provide relief from the symptoms. However, no drug yet can stop the progression of the disease, and in many cases medications lose their benefit over time. In such cases, surgery, such as deep brain stimulation, pallidotomy, or transplantation, may be considered (Volkmann 2007).

One study reports that the rate of neurogenesis, measured by BrdU labeling, is stimulated in the SN following lesion induced by a systemic dose of MPTP (1-methyl-4-phenyl-1,2,3,6-tetrahydropyridine) (Zhao, Momma, Delfani et al. 2003). Another study reports no evidence of new dopaminergic neurons in the SN of 6-hydroxydopamine-lesioned hemi-parkinsonian rodents (Frielingsdorf, Schwarz, Brundin et al. 2004).

Hence, neurogenesis in the SN is the source of debate and controversy. Therefore, reports that neurogenesis can be stimulated in the SN must be approached with caution, and need to be confirmed.

In all, neurogenesis is enhanced in many neurological diseases and disorders. However, these data remain to be further evaluated and confirmed. The role, contribution, and significance of enhanced neurogenesis in the etiology and pathogenesis of neurological diseases and disorders remain to be established.

Therapeutic Potential of Adult Neural Stem Cells

Cellular therapy is the replacement of unhealthy or damaged cells or tissues by new ones. Because of their potential to generate the different cell types of the nervous system, NSCs hold the promise to cure a broad range of CNS diseases and injuries. The recent confirmation that neurogenesis occurs in the adult brain and that NSCs reside in the adult mammalian CNS suggests that the CNS may be amenable to repair, and offers new opportunities for cellular therapy in the CNS (Taupin 2006a). Cell therapeutic intervention may involve the stimulation or transplantation of neural progenitor and stem cells of the adult CNS.

Stimulation of Neural Progenitor or Stem Cells of the Adult CNS

Self-renewing multipotent neural progenitor and stem cells have been isolated and characterized in vitro from various regions of the adult mammalian CNS, including the spinal cord (Reynolds, Weiss 1992; Gage, Coates, Palmer et al. 1995; Gritti, Parati, Cova et al. 1996; Palmer, Takahashi, Gage et al. 1997; Shihabuddin, Horner, Ray et al. 2000). This suggests that neural progenitor and stem cells reside throughout the adult CNS in mammals. The stimulation of endogenous neural progenitor or stem cells locally would represent a strategy to promote regeneration of the diseased and/or injured nervous system. The administration of platelet-derived growth factor (PDGF) and brain-derived neurotrophic factor (BDNF) induces neurogenesis in the striatum in adult rats with 6-hydroxydopamine lesions, with no indications of any newborn neuronal cells displaying a dopaminergic phenotype (Mohapel, Frielingsdorf, Haggblad et al. 2005). The administration of glial cell line–derived neurotrophic factor (GDNF) increases cell proliferation in the SN significantly, with new cells displaying glial features, and none of the newborn BrdU-positive cells co-label for the dopamine neuronal marker tyrosine hydroxylase (TH) (Chen, Ai, Slevin et al. 2005). The increase in TH activity observed after administration of GDNF results not from neurogenic activity but from a restorative activity of GDNF (Slevin, Gerhardt, Smith et al. 2005). Hence, stimulation of endogenous neural progenitor and stem cells locally remains to be validated as a strategy for repairing the nervous system.

New neuronal cells are generated at sites of degeneration in the diseased brain and after CNS injuries, such as in HD and experimental models of cerebral strokes (Arvidsson, Collin, Kirik et al. 2002; Curtis, Penney, Pearson et al. 2003; Jin, Sun, Xie et al. 2003). These cells originate from the SVZ and migrate partially through the RMS to the sites of degeneration. This suggests that strategies to promote regeneration and repair may focus on stimulating SVZ neurogenesis. The intracerebroventricular administration of trophic factors provides a strategy to promote SVZ neurogenesis in the diseased or injured nervous system (Craig, Tropepe, Morshead et al. 1996; Kuhn, Winkler, Kempermann et al. 1997). Newborn neuronal cells in the adult brain undergo programmed cell death before achieving maturity (Morshead, van der Kooy 1992; Cameron, McKay 2001). Thus, administration of factors preventing cell death, such as caspases, would also be potentially beneficial for cellular therapy to promote SVZ neurogenesis, alone or in combination with the administration of trophic factors (Ekdahl, Mohapel, Elmer et al. 2001).

Table 2. Stimulation of endogenous neural progenitor or stem cells in the adult brain

Trophic factors	Neurogenic activity	References
PDGF/BDNF	Neurogenesis in striatum, after 6-hydroxydopamine lesions	Mohapel (2005)
GDNF	Proliferation in substantia nigra	Chen (2005)
GDNF	Increased TH activity	Slevin2005
EGF	SVZ neurogenesis	Craig (1996), Kuhn (1997)

To summarize, various strategies can be considered to stimulate endogenous neurogenesis to promote brain repair in the diseased and/or injured brain (Table 2). These strategies have yet to be experimentally validated before their potential use for therapeutic applications can be proved. However, two trophic factors/cytokines, human chorionic gonadotropin and erythropoietin, are currently in clinical trial (phase IIa) in Canada for the treatment of cerebral strokes. The aim of this clinical trial is to promote the proliferation and differentiation of endogenous neural progenitor and stem cells into mature nerve cells, to promote functional recovery in patients suffering from cerebral stroke. This study carries a lot of hope for cellular therapy particularly that aimed at stimulating endogenous neural progenitor and stem cells to promote functional recovery.

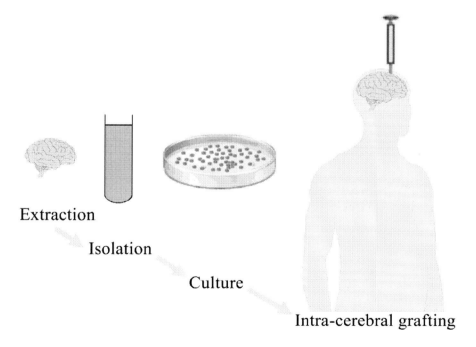

Figure 3. Adult neural stem cells and cellular therapy. Neural progenitor and stem cells can be isolated from the adult brain and cultured in vitro from various regions of the CNS, providing valuable sources of tissue for cellular therapy. Adult-derived neural progenitor and stem cells engraft the host tissues and express mature neuronal and glial markers when transplanted in the brain, providing proof of principle of the potential of adult-derived neural progenitor and stem cells for therapy.

The stimulation of endogenous neural progenitor or stem cells represents a strategy to promote regeneration of the diseased and injured nervous system. Various trophic factors and cytokines have been studied for their activity in promoting endogenous neurogenesis in the adult brain and in animal models of neurological diseases.

BDNF, brain-derived neurotrophic factor; EGF, epidermal growth factor; GDNF, glial cell line-derived neurotrophic factor; PDGF, platelet-derived growth factor.

Transplantation of Neural Progenitor and Stem Cells of the Adult CNS

Neural progenitor and stem cells can be isolated from the adult brain and cultured in vitro from various regions of the CNS, including from human biopsies and post-mortem tissues (Roy, Wang, Jiang et al. 2000; Palmer, Schwartz, Taupin et al. 2001), providing valuable sources of tissue for cellular therapy. Experimental studies reveal that adult-derived neural progenitor and stem cells engraft the host tissues and express mature neuronal and glial markers when transplanted in the brain (Gage, Coates, Palmer et al. 1995; Shihabuddin, Horner, Ray et al. 2000), providing proof of principle of the potential of adult-derived neural progenitor and stem cells for therapy.

Intracerebral transplantation aims at replacing unhealthy or damaged tissues at sites of degeneration (Figure 3). Such a strategy may not be applicable for injuries or diseases where the degeneration is widespread, particularly for neurodegenerative diseases such as AD, HD, and multiple sclerosis. Neural progenitor and stem cells, administered intravenously, migrate to diseased and injured sites of the brain (Brown, Yang, Schmidt et al. 2003; Pluchino, Quattrini, Brambilla et al. 2003). Experimental studies reveal that systemic injection of neural progenitors and stem cells promote functional recovery in an animal model of multiple sclerosis (Pluchino, Quattrini, Brambilla et al. 2003). This shows that systemic injection provides a model of choice for delivering adult-derived neural progenitor and stem cells for the treatment of neurological diseases and injuries where the degeneration is widespread. Hence, adult-derived neural progenitor and stem cells provide a promising model for cellular therapy for a broad range of neurological diseases and injuries. In addition, systemic injection provides a non-invasive strategy for delivering neural progenitor and stem cells in the adult CNS.

The potential of neural progenitor and stem cells to promote functional recovery has been studied in animal models, mostly with fetal-derived neural progenitor and stem cells. Studies from fetal tissues have revealed that grafted neural progenitor and stem cells induce functional recovery in animal models. In this process, the release of trophic factors by the grafted neural progenitor and stem cells is believed to play a major role in the recovery process (Ourednik, Ourednik, Lynch et al. 2002; Yan, Welsh, Bora et al. 2004; Bjugstad, Redmond, Teng et al. 2005). In a study where human fetal-derived neural progenitor and stem cells were injected after spinal cord injury in mice, the improvements in walking disappeared following treatment with diphtheria toxin, which kills only human cells and not mouse cells (Cummings, Uchida, Tamaki et al. 2005). This shows that neural progenitor and stem cells have a beneficial effect after transplantation and that the grafted cells themselves contribute to the recovery process, by both trophic activities and their integration to the network. However, ex vivo studies have revealed that grafted neural progenitor and stem cells derived from the spinal cord adopt the fate of the stem cells in the niches into which they are transplanted (Shihabuddin, Horner, Ray et al. 2000). Hence, the microenvironment is also a determining factor for the efficiency of transplantation (Taupin 2006b). The understanding of all these mechanisms will contribute to the optimization of therapeutic applications involving the transplantation of neural progenitor and stem cells.

Neural stem and progenitor cells derived from human fetal tissues are currently in clinical trial for the treatment of Batten's disease, a childhood neurodegenerative disorder (Taupin 2006c). Preclinical data reveal that grafted neural progenitor and stem cells survive in damaged brain tissues and migrate to specific sites of degeneration, where they differentiate into neural lineages. This study carries a lot of hope for cellular therapy. However, the use of human fetal tissue is associated with ethical and political constraints. Hence, adult-derived neural progenitor and stem cells offer an alternative to the use of fetal-derived neural progenitor and stem cells for therapy. Adult-derived neural progenitor and stem cells can be isolated from post-mortem tissues, providing multiple sources or tissues for therapy (Palmer, Schwartz, Taupin et al. 2001).

In summary, adult-derived neural progenitor and stem cells provide a promising strategy for cellular therapy to treat a broad range of neurological diseases and injuries. However, the mechanisms underlying the integration of neural progenitor and stem cells in the host and their potential for recovery remain to be established.

Neuroinflammation and the Therapeutic Potential of Adult NSCs

Neuroinflammation in Neurological Diseases and Injuries

Inflammation is a process in which the body's white blood cells and chemicals protect the individual from infections, foreign substances, and injuries. In the CNS, neuroinflammation occurs following traumatic brain injuries, spinal cord injuries, and cerebral strokes (Ghirnikar, Lee, Eng 1998; Stoll, Jander, Schroeter 1998; Nencini, Sarti, Innocenti et al. 2003; Schmidt, Heyde, Ertel et al. 2005). There are two types of immune cells that are activated following injury to the CNS: microglial cells, a population of glial cells of the CNS (Stoll, Jander 1999; Streit, Walter, Pennell 1999), and cells from the hematopoietic system, such as lymphocytes, monocytes, and macrophages. Neuroinflammation disrupts the blood–brain barrier (BBB), allowing cells from the hematopoietic system to leave the blood stream and come in contact with the injury site (Lossinsky, Shivers 2004). The immune cells respond to injury by eliminating debris and releasing a host of powerful regulatory substances, such as the complements, glutamate, interleukins, nitric oxide, reactive oxygen species, and transforming growth factors (Ghirnikar, Lee, Eng 1998; Stoll, Jander 1999; Jander, Schroeter, Stoll 2002; Stoll, Schroeter, Jander et al. 2004; Hensley, Mhatre, Mou et al. 2006; Bonifati, Kishore 2007). These chemicals are both beneficial and harmful to the cellular environment, thereby creating further damage to the CNS (Stoll Jander, Schroeter 2002). Mature astrocytes are also activated following injury to the CNS (Latov, Nilaver, Zimmerman et al. 1979; Miyake, Hattori, Fukuda et al. 1988). Astrocytic activation is believed to be necessary for containing the immune response, repairing the BBB, and attenuating further neuronal death (Bush, Puvanachandra, Horner et al. 1999; Lossinsky, Shivers 2004).

It is now well documented that neuroinflammation is actively involved in neurological diseases and disorders such as AD, depression, HD, PD, amyotrophic lateral sclerosis, and multiple sclerosis (Minghetti 2005; Arnaud, Robakis, Figueiredo-Pereira 2006; Eikelenboom, Veerhuis, Scheper et al. 2006; Hensley, Mhatre, Mou et al. 2006; Sivaprakasam 2006; Klegeri, Schulzer, Harper et al. 2007). In AD, there is a correlation between local inflammation and amyloid plaques and neurofibrillary tangles (Zilka, Ferencik, Hulin 2006). Chronic inflammation is considered as a causative factor in the pathogenesis of neurological diseases and disorders (Eikelenboom, Veerhuis, Scheper et al. 2006; Zilka, Ferencik, Hulin 2006; Whitton 2007). It is proposed that the immune cells and proinflammatory chemicals involved in neuroinflammation underlie the mechanisms of neurodegeneration. The activation or over activation of immune cells involved in neuroinflammation and release of proinflammatory chemicals would result in reduced neuroprotection and neuronal repair, and increased neurodegeneration, leading to neurodegenerative diseases (Bonifati, Kishore 2007; Donnelly, Popovich 2008). Interestingly, depression is a common antecedent to many neurological diseases, particularly AD and PD (Karceski 2007; Potter, Steffens 2007). Hence, chronic inflammation during depressive episodes could predispose depressive patients to neurodegenerative diseases later in life (Leonard 2007).

Neuroinflammation in Adult Neurogenesis

Neuroinflammation inhibits neurogenesis in the adult hippocampus (Ekdahl, Mohapel, Elmer et al. 2003; Monje, Toda, Palmer 2003) (Table 3). The function, significance, and mechanisms of the modulation of neurogenesis during inflammatory processes remain to be elucidated. The function and significance of the modulation of neurogenesis during inflammatory processes remain to be particularly elucidated during neurological diseases and disorders, such as AD and depression. On the cellular level, neurological diseases and disorders are associated with microglia activation (Stoll, Jander 1999), a component of the inflammation reaction known to impair hippocampal neurogenesis in adult rats (Ekdahl, Mohapel, Elmer et al. 2003; Monje, Toda, Palmer 2003). On the molecular level, substances such as interleukin (Vallieres, Campbell, Gage et al. 2002) and nitric oxide (Packer, Stasiv, Benraiss et al. 2003), released by the immune cells, regulate adult neurogenesis negatively. Hence, neuroinflammation may contribute to the effects of neurological diseases and disorders on adult neurogenesis. The contribution and involvement of neuroinflammation with regard to the effects of neurological diseases and disorders on adult neurogenesis remain to be determined.

Table 3. Adult neurogenesis and neuroinflammation

Disease/Model	Regulation	References
Neuroinflammation	decrease	Ekdahl (2003), Monje (2003)
Microglia activation	decrease	Ekdahl (2003), Monje (2003)
Interleukins	decrease	Vallieres (2002)
Nitric oxide	decrease	Packer (2003)

Neuroinflammation inhibits neurogenesis in the adult hippocampus. Chronic inflammation is associated with neurological diseases and disorders, such as Alzheimer's and Parkinson's diseases, and is thought to be a causative factor for these diseases. The involvement and significance of the modulation of adult neurogenesis in neurological diseases and disorders remain to be established.

X-ray irradiation has been used to study the function and involvement of adult neurogenesis in various neurological diseases and disorders, such as epilepsy and depression (Parent, Tada, Fike et al. 1999; Santarelli, Saxe, Gross et al. 2003). Brain irradiation induces inflammatory responses. The effect of brain irradiation on adult neurogenesis in animal models, particularly of neurological diseases and disorders, is therefore difficult to interpret in light of these data.

Neuroinflammation and Neural Progenitor and Stem Cell Transplantation

Neural progenitor and stem cells express receptors and respond to trophic factors and cytokines. Hence, the inflammatory process involved in the pathological processes to be treated by the transplantation of neural progenitor and stem cells may have adverse effects on the success of the graft. On the one hand, adult-derived neural progenitor and stem cells promote neuroprotection via an immunomodulatory mechanism (Pluchino, Zanotti, Rossi et al. 2005). This shows that grafted neural progenitor and stem cells interact with the host to promote functional recovery. This also suggests that neural progenitor and stem cells may provide clinical benefit for the treatment of autoimmune diseases. On the other hand, the timing of transplantation in the diseased brain or after injuries may be critical for successful transplantation of neural progenitor and stem cell therapy (Mueller, McKercher, Imitola et al. 2005). This suggests that preclinical studies involving immunosuppressed mice to study the engraftment of neural progenitor and stem cells for future therapy may not represent an appropriate model to characterize and validate sources of human-derived neural progenitor and stem cells for therapy (Taupin 2006c).

In summary, neuroinflammation is involved in the pathogenesis of neurological diseases and disorders, but its contribution and involvement with regard to these pathological processes remain to be elucidated. It may be involved in the modulation of neurogenesis in neurological diseases and disorders, but the contribution and significance of this modulation remain to be understood. Neuroinflammation may affect the success of therapeutic strategies involving the transplantation of neural progenitor and stem cells. Hence, therapeutic strategies for promoting neurogenesis after injuries or in neurological diseases and disorders and for promoting the engraftment of neural progenitor and stem cells may involve the use of anti-inflammatory treatments to reduce the adverse effects of neuroinflammation on adult neurogenesis and transplants, respectively (Craft, Watterson, Van Eldik 2005; Hernan, Logroscino, Garcia Rodriguez 2006; Ho, Qin, Stetka et al. 2006; Vardy, Hussain, Hooper 2006).

Limitations and Pitfalls of BrdU Labelling for Studying Neurogenesis

BrdU is a thymidine analogue that incorporates DNA of dividing cells during the S-phase of the cell cycle and is used for birthdating and monitoring cell proliferation (Miller, Nowakowski 1988). There are limitations and pitfalls regarding the use of BrdU for studying neurogenesis. BrdU is a toxic and mutagenic substance (Nowakowski, Hayes 2001; Taupin 2007). It triggers cell death and formation of teratomes. It alters DNA stability, lengthens the cell cycle. It also has mitogenic, transcriptional, and translational effects on cells that incorporate it. BrdU is not a marker for cell proliferation but a marker for DNA synthesis. In addition, many physiological and pathological processes affect the permeability of the BBB and cerebral flow, particularly exercise; neurological diseases and injuries such as AD, PD, and cerebral strokes; and neuroinflammation and drug treatments (Lossinsky, Shivers 2004; Deane, Zlokovic 2007; Desai, Monahan, Carvey et al. 2007; Pereira, Huddleston, Brickman et al. 2007), all of which can affect the bioavailability of BrdU in the brain. Hence, studies involving the use of BrdU for studying adult neurogenesis must be carefully assessed, and their conclusions carefully weighted (Taupin 2007).

Conclusions and Perspectives

The confirmation that adult neurogenesis occurs in the adult brain and that NSCs reside in the adult CNS suggests that the adult brain may be amenable to repair and raises the question of the function of newborn neuronal cells in the physiology and pathology of the adult nervous system. The modulation of adult neurogenesis in neurological diseases and disorders suggests that it may be involved in the etiology and pathogenesis of the diseases. The contribution and significance of this modulation is yet to be elucidated. Newborn neuronal cells may be involved in regenerative attempts and plasticity of the nervous system. The stimulation of endogenous neural progenitor or stem cells or the transplantation of adult-derived neural progenitor and stem cells offers new opportunities for cellular therapy. Particularly, intrinsic properties of adult NSCs provide new strategies to treat a broad range of neurological diseases and injuries, as well as brain tumors. However, NSCs are still elusive cells, and will have to be fully and unequivocally characterized before adult NSCs are brought to therapy.

Chronic inflammation is associated with neurological diseases and disorders such as AD and PD, and is thought to be a causative factor for these diseases. Neuroinflammation modulates adult neurogenesis, particularly in the hippocampus. However, the significance of this modulation and its impact on adult neurogenesis in neurological diseases remain to be established. Chronic inflammation and proinflammatory substances have tremendous implications for cellular therapy involving adult NSCs, both in vivo and ex vivo. Neuroinflammation may affect the potential of NSC therapy and provide new perspectives for NSC therapy. Therapeutic strategies for promoting neurogenesis after injuries or in neurological diseases and disorders and for promoting the engraftment of neural progenitor and stem cells may involve the use of anti-inflammatory treatments to reduce the adverse effects of neuroinflammation on adult neurogenesis and NSC transplants. Future studies will aim at elucidating the contribution and involvement of chronic inflammation with regard to neurological diseases, disorders, and injuries; its underlying mechanism; and its potential for cellular therapy. These investigations will result in new therapeutic strategies to treat neurological diseases, disorders, and injuries.

Acknowledgments

Reproduced from: Taupin P. Adult neurogenesis, neuroinflammation and therapeutic potential of adult neural stem cells. Neurovascular Medicine: Pursuing Cellular Longevity for Healthy Aging. Oxford University Press (2008), pp 255-268, chpt. 10, by permission of Oxford University Press, Inc.

References

Arnaud L, Robakis NK, Figueiredo-Pereira ME. 2006. It may take inflammation, phosphorylation and ubiquitination to "tangle" in Alzheimer's disease. *Neurodegener Dis.* 3(6):313–319.

Arvidsson A, Collin T, Kirik D, Kokaia Z, Lindvall O. 2002. Neuronal replacement from endogenous precursors in the adult brain after stroke. *Nat Med.* 8(9):963–970.

Belluzzi O, Benedusi M, Ackman J, LoTurco JJ. 2003. Electrophysiological differentiation of new neurons in the olfactory bulb. *J Neurosci.* 23(32):10411–10418.

Bjugstad KB, Redmond DE Jr, Teng YD et al. 2005. Neural stem cells implanted into MPTP-treated monkeys increase the size of endogenous tyrosine hydroxylase-positive cells found in the striatum: A return to control measures. *Cell Transplant.* 14(4):183–192.

Bonifati DM, Kishore U. 2007. Role of complement in neu-rodegeneration and neuroinfl ammation. *Mol Immunol.* 44(5):999–1010.

Brown AB, Yang W, Schmidt NO et al. 2003. Intravascular delivery of neural stem cell lines to target intracranial and extracranial tumors of neural and non-neural origin. *Hum Gene Ther.* 14(18):1777–1785.

Bush TG, Puvanachandra N, Horner CH et al. 1999. Leukocyte infiltration, neuronal degeneration, and neurite outgrowth after ablation of scar-forming, reactive astrocytes in adult transgenic mice. *Neuron.* 23(2):297–308.

Cajal Santiago Ramon y. 1928. *Degeneration and Regeneration of the Nervous System.* New York: Hafner.

Cameron HA, Woolley CS, McEwen BS, Gould E. 1993. Differentiation of newly born neurons and glia in the dentate gyrus of the adult rat. *Neuroscience.* 56(2):337–344.

Cameron HA, McKay RD. 2001. Adult neurogenesis produces a large pool of new granule cells in the dentate gyrus. *J Comp Neurol.* 435(4):406–417.

Campbell S, Macqueen G. 2004. The role of the hippocampus in the pathophysiology of major depression. *J Psychiatry Neurosci.* 29(6):417–426.

Caselli RJ, Beach TG, Yaari R, Reiman EM. 2006. Alzheimer's disease a century later. *J Clin Psychiatry.* 67(11):1784–1800.

Chen Y, Ai Y, Slevin JR, Maley BE, Gash DM. 2005. Progenitor proliferation in the adult hippocampus and substantia nigra induced by glial cell line-derived neurotrophic factor. *Exp Neurol.* 196(1):87–95.

Chiasson BJ, Tropepe V, Morshead CM, van der Kooy D. 1999. Adult mammalian forebrain ependymal and subependymal cells demonstrate proliferative potential but only subependymal cells have neural stem cell characteristics. *J Neurosci.* 19(11):4462–4471.

Colla M, Kronenberg G, Deuschle M et al. 2007. Hippocampal volume reduction and HPA-system activity in major depression. *J Psychiatr Res.* 41(7):553–560.

Craft JM, Watterson DM, Van Eldik LJ. 2005. Neuroinflammation: a potential therapeutic target. *Expert Opin Ther Targets.* 9(5):887–900.

Craig CG, Tropepe V, Morshead CM, Reynolds BA, Weiss S, van der Kooy D. 1996. In vivo growth factor expansion of endogenous subependymal neural precursor cell populations in the adult mouse brain. *J Neurosci.* 16(8):2649–2658.

Cummings BJ, Uchida N, Tamaki SJ et al. 2005. Human neural stem cells differentiate and promote locomotor recovery in spinal cord-injured mice. *Proc Natl Acad Sci U S A.* 102(39):14069–14074.

Curtis MA, Penney EB, Pearson AG et al. 2003. Increased cell proliferation and neurogenesis in the adult human Huntington's disease brain. *Proc Natl Acad Sci U S A.* 100(15):9023–9027.

Curtis MA, Kam M, Nannmark U et al. 2007. Human neuroblasts migrate to the olfactory bulb via a lateral ventricular extension. *Science.* 315(5816):1243–1249.

Deane R, Zlokovic BV. 2007. Role of the blood-brain barrier in the pathogenesis of Alzheimer's disease. *Curr Alzheimer Res.* 4(2):191–197.

Desai BS, Monahan AJ, Carvey PM, Hendey B. 2007. Blood-brain barrier pathology in Alzheimer's and Parkinson's disease: implications for drug therapy. *Cell Transplant.* 16(3):285–99.

Doetsch F, Caille I, Lim DA, Garcia-Verdugo JM, Alvarez-Buylla A. 1999. Subventricular zone astrocytes are neural stem cells in the adult mammalian brain. *Cell.* 97(6):703–16.

Donnelly DJ, Popovich PG. 2008. Inflammation and its role in neuroprotection, axonal regeneration and functional recovery after spinal cord injury. *Exp Neurol.* 209(2):378–388.

Douglas MR, Lewthwaite AJ, Nicholl DJ. 2007. Genetics of Parkinson's disease and parkinsonism. *Expert Rev Neurother.* 7(6):657–666.

Eikelenboom P, Veerhuis R, Scheper W, Rozemuller AJ, van Gool WA, Hoozemans JJ. 2006. The signifi cance of neuroinflammation in understanding Alzheimer's disease. *J Neural Transm.* 113(11):1685–1695.

Ekdahl CT, Mohapel P, Elmer E, Lindvall O. 2001. Caspase inhibitors increase short-term survival of progenitor-cell progeny in the adult rat dentate gyrus following status epilepticus. *Eur J Neurosci.* 14(6):937–945.

Ekdahl CT, Claasen JH, Bonde S, Kokaia Z, Lindvall O. 2003. Inflammation is detrimental for neurogenesis in adult brain. *Proc Natl Acad Sci U S A.* 100(23):13632–13637.

Eriksson PS, Perfilieva E, Bjork-Eriksson T et al. 1998. Neurogenesis in the adult human hippocampus. *Nat Med.* 4(11):1313–1317.

Feng R, Rampon C, Tang YP et al. 2001. Defi cient neurogenesis in forebrain-specific presenilin-1 knockout mice is associated with reduced clearance of hippocampal memory traces. [published erratum appears in Neuron. 2002 33(2):313]. *Neuron.* 32(5):911–926.

Fernandez-Espejo E. 2004. Pathogenesis of Parkinson's disease: prospects of neuroprotective and restorative therapies. *Mol Neurobiol.* 29(1):15–30.

Fortunel NO, Out HH, Ng HH et al. 2003. Comment on " 'Stemness': transcriptional profiling of embryonic and adult stem cells" and "a stem cell molecular signature". *Science.* 302(5644):393.

Frielingsdorf H, Schwarz K, Brundin P, Mohapel P. 2004. No evidence for new dopaminergic neurons in the adult mammalian substantia nigra. *Proc Natl Acad Sci U S A.* 101(27):10177–10182.

Gage FH, Coates PW, Palmer TD et al. 1995. Survival and differentiation of adult neuronal progenitor cells transplanted to the adult brain. Proc Natl Acad Sci U S A. 92(25):11879–11883.

Gage FH. 2000. Mammalian neural stem cells. Science. 287(5457):1433–1438.

Garcia-Verdugo, JM, Alvarez-Buylla, A. Dodart JC, Mathis C, Bales KR, Paul SM 2002. Does my mouse have Alzheimer's disease? Genes Brain Behav. 1(3):142–155.

Ghirnikar RS, Lee YL, Eng LF. 1998. Infl ammation in traumatic brain injury: role of cytokines and chemokines. Neurochem Res. 23(3):329–340.

Gould E, Reeves AJ, Graziano MS, Gross CG. 1999. Neurogenesis in the neocortex of adult primates. Science. 286(5439):548–552.

Gould E, Tanapat P, McEwen BS, Flugge G, Fuchs E. 1998. Proliferation of granule cell precursors in the dentate gyrus of adult monkeys is diminished by stress. Proc Natl Acad Sci U S A. 95(6):3168–3171.

Gritti A, Parati EA, Cova L et al. 1996. Multipotential stem cells from the adult mouse brain proliferate and self-renew in response to basic fibroblast growth factor. J Neurosci. 16(3):1091–1100.

Gross CG. 2000. Neurogenesis in the adult brain: death of a dogma. Nat Rev Neurosci. 1(1):67–73.

Hensley K, Mhatre M, Mou S et al. 2006. On the relation of oxi-dative stress to neuroinflammation: lessons learned from the G93A-SOD1 mouse model of amyotrophic lateral sclerosis. Antioxid Redox Signal. 8(11–12):2075–2087.

Hernan MA, Logroscino G, Garcia Rodriguez LA. 2006. Nonsteroidalanti-inflammatory drugs and the incidence of Parkinson disease. Neurology. 66(7):1097–1099.

Herrup K, Neve R, Ackerman SL, Copani A. 2004. Divide and die: cell cycle events as triggers of nerve cell death. J Neurosci. 24(42):9232–9239.

Ho L, Qin W, Stetka BS, Pasinetti GM. 2006. Is there a future for cyclo-oxygenase inhibitors in Alzheimer's disease? CNS Drugs. 20(2):85–98.

Houser CR. 1990. Granule cell dispersion in the dentate gyrus of humans with temporal lobe epilepsy. Brain Res. 535(2):195–204.

Jacobs BL, Praag H, Gage FH. 2000. Adult brain neurogenesis and psychiatry: a novel theory of depression. Mol Psychiatry. 5(3):262–269.

Jander S, Schroeter M, Stoll G. 2002. Interleukin-18 expression after focal ischemia of the rat brain: association with the late-stage inflammatory response. J Cereb Blood Flow Metab. 22(1):62–70.

Jin K, Galvan V, Xie L et al. 2004. Enhanced neurogenesis in Alzheimer's disease transgenic (PDGF-APPSw, Ind) mice. Proc Natl Acad Sci U S A. 101(36):13363–13367.

Jin K, Peel AL, Mao XO et al. 2004. Increased hippocampal neurogenesis in Alzheimer's disease. Proc Natl Acad Sci U S A. 101(1):343–347.

Jin K, Sun Y, Xie L et al. 2003. Directed migration of neuronal precursors into the ischemic cerebral cortex and striatum. Mol Cell Neurosci. 24(1):171–189.

Johansson CB, Momma S, Clarke DL, Risling M, Lendahl U, Frisen J. 1999. Identification of a neural stem cell in the adult mammalian central nervous system. *Cell.* 96(1):25–34.

Kaplan MS. 2001. Environment complexity stimulates visual cortex neurogenesis: death of a dogma and a research career. *Trends Neurosci.* 24(10):617–620.

Karceski, S. 2007. Early Parkinson disease and depression. *Neurology.* 69(4):E2–E3.

Kato T, Yokouchi K, Fukushima N, Kawagishi K, Li Z, Moriizumi T. 2001. Continual replacement of newly-generated olfactory neurons in adult rats. *Neurosci Lett.* 307(1):17–20.

Kempermann G, Kuhn HG, Gage FH. 1997. More hippocampal neurons in adult mice living in an enriched environment. *Nature.* 386(6624):493–495.

Kessler RC, McGonagle KA, Zhao S et al. 1994. Lifetime and 12-month prevalence of DSM-III-R psychiatric disorders in the United States. Results from the National Comorbidity Survey. *Arch Gen Psychiatry.* 51(1):8–19.

Klegeris A, Schulzer M, Harper DG, McGeer PL. 2007. Increase in core body temperature of Alzheimer's disease patients as a possible indicator of chronic neuroinflammation: a meta-analysis. *Gerontology.* 53(1):7–11.

Kornack DR, Rakic P. 1999. Continuation of neurogenesis in the hippocampus of the adult macaque monkey. *Proc Natl Acad Sci U S A.* 96(10):5768–5773.

Kornack DR, Rakic P. 2001. Cell proliferation without neurogenesis in adult primate neocortex. *Science.* 294(5549):2127–2130.

Kornblum HI, Geschwind DH. 2001. Molecular markers in CNS stem cell research: hitting a moving target. *Nat Rev Neurosci.* 2(11):843–846.

Kuhn HG, Winkler J, Kempermann G, Thal, LJ, Gage FH. 1997. Epidermal growth factor and fi broblast growth factor-2 have different effects on neural progenitors in the adult rat brain. *J Neurosci.* 17(15):5820–5829.

Latov N, Nilaver G, Zimmerman EA et al. 1979. Fibrillary astrocytes proliferate in response to brain injury: a study combining immunoperoxidase technique for glial fibrillary acidic protein and radioautography of tritiated thymidine. *Dev Biol.* 72(2):381–384.

Lazic SE, Grote H, Armstrong RJ et al. 2004. Decreased hippocampal cell proliferation in R6/1 Huntington's mice. *Neuroreport.* 15(5):811–813.

Leonard BE. 2007. Inflammation depression and dementia: are they connected? *Neurochem Res.* 32(10):1749–1756.

Li SH, Li XJ. 2004. Huntingtin-protein interactions and the pathogenesis of Huntington's disease. *Trends Genet.* 20(3):146–154.

Lois C, Alvarez-Buylla A. 1994. Long-distance neuronal migration in the adult mammalian brain. *Science.* 264(5162):1145–1148.

Lossinsky AS, Shivers RR. 2004. Structural pathways for macromolecular and cellular transport across the blood-brain barrier during inflammatory conditions. *Histol Histopathol.* 19(2):535–564.

Luskin MB. 1993. Restricted proliferation and migration of postnatally generated neurons derived from the forebrain subventricular zone. *Neuron.* 11(1):173–189.

Malberg JE, Eisch AJ, Nestler EJ, Duman RS. 2000. Chronic antidepressant treatment increases neurogenesis in adult rat hippocampus. *J Neurosci.* 20(24):9104–9110.

Malberg JE, Duman RS. 2003. Cell proliferation in adult hippocampus is decreased by inescapable stress: reversal by fluoxetine treatment. *Neuropsychopharmacol.* 28(9):1562–1571.

Markakis EA, Gage FH. 1999. Adult-generated neurons in the dentate gyrus send axonal projections to fi eld CA3 and are surrounded by synaptic vesicles. *J Comp Neurol.* 406(4):449–460.

Miller MW, Nowakowski RS. 1988. Use of bromodeoxyu-ridine-immunohistochemistry to examine the proliferation, migration and time of origin of cells in the central nervous system. *Brain Res.* 457(1):44–52.

Minghetti L. 2005. Role of inflammation in neurodegenerative diseases. *Curr Opin Neurol.* 18(3):315–321.

Miyake T, Hattori T, Fukuda M, Kitamura T, Fujita S. 1988. Quantitative studies on proliferative changes of reactive astrocytes in mouse cerebral cortex. *Brain Res.* 451(1–2):133–138.

Mohapel P, Frielingsdorf H, Haggblad J, Zachrisson O, Brundin P. 2005. Platelet-derived growth factor (PDGF-BB) and brain-derived neurotrophic factor (BDNF) induce striatal neurogenesis in adult rats with 6-hydroxydopamine lesions. *Neurosci.* 132(3):767–776.

Monje ML, Toda H, Palmer TD. 2003. Infl ammatory blockade restores adult hippocampal neurogenesis. *Science.* 302(5651):1760–1765.

Morshead CM, van der Kooy D. 1992. Postmitotic death is the fate of constitutively proliferating cells in the sub-ependymal layer of the adult mouse brain. *J Neurosci.* 12(1):249–256.

Mueller FJ, McKercher SR, Imitola J et al. 2005. At the interface of the immune system and the nervous system: how neuroinflammation modulates the fate of neural progenitors in vivo. *Ernst Schering Res Found Workshop.* (53):83–114.

Nencini P, Sarti C, Innocenti R, Pracucci G, Inzitari D. 2003. Acute inflammatory events and ischemic stroke subtypes. *Cerebrovasc Dis.* 15(3):215–221.

Nowakowski RS, Hayes NL. 2001. Stem cells: the promises and pitfalls *Neuropsychopharmacol.* 25(6):799–804.

Ourednik J, Ourednik V, Lynch WP, Schachner M, Snyder EY. 2002. Neural stem cells display an inherent mechanism for rescuing dysfunctional neurons. *Nat Biotechnol.* 20(11):1103–1110.

Packer MA, Stasiv Y, Benraiss A et al. 2003. Nitric oxide negatively regulates mammalian adult neurogenesis. *Proc Natl Acad Sci U S A.* 100(16):9566–9571.

Palmer TD, Takahashi J, Gage FH. 1997. The adult rat hip-pocampus contains primordial neural stem cells. *Mol Cell Neurosci.* 8(6):389–404.

Palmer TD, Schwartz PH, Taupin P, Kaspar B, Stein SA, Gage FH. 2001. Cell culture. Progenitor cells from human brain after death. *Nature.* 411(6833):42–43.

Parent JM, Yu TW, Leibowitz RT, Geschwind DH, Sloviter RS, Lowenstein DH. 1997. Dentate granule cell neurogenesis is increased by seizures and contributes to aberrant network reorganization in the adult rat hippocampus. *J Neurosci.* 17(10):3727–3738.

Parent JM, TadaE, FikeJR,Lowenstein DH. 1999. Inhibitionof dentate granule cell neurogenesis with brain irradiation does not prevent seizure-induced mossy fi ber synaptic reorganization in the rat. *J Neurosci.* 19(11):4508–4519.

Pereira AC, Huddleston DE, Brickman AM et al. 2007. An in vivo correlate of exercise-induced neurogenesis in the adult dentate gyrus. *Proc Natl Acad Sci U S A.* 104(13):5638–5643.

Pluchino S, Quattrini A, Brambilla E et al. 2003. Injection of adult neurospheres induces recovery in a chronic model of multiple sclerosis. *Nature.* 422(6933):688–694.

Pluchino S, Zanotti L, Rossi B et al. 2005. Neurospherederived multipotent precursors promote neuroprotection by an immunomodulatory mechanism. *Nature.* 436(7048):266–271.

Potter GG, Steffens DC. 2007. Contribution of depression to cognitive impairment and dementia in older adults. *Neurologist.* 13(3):105–117.

Raber J, Huang Y, Ashford JW. 2004. ApoE genotype accounts for the vast majority of AD risk and AD pathology. *Neurobiol Aging.* 25(5):641–650.

Rakic P. 1985. Limits of neurogenesis in primates. *Science.* 227(4690):1054–1056.

Reif A, Fritzen S, Finger M. 2006. Neural stem cell proliferation is decreased in schizophrenia, but not in depression. *Mol Psychiatry.* 11(5):514–522.

Represa A, Tremblay E, Ben-Ari Y. 1990. Sprouting of mossy fibers in the hippocampus of epileptic human and rat. *Adv Exp Med Biol.* 268:419–424.

Reynolds BA, Weiss S. 1992. Generation of neurons and astrocytes from isolated cells of the adult mammalian central nervous system. *Science.* 255(5052):1707–1710.

Rietze R, Poulin P, Weiss S. 2000. Mitotically active cells that generate neurons and astrocytes are present in multiple regions of the adult mouse hippocampus. *J Comp Neurol.* 424(3):397–408.

Rogaeva E, Meng Y, Lee JH et al. 2007. The neuronal sorti-lin-related receptor SORL1 is genetically associated with Alzheimer disease. *Nat Genet.* 39(2):168–177.

Roy NS, Wang S, Jiang L et al. 2000. In vitro neurogenesis by progenitor cells isolated from the adult human hippocampus. *Nat Med.* 6(3):271–277.

Santarelli L, Saxe M, Gross C et al. 2003. Requirement of hippocampal neurogenesis for the behavioral effects of antidepressants. *Science.* 301(5634):805–809.

Sawa A, Tomoda T, Bae BI. 2003. Mechanisms of neuronal cell death in Huntington's disease. *Cytogenet Genome Res.* 100(1–4):287–295.

Schmidt OI, Heyde CE, Ertel W, Stahel PF. 2005. Closed head injury—An inflammatory disease? *Brain Res Brain Res Rev.* 48(2):388–399.

Seri B, Garcia-Verdugo JM, McEwen BS, Alvarez-Buylla A. 2001. Astrocytes give rise to new neurons in the adult mammalian hippocampus. *J Neurosci.* 21(18):7153–7160.

Sheline YI, Wang PW, Gado MH, Csernansky JG, Vannier MW. 1996. Hippocampal atrophy in recurrent major depression. *Proc Natl Acad Sci U S A.* 93(9):3908–3913.

Shihabuddin LS, Horner PJ, Ray J, Gage FH. 2000. Adult spinal cord stem cells generate neurons after transplantation in the adult dentate gyrus. *J Neurosci.* 20(23):8727–8735.

Sivaprakasam K. 2006. Towards a unifying hypothesis of Alzheimer's disease: cholinergic system linked to plaques, tangles and neuroinfl ammation. *Curr Med Chem.* 13(18):2179–2188.

Slevin JT, Gerhardt GA, Smith CD, Gash DM, Kryscio R, Young B. 2005. Improvement of bilateral motor functions in patients with Parkinson disease through the unilateral intraputaminal infusion of glial cell line-derived neurotrophic factor. *J Neurosurg.* 102(2):216–222.

St George-Hyslop PH, Petit A. 2005. Molecular biology and genetics of Alzheimer's disease. *C R Biol.* 328(2):119–130.

Stanfield BB, Trice JE. 1988. Evidence that granule cells generated in the dentate gyrus of adult rats extend axonal projections. *Exp Brain Res.* 72(2):399–406.

Stoll G, Jander S, Schroeter M. 1998. Inflammation and glial responses in ischemic brain lesions. *Prog Neurobiol.* 56(2):149–171.

Stoll G, Jander S. 1999. The role of microglia and macrophages in the pathophysiology of the CNS. *Prog Neurobiol.* 58(3):233–247.

Stoll G, Jander S, Schroeter M. 2002. Detrimental and beneficial effects of injury-induced inflammation and cytokine expression in the nervous system. *Adv Exp Med Biol.* 513:87–113.

Stoll G, Schroeter M, Jander S et al. 2004. Lesion-associated expression of transforming growth factor-beta-2 in the rat nervous system: evidence for down-regulating the phagocytic activity of microglia and macrophages. *Brain Pathol.* 14(1):51–58.

Streit WJ, Walter SA, Pennell NA. 1999. Reactive microgliosis. *Prog Neurobiol.* 57(6):563–581.

Suslov ON, Kukekov VG, Ignatova TN, Steindler DA. 2002. Neural stem cell heterogeneity demonstrated by molecular phenotyping of clonal neurospheres. *Proc Natl Acad Sci U S A.* 99(22):14506–14511.

Sutula T, Cascino G, Cavazos J, Parada I, Ramirez L. 1989. Mossy fiber synaptic reorganization in the epileptic human temporal lobe. *Ann Neurol.* 26(3):321–330.

Tada E,Parent JM, LowensteinDH,Fike JR. 2000. X-irradiation causes a prolonged reduction in cell proliferation in the dentate gyrus of adult rats. *Neuroscience.* 99(1):33–41.

Tattersfield AS, Croon RJ, Liu YW, Kells AP, Faull RL, Connor B. 2004. Neurogenesis in the striatum of the quinolinic acid lesion model of Huntington's disease. *Neuroscience.* 127(2):319–332.

Taupin P. 2006a. The therapeutic potential of adult neural stem cells. *Curr Opin Mol Ther.* 8(3):225–231.

Taupin. P. 2006b. Adult neural stem cells, neurogenic niches and cellular therapy. *Stem Cell Reviews.* 2(3):213–220.

Taupin P. 2006c. HuCNS-SC (StemCells). *Curr Opin Mol Ther.* 8(2):156–163.

Taupin P. 2007. BrdU immunohistochemistry for studying adult neurogenesis: paradigms, pitfalls, limitations, and validation. *Brain Res Rev.* 53(1):198–214.

Taupin P, Gage FH. 2002. Adult neurogenesis and neural stem cells of the central nervous system in mammals. *J Neurosci Res.* 69(6):745–749.

Toni N, Teng EM, Bushong EA et al. 2007. Synapse formation on neurons born in the adult hippocampus. *Nat Neurosci.* 10(6):727–734.

Vallieres L, Campbell IL, Gage FH, Sawchenko PE. 2002. Reduced hippocampal neurogenesis in adult transgenic mice with chronic astrocytic production of interleukin-6. *J Neurosci.* 22(2):486–492.

van Praag H, Schinder AF, Christie BR, Toni N, Palmer TD, Gage FH. 2002. Functional neurogenesis in the adult hippocampus. *Nature.* 415(6875):1030–1034.

Vardy ER, Hussain I, Hooper NM. 2006. Emerging therapeutics for Alzheimer's disease. *Expert Rev Neurother.* 6(5):695–704.

Volkmann J. 2007. Update on surgery for Parkinson's disease. *Curr Opin Neurol.* 20(4):465–469.

Wen PH, Shao X, Shao Z et al. 2002. Overexpression of wild type but not an FAD mutant presenilin-1 promotes neurogenesis in the hippocampus of adult mice. *Neurobiol Dis.* 10(1):8–19.

White JK, Auerbach W, Duyao MP et al. 1997. Huntingtin is required for neurogenesis and is not impaired by the Huntington's disease CAG expansion. *Nat Genet.* 17(4):404–410.

Whitton PS. 2007. Inflammation as a causative factor in the aetiology of Parkinson's disease. *Br J Pharmacol.* 150(8):963–976.

Wong ML, Licinio J. 2001. Research and treatment approaches to depression. *Nat Rev Neurosci.* 2(5):343–351.

Yan J, Welsh AM, Bora SH, Snyder EY, Koliatsos VE. 2004. Differentiation and tropic/trophic effects of exogenous neural precursors in the adult spinal cord. *J Comp Neurol.* 480(1):101–114.

Yang Y, Geldmacher DS, Herrup K. 2001. DNA replication precedes neuronal cell death in Alzheimer's disease. *J Neurosci.* 21(8):2661–2668.

Zhao M, Momma S, Delfani K et al. 2003. Evidence for neu-rogenesis in the adult mammalian substantia nigra. *Proc Natl Acad Sci U S A.* 100(13):7925–7930.

Zilka N, Ferencik M, Hulin I. 2006. Neuroinflammation in Alzheimer's disease: protector or promoter? *Bratisl Lek Listy.* 107(9–10):374–383.

Chapter VIII

A Dual Activity of ROS and Oxidative Stress on Adult Neurogenesis and Alzheimer's Disease[*]

Abstract

Oxidative stress is a deleterious condition leading to cellular death. It plays a key role in the development and pathology of neurodegenerative diseases, like Alzheimer's disease (AD). AD is the most common form of dementia among elderly. Genetic mutations and genetic, acquired and environmental risk factors, particularly neuroinflammation and oxidative stress, are the main causes of AD. Neurogenesis occurs in the adult brain of mammals, particularly in the hippocampus, and is enhanced in the brain of patients with AD. Enhanced neurogenesis in AD may represent an attempt by the central nervous system to compensate for the neuronal loss and repair itself. Reactive oxygen species (ROS) promote cell death and the nondisjunction of chromosomes, leading to aneuploidy. The activity of ROS on newly generated neuronal cells in the adult brain may contribute to the pathogenesis of AD. Antioxidant may be used to reduce the deleterious activity of ROS, particularly on newly generated neuronal cells of the adult brain, potentially delaying the development of AD and promoting the regenerative capacity of the adult brain.

Introduction

Reactive oxygen species (ROS) are highly reactive substances formed by the incomplete reduction of oxygen. They include superperoxide (O_2-), a product of the mitochondrial respiratory chain, hydrogen peroxide (H_2O_2), generated from the conversion of superperoxide by the enzyme superoxide dismutase, hydroxyl radical (OH), a product of the

---

[*] Copyright notice. Reproduced with permission from Bentham Science Publishers, Ltd.: Taupin P. A dual activity of ROS and oxidative stress on adult neurogenesis and Alzheimer's disease. Central Nervous System Agents in Medicinal Chemistry. (2010) 10(1):16-21. Copyright 2010, Bentham Science Publishers, Ltd.

reduction of hydrogen peroxide, and peroxynitrite anions (ONOO-), generated by the reaction of superperoxide with nitric oxide. ROS are produced under physiological conditions by the cells and are involved in cell signaling and metabolism [1]. ROS are toxic and damaging to the cells. They oxidize the components of the cells; membrane and cytoplasmic proteins, lipids and nucleic acids. Protein and nucleic acid oxidation and lipid peroxidation compromise cellular functions. The cells are protected against the toxicity of ROS, by enzymes, like superoxide dismutase, catalase and glutathione. These enzymes act as natural antioxidants. Under normal conditions, the balance between the generation and degradation of ROS by the cells and organisms is highly regulated [2].

Oxidative stress occurs when the levels of ROS exceed the antioxidant capacity of the cells. Oxidative stress results from an elevation of the production of free radicals or a decrease in the scavenging of free radicals or in the mechanisms used to repair oxidized macromolecules. This leads to cellular dysfunction and cell death. Excessive production of ROS can lead to cell death via apoptosis or necrosis [3]. Oxidative stress plays a key role in the development of numerous pathologies, particularly neurodegenerative diseases like Alzheimer's disease (AD) [4]. Proteins and nucleic acids elicit high rate of oxidation and lipids of peroxidation in patients with AD, particularly in regions containing senile plaques and neurofibrillary tangles in the brain [5, 6]. The level of DNA damage and oxidized DNA bases (pyrimidines and purines) is increased by 2-fold in leukocytes of individuals with mild cognitive impairment (MCI) and AD, compared to individuals not diagnosed with the diseases [7, 8]. Patients with MCI have a probability to develop AD of 12% per year or 50% within 4 years [9]. Hence, oxidative damage occurs at the early stages of AD and oxidative stress contributes to the pathogenesis of the disease [10].

In this manuscript, we will review and discuss the contribution of oxidative stress to the pathogenesis and pathology of AD. We will particularly review and discuss the mechanisms underlying neuronal death and the contribution of newly generated neuronal cells of the adult brain to the pathogenesis of AD, under conditions of oxidative stress.

Alzheimer's Disease Is Caused by Excessive Rate of Genome Damage

AD is an irreversible progressive neurodegenerative disease, leading to severe incapacity and death. It is the most common form of dementia among elderly, affecting 30% of individuals of age over 80 [11]. There are two forms of the disease, the sporadic form and the familial form. The sporadic form of AD is the most common form of the disease. It is believed to be caused by a combination of genetic, acquired and environmental risk factors [12]. These include the presence of the ApoE varepsilon 4 allele (ApoE4), the presence of variants in at least two different clusters of intronic sequences in the neuronal sortilin-related receptor (SORL1) gene, hypertension, diabetes, neuroinflammation and oxidative stress [13-16]. Inherited form of AD, also known as familial Alzheimer's disease (FAD), is a rare form of the disease. It is caused by mutations in so-called familial Alzheimer genes, like the gene of β-amyloid precursor protein (APP), the presenilin-1 (PSEN-1) gene and the presenilin-2 (PSEN-2) gene [17]. The late-onset AD (LOAD) refers to cases of AD diagnosed after the age of 65. The early-onset AD (EOAD) refers to cases of AD diagnosed at younger age. LOAD accounts for the majority, over 93%, of all cases of AD. The sporadic form of AD accounts for most cases of LOAD, whereas inherited form of AD accounts for most cases of EOAD. AD affects more than 26 millions of patients worldwide, a number expected to quadruple by 2050 as population age [18].

Amyloid plaques and neurofibrillary tangles are the histological hallmarks of AD and two of the probable causes of the pathogenesis of AD. They are deposits of proteins distributed throughout the brain of patients with AD, particularly in the entorhinal cortex, hippocampus, temporal, frontal and inferior parietal lobes [19, 20]. Amyloid plaques are primarily composed of aggregates of protein β-amyloid and neurofibrillary tangles of aggregates of protein Tau hyperphosphorylated. Protein β-amyloid is a 42 amino acid β-peptide originating from the post-transcriptional maturation of APP [21]. The abnormal processing of APP results in the aggregation of protein amyloid and the formation of amyloid plaques. Tau protein is a microtubule-associated phosphoprotein. The hyperphosphorylation of Tau protein by kinases results in the aggregation of Tau protein and the breakdown of microtubules [22]. Amyloid plaques and neurofibrillary tangles would cause cell death in the brain [23].

AD is associated with the loss of nerve cells in areas of the brain that are vital to memory and other mental abilities, like the entorhinal cortex, hippocampus and neocortex. A substantial number of neurons, 4 to 10%, in regions of degeneration, like the hippocampus, express proteins of the cell cycle and some at-risk neurons are aneuploid in the brain of AD patients [24, 25]. It is proposed that the genetic imbalance in aneuploid cells signifies that they are fated to die [26]. Their relatively high percentage at any one time in regions of degeneration in AD brains suggests that they will undergo a slow death process. Unlike apoptosis, these cells may live in this state for months, possibly up to 1 year [26]. The deregulation and/or re-expression of proteins controlling the cell cycle of nerve cells and genetic imbalance in aneuploid cells would underlie the neurodegenerative process and pathogenesis of AD. The nuclear and mitochondrial DNA in diseased regions of the brain of AD patients also elicits lesions and mutational events, like DNA oxidation, as evidenced by the presence of the modified base 8-hydroxydeoxyguanosine, strand breaks and large deletions [27].

In all, AD is a neurodegenerative disease caused by an excessive rate of damage in the genome [28].

Enhanced Neurogenesis in Alzheimer's Disease

Most nerve cells in the central nervous system (CNS) of adult mammals are terminally differentiated post-mitotic cells. They are maintained in the quiescent phase G0 of the cell cycle and no longer divide. They are born from primordial neural stem cells (NSCs) during development. NSCs are the self-renewing multipotent cells that generate the main phenotypes of the nervous system, neuronal, astroglial and oligodendroglial. It was believed that the adult brain was devoid of stem cells, hence lacks the capacity to generate new nerve cells and regenerate after injury. Studies in the 1960s and, mostly in the 1980s and 90s, have reported and confirmed that contrary to a long-held dogma, neurogenesis occurs throughout adulthood in the brain and NSCs reside in the adult CNS of mammals [29].

Neurogenesis occurs primarily in two regions of the adult mammalian brain, the dentate gyrus (DG) of the hippocampus and the subventricular zone (SVZ) along the ventricles, in various species including humans. In the DG, newly generated neuronal cells in the subgranular zone migrate to the granule cell layer, where they differentiate into granule-like cells and extend axonal projections to the CA3 region of the Ammon's horn [30]. Newly generated neuronal cells in the anterior part of the SVZ migrate through the rostro-migratory stream to the olfactory bulb, where they differentiate into interneurons, granule and periglomerular neurons [31].

The expression of markers of immature neuronal cells, like doublecortin and polysialylated nerve cell adhesion molecule, is increased in hippocampal regions, particularly the DG, of the brain of patients with clinical diagnosis of AD [32]. Neurogenesis is decreased in the DG of PDAPP adult transgenic mice, a model of AD with age-dependent accumulation of protein β-amyloid [33]. It is enhanced in the DG of adult mice that express the Swedish and Indiana APP mutations, a mutant form of human APP [34]. It is impaired in the DG and SVZ of adult mice deficient for PSEN-1 and/or APP and in transgenic mice over expressing variants of APP or PSEN-1 [35-37].

The discrepancies between the data observed in the various studies may originate from the validity of the animal models, as representative of AD and to study adult phenotypes. Mice deficient for APP and PSEN-1 provide information on the activities and functions of the proteins involved in familial forms of AD. The effects of genetic mutations during development in transgenic mice may have adverse effects on adult phenotypes, particularly adult neurogenesis. In addition, most studies use bromodeoxyuridine (BrdU) labeling and/or immuno-histochemistry for proteins of the cell cycle, as paradigms to study and assess adult neurogenesis. BrdU is a thymidine analog that incorporates DNA of dividing cells during the S-phase of the cell cycle. It is used for birth dating and monitoring cell proliferation, by immunohistology and confocal microscopy [38]. There are pitfalls and limitations over the use of thymidine analogs, and particularly BrdU, for studying neurogenesis. BrdU is not a marker for cell proliferation, but a marker for DNA synthesis. Studying neurogenesis with BrdU requires distinguish cell proliferation and neurogenesis from other events involving DNA synthesis, like abortive cell cycle re-entry leading to apoptosis and cell cycle re-entry and gene duplication, without cell division, leading to aneuploidy [39-41].

Some at-risk neurons in regions of degeneration are aneuploid [24,25]. Abortive cell cycle re-entry and gene duplication without cell division precede neuronal death in degenerating regions in the brain of patients with AD [24, 25]. The use of BrdU labeling and immuno-histochemistry for proteins of the cell cycle, as paradigms for studying cell proliferation and adult neurogenesis in neurological diseases and disorders, does not allow to discriminate between cells re-entering the cell cycle as prelude to apoptosis, cells undergoing DNA duplication without cell division, as part of their pathological fate, and the genesis of neuronal cells [40, 41]. In addition, the permeability of the blood-brain barrier is affected in AD [42]. In these conditions, an increase in BrdU-labeling in the brain could originate from an increase in BrdU uptake rather than an increase in cell proliferation and neurogenesis. Hence, studies involving the use of BrdU labeling and immunohistochemistry for proteins of the cell cycle must be carefully addressed and discussed in light of these limitations and pitfalls [40, 41].

In all, neurogenesis may be enhanced in the brain of patients with AD. It would result from damaged or stimulation induction of neurogenesis and may be a consequence, rather than a cause, of the disease [43]. Enhanced neurogenesis in AD would contribute to a regenerative attempt, to compensate for the neuronal loss.

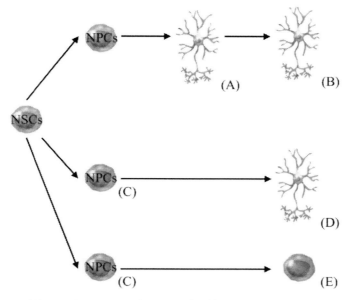

(A): newly generated neuronal cells
(B): aneuploid nerve cells
(C): aneuploid neural progenitor cells
(D): aneuploid newly generated neuronal cells
(E): aneuploid neural progenitor cells not proceeding with developmental program

Figure 1. Fate of newly generated neuronal cells in the adult brain of patients with AD. Neurogenesis occurs in the adult brain. Newly generated neuronal cells in the adult brain originate from a population of stem cells; neural stem cells (NSCs). NSCs generate a large number of progenies through an intermediate population of cells; neural progenitor cells (NPCs). The process of adult neurogenesis holds the potential to generate populations of aneuploid cells particularly in the neurogenic regions. (A) Newly generated neuronal cells of the adult brain originating from the proliferation and maturation of neural progenitor and stem cells. (B) Aneuploid nerve cells in the adult brain could originate from mature nerve cells born during development or from newly generated neuronal cells of the adult brain re-entering the cell cycle and undergoing DNA replication, but not completing the cell cycle. (C) Aneuploid NPCs cells in the adult brain could originate from the nondisjunction of chromosomes during the process of cell division of NSCs, leading to (D) newly generated neuronal cells that are aneuploid or to (E) a population of aneuploid NPCs that would not proceed with their developmental program [56, 63]. Oxidative stress promotes aneuploidy for chromosome 17, the chromosome carrying the gene for TAU. ROS decreases neurogenesis in the adult brain. Although oxidative stress could promote the formation of neurofibrillary tangles and aneuploidy in the neurogenic regions of the adult brain, contributing to the pathogenesis of AD, this activity may be limited by the decrease in neurogenesis.

Oxidative Stress Contributes to the Pathogenesis of Alzheimer's Disease

Oxidative stress is a risk factor for developing AD and individuals with MCI and AD elicit high level of DNA damage and oxidized DNA bases [7, 8, 14]. Protein β-amyloid promotes the generation of ROS in the brain of AD patients [44]. Rat embryonic cortical neurons cultured with toxic concentrations of protein β-amyloid re-enter the cell cycle and die by apoptosis in vitro [45]. Hence, ROS, particularly generated by protein β-amyloid, and oxidative stress would contribute to cell death and neurodegeneration in the pathogenesis of AD. The forced expression of oncogenes in post-mitotic nerve cells, causes cell death rather than cell proliferation and a substantial number of neurons in regions of degeneration, like the hippocampus, of the brain of AD patients express proteins of the cell cycle, including proliferating nuclear antigen, Ki-67, cyclin D, cyclin-dependent kninase 4 and cyclin B1 [46-48]. The deregulation and/or re-expression of proteins controlling the cell cycle in post-mitotic nerve cells signify that these cells undergo a process of abortive cell cycle re-entry, leading to apoptosis, in regions of degeneration in the brain of AD patients [26]. A wide range of cells elicit aneuploidy in patients with AD, particularly for chromosome 21 [49, 50]. Cells that are the most likely to develop aneuploidy are dividing cells. The nondisjunction of chromosomes in populations of somatic cells that retain their ability to divide is most likely at the origin of aneuploidy in patients with AD [51]. In the brain of patients with AD, some at-risk neurons are also aneuploid [24, 25]. Cell cycle re-entry and gene duplication, without cell division, is most likely at the origin of aneuploidy in post-mitotic nerve cells in the brain of AD patients [26]. Oxidative stress promotes aneuploidy, particularly for chromosome 17 [52]. Hence, ROS and oxidative stress contribute to the pathogenesis of AD by inducing cell cycle re-entry of post-mitotic nerve cells, and neuronal death, and gene duplication, without cell division, at the origin of aneuploidy in post-mitotic nerve cells in the brain of AD patients [53, 54].

A "two-hit hypothesis" has been proposed to conciliate the activity of oxidative stress and abnormal mitotic signaling, like abortive cell cycle re-entry leading to apoptosis and gene duplication without cell division leading to aneuploidy, as causative factors of AD. Oxidative stress and abnormal mitotic signaling can act independently as initiators, however both processes are necessary to propagate the pathogenesis of AD [55]. Abnormal mitotic signaling may lead to a small population of aneuploid cells that over-express genes that contribute to the development of the disease, like APP and TAU. As these cells undergo cell death, they trigger an inflammatory reaction in the regions of amyloid and neurotic plaques formation. This further promotes the development of the disease. In this model, individuals may eventually develop the disease, over a longer period of time.

Table 1. Experimental studies. Drug treatments for Alzheimer's disease and oxidative stress on adult neurogenesis in rodents

Drug	Family	Dose administered	References
Alzheimer's disease			
Galantamine	AChE inhibitor	5 mg/kg for 14 days	[62]
Memantine	NMDA-R antagonist	7.5 mg/kg for 14 days	[62]
Tacrine	AChE inhibitor	5 mg/kg for 14 days	[62]
Oxidative stress			
Curcumin	Ginger	500 nmol/kg for 4 days	[59]

Experiments were performed in rodents. Galantamine, tacrine and curcumin were administered intraperitoneally. The administration of memantine was intragastric. Abbreviations: AChE, acetylcholinesterase; NMDA-R, N-methyl-D-aspartate-glutamate receptor.

A Dual Activity of ROS and Oxidative Stress on Adult Neurogenesis and on the Pathogenesis of Alzheimer's Disease

Stem cells and somatic cells that retain the ability to divide are the most likely to develop aneuploidy. Since newly generated neuronal cells of the adult brain originate from stem cells, they are most likely to develop aneuploidy, (Figure (1)). The nondisjunction of chromosomes during the process of cell division of newly generated progenitor cells of the adult brain, particularly in the hippocampus, would lead to newly generated neuronal cells that are aneuploid or to a population of aneuploid neural progenitor cells that would not proceed with their developmental program [56]. The APP, PSEN1 and TAU genes are located on chromosomes 21, 14 and 17, respectively [17, 57, 58]. Aneuploidy for these chromosomes contributes to the pathogenesis of AD, by promoting the aggregation of protein β-amyloid and Tau protein [51]. Oxidative stress promotes aneuploidy, particularly for chromosome 17 [52]. Hence, ROS and oxidative stress would increase the risk of the generation of newly generated neuronal cells that are aneuploid for chromosome 17, or of a population of neural progenitor cells that are aneuploid for chromosome 17 and would not proceed with their developmental program. The TAU gene is located on chromosome 17 [58]. Aneuploidy for chromosome 17 in newly generated cells of the adult brain would promote the expression of Tau proteins in the hippocampus, particularly. The hyperphosphorylation of Tau proteins produced by these cells would result in the formation of neurofibrillary tangles and the breakdown of microtubules locally in the adult brain of AD patients, leading to further aneuploidy in newly generated neuronal cells [55]. Hence, oxidative stress would promote aneuploidy and the formation of neurofibrillary tangles, in the neurogenic regions of the adult brain, contributing to neurodegeneration and to the pathogenesis of AD.

Antioxidants, like curcumin, increase neurogenesis in the hippocampus of adult rodents (Table 1) [59]. Hence, ROS may decrease neurogenesis in the adult brain. On the one hand, such decrease would reduce the deleterious activity of ROS in inducing aneuploidy in newly generated adult neuronal cells of the adult brain. On the other hand, it may limit the regenerative potential of adult neurogenesis. This reveals that the activity of ROS and oxidative stress elicit a dual activity on newly generated neuronal cells of the adult brain and on the pathogenesis of AD, promoting aneuploidy and decreasing neurogenesis.

ROS and Oxidative Stress Control the Cell Cycle and Genomic Stability

ROS and oxidative stress promote abortive cell cycle re-entry, leading to apoptosis, of nerve cells of the adult brain, cell cycle re-entry and gene duplication without cell division, leading to aneuploidy, and DNA damage [53]. The mechanisms by which ROS and oxidative stress increase the risk of developing AD remain mostly unknown. ROS and oxidative stress would contribute to the pathogenesis of AD through their activity in controlling the cell cycle.

It would increase the risk of developing AD, directly or indirectly, through their oxidative activity on DNA and on various enzymatic and mitogenic pathways, like the EGF and VEGF pathways, the stress-activated protein kinases JNK and p38, JAK/STAT, protein kinase C pathways and histone deacetylase and through mutational events including strand breaks and large deletions [60]. If the oxidation of DNA surpasses the DNA-repair capacity of the cell, mutations could accumulate, leading to the loss of genome stability, a landmark of AD pathology. Studies show that whether ROS-exposed cells undergo proliferation, growth arrest or apoptosis depends in part on where the cell resides in the cell cycle when insulted [61]. This has implications on the mechanisms by which oxidative stress may affect neuronal cells in the adult brain, whether and how it affects mature neurons or newly generated neuronal cells in regions of neurodegeneration, like the hippocampus.

Concluding Remarks

Oxidative stress is an environmental risk factor for developing AD. Oxidative stress and ROS are candidates for causal factors for cycle re-entry-induced neuronal death and gene duplication without cell division, leading to aneuploidy, in the adult brain of patients with AD. ROS may decrease neurogenesis in the adult brain, reducing the risk of generating aneuploid newly generated neuronal cells and aneuploid neural progenitor cells that would not proceed with their developmental program in the adult brain. Adult neurogenesis is enhanced in the brain of patients with AD. The decrease of neurogenesis induced by ROS would limit the regenerative capacity of the adult brain. It has been proposed to use antioxidant for the treatment of AD. These drugs may not only reduce the deleterious activities of ROS and oxidative stress, but also promote the regenerative capacity of the adult brain. Further studies will aim at identifying and validating the use and benefits of antioxidants for treating AD, particularly in relation to their activities on adult neurogenesis.

References

[1] Starkov, A.A. The role of mitochondria in reactive oxygen species metabolism and signaling. Ann. N. Y. *Acad. Sci.,* 2008, 1147, 37 52.

[2] Klein, J.A.; Ackerman, S.L. Oxidative stress, cell cycle, and neurodegeneration. *J. Clin. Invest.,* 2003, 111, 785-793.

[3] Kannan, K.; Jain, S.K. Oxidative stress and apoptosis. *Pathophysiology,* 2000, 7, 153-163.

[4] Sayre, L.M.; Smith, M.A.; Perry, G. Chemistry and biochemistry of oxidative stress in neurodegenerative disease. *Curr. Med. Chem.,* 2001, 8, 721-738.

[5] Mecocci, P.; Polidori, M.C.; Ingegni, T.; Cherubini, A.; Chionne, F.; Cecchetti, R.; Senin, U. Oxidative damage to DNA in lymphocytes from AD patients. *Neurology,* 1998, 51, 1014-1017.

[6] Lovell, M.A.; Gabbita, S.P.; Markesbery, W.R. Increased DNA oxidation and decreased levels of repair products in Alzheimer's disease ventricular CSF. *J. Neurochem.,* 1999, 72, 771-776.

[7] Beal, M.F. Oxidative damage as an early marker of Alzheimer's disease and mild cognitive impairment. *Neurobiol. Aging,* 2005, 26, 585-586.

[8] Lovell, M.A.; Markesbery, W.R. Oxidative damage in mild cognitive impairment and early Alzheimer's disease. *J. Neurosci. Res.,* 2007, 85, 3036-3040.

[9] Mitchell, A.J.; Shiri-Feshki, M. Temporal trends in the long term risk of progression of mild cognitive impairment: a pooled analysis. *J. Neurol. Neurosurg. Psychiatry,* 2008, 79, 1386-1391.

[10] Mecocci, P. Oxidative stress in mild cognitive impairment and Alzheimer disease: a continuum. *J. Alzheimers Dis.,* 2004, 6, 159 163.

[11] Burns, A.; Byrne, E.J.; Maurer, K. Alzheimer's disease. *Lancet,* 2002, 360, 163-165.

[12] Cankurtaran, M.; Yavuz, B.B.; Cankurtaran, E.S.; Halil, M.; Ulger, Z.; Ariogul, S. Risk factors and type of dementia: Vascular or Alzheimer? *Arch. Gerontol. Geriatr.,* 2008, 47, 25-34.

[13] Goedert, M.; Strittmatter, W.J.; Roses, A.D. Alzheimer's disease. Risky apolipoprotein in brain. *Nature,* 1994, 372, 45-46.

[14] Onyango, I.G.; Khan, S.M. Oxidative stress, mitochondrial dysfunction, and stress signaling in Alzheimer's disease. *Curr. Alz-heimer Res.,* 2006, 3, 339-349.

[15] Zilka, N.; Ferencik, M.; Hulin, I. Neuroinflammation in Alz-heimer's disease: protector or promoter? *Bratisl. Lek. Listy,* 2006, 107, 374-383.

[16] Rogaeva, E.; Meng, Y.; Lee, J.H.; Gu, Y.; Kawarai, T.; Zou, F.; Katayama, T.; Baldwin, C.T.; Cheng, R.; Hasegawa, H.; Chen, F.; Shibata, N.; Lunetta, K.L.; Pardossi-Piquard, R.; Bohm, C.; Wakutani, Y.; Cupples, L.A.; Cuenco, K.T.; Green, R.C.; Pinessi, L.; Rainero, I.; Sorbi, S.; Bruni, A.; Duara, R.; Friedland, R.P.; Inzel berg, R.; Hampe, W.; Bujo, H.; Song, Y.Q.; Andersen, O.M.; Will-now, T.E.; Graff-Radford, N.; Petersen, R.C.; Dickson, D.; Der, S.D.; Fraser, P.E.; Schmitt-Ulms, G.; Younkin, S.; Mayeux, R.; Farrer, L.A.; St George-Hyslop, P. The neuronal sortilin-related receptor SORL1 is genetically associated with Alzheimer disease. *Nat. Genet.,* 2007, 39, 168-177.

[17] Schellenberg, G.D.; Bird, T.D.; Wijsman, E.M.; Orr, H.T.; Anderson, L.; Nemens, E.; White, J.A.; Bonnycastle, L.; Weber, J.L.; Alonso, M.E.; et al. Genetic linkage evidence for a familial Alzheimer's disease locus on chromosome 14. *Science,* 1992, 258, 668-671.

[18] Brookmeyer, R.; Johnson, E.; Ziegler-Graham, K.; Arrighi, H.M. Forecasting the Global Burden of Alzheimer's Disease; Johns Hopkins University, Department of Biostatistics Working Papers, 2007, Working Paper 130. http://www.bepress. com/jhubiostat/paper130.

[19] Fukutani, Y.; Kobayashi, K.; Nakamura, I.; Watanabe, K.; Isaki, K.; Cairns, N.J. Neurons, intracellular and extra cellular neurofi-brillary tangles in subdivisions of the hippocampal cortex in normal ageing and Alzheimer's disease. *Neurosci. Lett.,* 1995, 200, 57-60.

[20] Anderson, D.H.; Talaga, K.C.; Rivest, A.J.; Barron, E.; Hageman, G.S.; Johnson, L.V. Characterization of beta amyloid assemblies in drusen: the deposits associated with aging and age-related macular degeneration. *Exp. Eye Res.,* 2004, 78, 243-256.

[21] Kang, J.; Lemaire, H.G.; Unterbeck, A.; Salbaum, J.M.; Masters, C.L.; Grzeschik, K.H.; Multhaup, G.; Beyreuther, K.; Müller-Hill, B. The precursor of Alzheimer's

disease amyloid A4 protein resembles a cell-surface receptor. *Nature,* 1987, 325, 733-736.

[22] Alonso, A.; Zaidi, T.; Novak, M.; Grundke-Iqbal, I.; Iqbal, K. Hyperphosphorylation induces self-assembly of tau into tangles of paired helical filaments/straight filaments. *Proc. Natl. Acad. Sci. USA,* 2001, 98, 6923-6928.

[23] Hardy, J.; Selkoe, D.J. The amyloid hypothesis of Alzheimer's disease: progress and problems on the road to therapeutics. Science, 2002, 297, 353-356. Erratum in: *Science,* 2002, 297, 2209.

[24] Busser, J.; Geldmacher, D.S.; Herrup, K. Ectopic cell cycle proteins predict the sites of neuronal cell death in Alzheimer's disease brain. *J. Neurosci.,* 1998, 18, 2801-2807.

[25] Yang, Y.; Geldmacher, D.S.; Herrup, K. DNA replication precedes neuronal cell death in Alzheimer's disease. *J. Neurosci.,* 2001, 21, 2661-2668.

[26] Herrup, K.; Neve, R.; Ackerman, S.L.; Copani, A. Divide and die: cell cycle events as triggers of nerve cell death. *J. Neurosci.,* 2004, 24, 9232-9239.

[27] Sekiguchi, M.; Tsuzuki, T. Oxidative nucleotide damage: consequences and prevention. *Oncogene,* 2002, 21, 8895-8804.

[28] Thomas, P.; Fenech, M. A review of genome mutation and Alzheimer's disease. *Mutagenesis,* 2007, 22, 15-33.

[29] Kaplan, M.S. Environment complexity stimulates visual cortex neurogenesis: death of a dogma and a research career. *Trends Neurosci.,* 2001, 24, 617-620.

[30] Taupin, P. Characterization and isolation of synapses of newly generated neuronal cells of the adult hippocampus at early stages of neurogenesis. *J. Neurodegener. Regen.,* 2009, 2, 9-17.

[31] Taupin, P. Neurogenesis in the adult central nervous system. C. R. *Biol.,* 2006, 329, 465-475.

[32] Jin, K.; Peel, A.L.; Mao, X.O.; Xie, L.; Cottrell, B.A.; Henshall, D.C, ; Greenberg, D.A. Increased hippocampal neurogenesis in Alzheimer's disease. *Proc. Natl. Acad. Sci. USA,* 2004, 101, 343-347.

[33] Donovan, M.H.; Yazdani, U.; Norris, R.D.; Games, D.; German, D.C.; Eisch, A.J. Decreased adult hippocampal neurogenesis in the PDAPP mouse model of Alzheimer's disease. *J. Comp. Neurol.,* 2006, 495, 70-83.

[34] Jin, K.; Galvan, V.; Xie, L.; Mao, X.O.; Gorostiza, O.F.; Bredesen, D.E.; Greenberg, D.A. Enhanced neurogenesis in Alzheimer's disease transgenic (PDGF-APPSw,Ind) mice. *Proc. Natl. Acad. Sci. USA,* 2004, 101, 13363-13367.

[35] Feng, R.; Rampon, C.; Tang, Y.P.; Shrom, D.; Jin, J.; Kyin, M.; Sopher, B.; Miller, M.W.; Ware, C.B.; Martin, G.M.; Kim, S.H.; Langdon, R.B.; Sisodia, S.S.; Tsien, J.Z. Deficient neurogenesis in forebrain-specific presenilin-1 knockout mice is associated with re-duced clearance of hippocampal memory traces. Neuron, 2001, 32, 911-926. Erratum in: *Neuron,* 2002, 33, 313.

[36] Zhang, C.; McNeil, E.; Dressler, L.; Siman, R. Long-lasting impairment in hippocampal neurogenesis associated with amyloid deposition in a knock-in mouse model of familial Alzheimer's disease. *Exp. Neurol.,* 2007, 204, 77-87.

[37] Rodríguez, J.J.; Jones, V.C.; Tabuchi, M.; Allan, S.M.; Knight, E.M.; LaFerla, F.M.; Oddo, S.; Verkhratsky, A. Impaired adult neurogenesis in the dentate gyrus of a triple transgenic mouse model of Alzheimer's disease. *PLoS ONE,* 2008, 3, e2935.

[38] Miller, M.W.; Nowakowski, R.S. Use of bromodeoxyuridineimmunohistochemistry to examine the proliferation, migration and time of origin of cells in the central nervous system. *Brain Res.*, 1988, 457, 44-52.

[39] Nowakowski, R.S.; Hayes, N.L. Stem cells: the promises and pitfalls. *Neuropsychopharmacology*, 2001, 25, 799-804.

[40] Taupin, P. BrdU Immunohistochemistry for studying adult neurogenesis: paradigms, pitfalls, limitations, and validation. *Brain Res. Rev.*, 2007, 53, 198-214.

[41] Taupin, P. Protocols for studying adult neurogenesis: insights and recent developments. *Reg. Med.*, 2007, 2, 51-62.

[42] Desai, B.S.; Monahan, A.J.; Carvey, P.M.; Hendey, B. Blood-brain barrier pathology in Alzheimer's and Parkinson's disease: implications for drug therapy. *Cell Transplant.*, 2007, 16, 285-299.

[43] Taupin, P. Adult neurogenesis pharmacology in neurological diseases and disorders. *Expert. Rev. Neurother.*, 2008, 8, 311-320.

[44] Hensley, K.; Carney, J.M.; Mattson, M.P.; Aksenova, M.; Harris, M.; Wu, J.F.; Floyd, R.A.; Butterfield, D.A. A model for beta-amyloid aggregation and neurotoxicity based on free radical gen-eration by the peptide: relevance to Alzheimer disease. *Proc. Natl. Acad. Sci. USA*, 1994, 91, 3270-3274.

[45] Copani, A.; Condorelli, F.; Caruso, A.; Vancheri, C.; Sala, A.; Giuffrida Stella, A.M.; Canonico, P.L.; Nicoletti, F.; Sortino, M.A. Mitotic signaling by beta-amyloid causes neuronal death. *FASEB J.*, 1999, 13, 2225-2234.

[46] McShea, A.; Harris, P.L.; Webster, K.R.; Wahl, A.F.; Smith, M.A. Abnormal expression of the cell cycle regulators P16 and CDK4 in Alzheimer's disease. *Am. J. Pathol.*, 1997, 150, 1933-1939.

[47] Nagy, Z.; Esiri, M.M.; Smith, A.D. Expression of cell division markers in the hippocampus in Alzheimer's disease and other neurodegenerative conditions. *Acta. Neuropathol.* (Berl), 1997, 93, 294-300.

[48] Feddersen, R.M.; Ehlenfeldt, R.; Yunis, W.S.; Clark, H.B.; Orr, H.T. Disrupted cerebellar cortical development and progressive degeneration of Purkinje cells in SV40 T antigen transgenic mice. *Neuron*, 1992, 9, 955-966.

[49] Geller, L.N.; Potter, H. Chromosome missegregation and trisomy 21 mosaicism in Alzheimer's disease. *Neurobiol. Dis.*, 1999, 6, 167-179.

[50] Migliore, L.; Botto, N.; Scarpato, R.; Petrozzi, L.; Cipriani, G.; Bonuccelli, U. Preferential occurrence of chromosome 21 malsegregation in peripheral blood lymphocytes of Alzheimer disease patients. *Cytogenet. Cell Genet.*, 1999, 87, 41-46.

[51] Potter, H. Review and hypothesis: Alzheimer disease and Down syndrome--chromosome 21 nondisjunction may underlie both disorders. *Am. J. Hum. Genet.*, 1991, 48, 1192-1200.

[52] Ramírez, M.J.; Puerto, S.; Galofré, P.; Parry, E.M.; Parry, J.M.; Creus, A.; Marcos, R.; Surrallés, J. Multicolour FISH detection of radioactive iodine-induced 17cen-p53 chromosomal breakage in buccal cells from therapeutically exposed patients. *Carcinogenesis*, 2000, 21, 1581-1586.

[53] Chen, Y.; McPhie, D.L.; Hirschberg, J.; Neve, R.L. The amyloid precursor protein-binding protein APP-BP1 drives the cell cycle through the S-M checkpoint and causes apoptosis in neurons. *J. Biol. Chem.*, 2000, 275, 8929-8935.

[54] Langley, B.; Ratan, R.R. Oxidative stress-induced death in the nervous system: cell cycle dependent or independent? *J. Neurosci. Res.,* 2004, 77, 621-629.

[55] Zhu, X.; Raina, A.K.; Perry, G.; Smith, M.A. Alzheimer's disease: the two-hit hypothesis. *Lancet Neurol.,* 2004, 3, 219-226.

[56] Taupin, P. Adult neurogenesis, neural stem cells and Alzheimer's disease: developments, limitations, problems and promises. *Curr. Alzheimer Res.,* 2009, 6, 461-470.

[57] Goldgaber, D.; Lerman, M.I.; McBridem, O.W.; Saffiotti, U.; Gajdusek, D.C. Characterization and chromosomal localization of a cDNA encoding brain amyloid of Alzheimer's disease. *Science,* 1987, 235, 877-880.

[58] Iqbal, K.; Grundke-Iqbal, I.; Smith, A.J.; George, L.; Tung, Y.C.; Zaidi, T. Identification and localization of a tau peptide to paired helical filaments of Alzheimer disease. *Proc. Natl. Acad. Sci. USA,* 1989, 86, 5646-5650.

[59] Kim, S.J.; Son, T.G.; Park, H.R.; Park, M.; Kim, M.S.; Kim, H.S.; Chung, H.Y.; Mattson, M.P.; Lee, J. Curcumin stimulates proliferation of embryonic neural progenitor cells and neurogenesis in the adult hippocampus. *J. Biol. Chem.,* 2008, 283, 14497-14505.

[60] Droge, W. Free radicals in the physiological control of cell function. *Physiol. Rev.,* 2002, 82, 47-95.

[61] Chen, Q.M.; Liu, J.; Merrett, J.B. Apoptosis or senescence-like growth arrest: influence of cell-cycle position, p53, p21 and bax in H2O2 response of normal human fibroblasts. *Biochem. J.,* 2000, 347, 543-551.

[62] Jin, K.; Xie, L.; Mao, X.O. Greenberg, DA. Alzheimer's disease drugs promote neurogenesis. *Brain Res.,* 2006, 1085, 183-188.

[63] Taupin, P. Adult neurogenesis in the pathogenesis of Alzheimer's disease. J. Neurodegener. *Regene.,* 2009, 2, 6-8.

Chapter IX

Adult Neurogenesis and Neural Stem Cells as a Model for the Discovery and Development of Novel Drugs

Abstract

Neurogenesis occurs in discrete regions of the adult brain, particularly the hippocampus. It is enhanced in the hippocampus of animal models and patients with neurological diseases and disorders, such as Alzheimer's disease (AD) and epilepsy. Adult hippocampal neurogenesis is modulated by drugs used for treating AD and depression, particularly galantamine, memantine and fluoxetine. This reveals that adult neurogenesis and newly generated neuronal cells of the adult hippocampus are involved in neurological diseases and disorders and that adult neurogenesis and neural stem cells (NSCs) of the adult hippocampus are the target of drugs used for treating AD and depression. Hence, adult neurogenesis and NSCs open new opportunities for our understanding of the pathology of the nervous system and new avenues to discover and develop novel drugs for treating neurogical diseases and disorders; drugs that would target specifically the NSCs of the neurogenic regions in the adult brain, or neurogenic drugs, and that would reverse or compensate deficits and impairments associated with neurological diseases and disorders, particularly those associated with the hippocampus. Adult NSCs represent a model to discover and develop novel drugs for treating neurological diseases and disorders. These drugs may also have potential for regenerative medicine and the treatment of brain tumors.

Introduction

Neurogenesis occurs throughout adulthood in the mammalian brain in various species including in humans [1]. It occurs in discrete regions or neurogenic niches of the adult brain, primarily in the dentate gyrus (DG) of the hippocampus and in the subventricular zone (SVZ), at the origin of newly generated neuronal cells in the olfactory bulb [2]. Neurogenic niches are specialized microenvironments in the adult brain that control the developmental potential of neural stem cells (NSCs). NSCs are the self-renewing multipotent cells that generate the main phenotypes of the nervous system. Newly generated neuronal cells in the adult brain would originate from a population of residual stem cells [3]. Because NSCs generate the main phenotypes of the nervous system, they hold the potential to treat and cure a broad range of neurological diseases and injuries, particularly neurodegenerative diseases, cerebral strokes and spinal cord injuries. They represent a promising model for cellular therapy and regenerative medicine. To this aim, the stimulation of endogenous neural progenitor or stem cells and the transplantation adult-derived neural progenitor and stem cells are proposed to repair and restore the degenerated or injured nerve pathways [4].

Neurogenesis is enhanced in the SVZ and hippocampus of the brain of patients with Huntington's disease (HD) and AD [5,6]. It is enhanced in the adult hippocampus of animal models of epilepsy and of animal models of AD, such as in transgenic mice that express the Swedish and Indiana amyloid precursor protein (APP) mutations [7,8]. It is reduced in the hippocampus of animal model of AD, such as in mice deficient for APP and presenilin-1, in transgenic mice overexpressing mutant genes for APP, presenilin-1 and tau protein, and in PDAPP transgenic mice [9-12]. In the brain of patients with depressive disorders, autopsy studies do not reveal any increase in neurogenesis in the hippocampus [13]. These studies show that neurogenesis is enhanced in the brain of animal models and of patients with AD, epilepsy and HD, but not of patients with episodes of depression. However, they report conflicting data, particularly in animal models of AD. The apparent discrepancies in the modulation of adult neurogenesis in neurodegenerative diseases and in the corresponding animal models may originate from the validity of these models as representative of the diseases and of transgenic mice to study adult phenotypes, such as adult neurogenesis. They may also originate from the facts that: i) there is no consensus on the term neurogenesis: some studies only present proliferation data, whereas others present only neuronal differentiation or survival data, and ii) in most studies, and in particular in the human post-mortem studies, only one time point along the pathology is analyzed. Indeed, neurogenesis might be differentially regulated along the pathogenesis.

Enhanced neurogenesis in neurological diseases would result from damage or stimulation induction of neurogenesis [14]. Hence, neurogenesis in the adult brain would contribute to the pathology of the nervous system, particularly to neurological diseases and disorders, such as AD, epilepsy and HD. It would contribute to regenerative attempts in the brain of patients with AD, epilepsy and HD, and to compensate for the neuronal loss in the hippocampus and SVZ. It may also contribute to the pathogenesis of neurological diseases and disorders, particularly in AD and but also schizophrenia [15,16]. In support of this contention, aneuploidy is a pathological landmark of AD and dividing cells are the most likely cells to develop aneuploidy. The process of adult neurogenesis holds the potential to generate populations of aneuploid cells particularly in the neurogenic areas such as the hippocampus, a region particularly affected in AD and, therefore, to contribute to the pathogenesis of AD [16]. Hence, adult neurogenesis and NSCs are involved in and contribute both beneficially and detrimentally, to the pathology of AD, the elucidation and determination of which will contribute to a better understanding of neurological diseases and disorders.

Drugs that are currently used for treating AD and depression, such as galantamine, memantine and fluoxetine, modulate adult neurogenesis in the hippocampus. Hence, adult neurogenesis and NSCs of the adult hippocampus that are involved in neurological diseases and disorders, such as AD and depression, are a target of drugs used for treating these diseases. Adult neurogenesis and NSCs represent a model of choice and a promising model to discover and develop novel drugs to treat neurological diseases and disorders.

Adult Neurogenesis and Drugs to Treat Neurological Diseases and Disorders

Adult Neurogenesis and NSCs Are Targets of Drugs Used for Treating Neurological Diseases and Disorders

Drugs that are currently used for the treatment of AD modulate neurogenesis in the hippocampus of adult rodents: galantamine, an inhibitor of acetylcholine esterase, and memantine, an antagonist of N-methyl-D-aspartate glutamate receptor, increase neurogenesis in the hippocampus and SVZ of adult rodents by 26 - 45% [17]. The activity of antidepressants has been assessed on adult neurogenesis in rodents and nonhuman primates. The chronic administration of fluoxetine (a serotoninergic antagonist) and of agomelatine (a melatonergic agonist) increases neurogenesis in the hippocampus, but not in the SVZ, of adult rats and non-human primates [18-20]. Antidepressants increase the number of neural progenitor cells in the hippocampus of adult humans [21]. Adult neurogenesis and NSCs contribute to and mediate the activities of these drugs [22,23], the role and mechanisms of which remain to be determined. Drugs may act directly or indirectly on newly generated neuronal cells of the adult brain. They may act via their pharmacological activities on messenger signaling pathways and/or via a neurogenic activity, by modulating neurogenesis [24]. However, others have reported that antidepressants, particularly fluoxetine, do not elicit pro-neurogenic effects [25-27]. Such discrepancies may originate from experimental paradigms, such as the use of certain strains of mice (BALB/cJ mice), anatomical differences and the age of the patients studied, such as in elderly patients. Hence, adult neurogenesis and NSCs are the target of drugs used for treating neurological diseases and disorders, particularly AD and depression [28]. Antidepressants may also produce their effects via distinct mechanisms, some independent of adult neurogenesis [14].

Neurogenic Drugs to Reverse or Compensate Deficits and Impairments Associated with the Hippocampus

The hippocampus is involved in various physio- and pathological conditions and processes, such as learning and memory, AD, depression and epilepsy. Adult neurogenesis is modulated in physio- and pathological processes particularly involving the hippocampus, such as learning and memory, AD and epilepsy, and is required for the activity of antidepressants, such as fluoxetine [6,7,22,23,29,30]. This reveals that adult neurogenesis and newly generated neuronal cells of the adult brain are involved in physio- and pathological conditions and processes of the nervous system, particularly associated with the hippocampus, including depression [31]. As a consequence, adult neurogenesis and NSCs may be the target of drugs used for treating deficits and impairments of neurological diseases and disorders, associated with the hippocampus, such as learning and memory deficits and impairments, AD, depression and epilepsy.

AD, epilepsy and depression are associated with neurodegeneration in the hippocampus that underlies deficits and impairments associated with these diseases and disorders [16,31]. The modulation - increase - of adult neurogenesis in the hippocampus by drugs used in the treatment of neurological diseases and disorders would signify a process to reverse or compensate those deficits and impairments associated with the hippocampus. Hence, drugs that target specifically the NSCs of the neurogenic regions in the adult brain, or neurogenic drugs, offer novel strategies for the treatment of neurological diseases and disorders: drugs that would target specifically the NSCs of the adult hippocampus and reverse or compensate deficits and impairments of neurological diseases and disorders, associated with this region of the adult brain. Adult neurogenesis and NSCs represent, therefore, a model to discover and develop novel drugs for treating neurological diseases and disorders.

Expert Opinion

Adult NSCs: A Promising Model to Discover and Develop Neurogenic Drugs

The process of drug discovery and development involves the screening of libraries of molecules and compounds to identify and select lead molecules. Assays used in these processes are primarily high-throughput screening and specific assays. Neural progenitor and stem cells have been isolated from the adult brain of mammals and characterized *in vitro* from various species and including from human biopsies and post-mortem tissues [32-35]. Adult-derived neural progenitor and stem cells provide, therefore, a model of choice for high-throughput screening of drugs *in vitro*, to identify and select lead molecules and compound candidates as neurogenic drugs. The read-out of the *in vitro* studies includes analytical and quantitative studies of proliferation, differentiation, survival, self-renewal and multipotentiality of the adult-derived neural progenitor and stem cells, particularly derived from human tissues [36-38]. To this aim, immunocytology for markers of neuronal, glial and oligodendrogial lineages, confocal microscopy and time lapse studies, as well as molecular biology techniques such as RT-PCR are most generally used to study and quantify adult neurogenesis *in vitro*. Candidate drugs identified and selected after high-throughput screening *in vitro* would then be submitted to assess their activity on adult neurogenesis *in vivo*, in controls and in animal models of neurological diseases and disorders. The read-out of the *in vivo* studies includes analytical and quantitative studies of proliferation, differentiation and survival of newly generated neuronal cells in the adult hippocampus, particularly. Bromodeoxyuridine (BrdU) labeling, immunohistology for markers of the cells cycle and confocal microscopy have been the paradigms the most used to study and quantify adult neurogenesis *in vivo*, in rodents and in primates. BrdU is a thymidine analog used for birth dating and monitoring cell proliferation [39]. Candidate drugs will be further submitted to physiological and behavioral studies, in animal models of neurological diseases and disorders, to correlate their biological activity with their *in vitro* and *in vivo* neurogenic activities, particularly in the Morris water maze and novel object recognition tasks. This is to determine the potential of the candidate drugs for treating learning and memory deficits and impairments and depression disorders, respectively; for example, based on their neurogenic activity. During the clinical trial process of these drugs, MTI technologies may be used in humans to correlate the activity of drugs to the cerebral flow volume as a mean to assess indirectly their neurogenic activities [40,41]. Hence, both *in vitro* and *in vivo* assays and models have been developed and may be used for discovering and developing neurogenic drugs. Adult NSCs represent, therefore, a promising model to discover and develop novel drugs for treating neurological diseases and disorders; drugs that target specifically the NSCs of the adult hippocampus and reverse or compensate deficits and impairments of neurological diseases and disorders, particularly learning and memory deficits and impairments and depressive disorders.

Limitations and Pitfalls of Adult NSCs for Discovering and Developing Neurogenic Drugs

There are limitations and pitfalls associated with the models currently developed and primarily used to study adult neurogenesis *in vitro* and *in vivo*. The current protocols established and used for isolating and propagating self-renewing multipotent NSCs *in vitro* yield to heterogeneous populations of neural progenitor and stem cells [42]. It has been reported that after 4 days *in vitro*, 62% of the adult derived-neural progenitor and stem cells in culture originate from 23% of the plated cells, revealing the existence of different populations of cells with different properties of growth in the culture [43]. Over time, the fast-dividing neural progenitor and stem cells represent a majority of the cells in culture reflecting the heterogeneity of adult derived-neural progenitor and stem cells *in vitro*. Other limitations to using NSCs for modeling *in vivo* neurogenesis and drug effect(s) include the accessibility of tissues, particularly human, and the ability to establish a robust baseline for *in vitro* differentiation [44,45]. Current protocols for studying and quantifying adult neurogenesis *in vivo* involve the use of the thymidine analog BrdU and of immunohistology for markers of the cells cycle and are subject to limitations and pitfalls [46]. BrdU is not a marker of cell proliferation and neurogenesis, but a marker of DNA synthesis. As such, studying neurogenesis with BrdU-labeling requires discriminating cell division and neurogenesis from other events involving DNA synthesis, such as abortive cell cycle re-entry, leading to apoptosis, and gene duplication, without cell division, leading to aneuploidy. The use of markers of the cell cycle for studying cell proliferation and neurogenesis is limited by their temporal expression and by the fact that such cell cycle markers reveal that quiescent cells have re-entered the cell cycle and resumed DNA synthesis, but not completed the cell cycle [47,48]. The drug discovery and development process to identify and select lead molecules and compound candidates as neurogenic drugs are, therefore, limited by the current protocols developed and used to study adult neurogenesis *in vitro* and *in vivo*. Hence, although adult NSCs represent a model of choice to discover and develop neurogenic drugs, the drug discovery and development process will need more stringent and more specific assays that target specifically the NSCs of the adult brain *in vitro*, *ex vivo* and *in vivo* to discover and develop novel drugs that are more potent and more specific for treating neurological diseases and disorders [49].

Neurogenic drugs are drugs that target specifically the NSCs of the neurogenic niches in the adult brain and reverse or compensate deficits and impairments of neurological diseases and disorders, such as those associated with the hippocampus [50]. They represent a novel class of drugs to treat neurological diseases and disorders. Adult neurogenesis and NSCs represent a model to discover and develop neurogenic drugs. However, limitations and pitfalls associated with protocols currently developed and used to study adultneurogenesis *in vitro* and *in vivo* limit the process of drug discovery and development. Adult neurogenesis and NSCs contribute, both beneficially and detrimentally, to the pathology of neurological diseases and disorders, particularly in AD. Hence, the process of drug discovery and development will aim at identifying candidate drugs that limit the potential deleterious effects of the drugs on adult neurogenesis, without disrupting its regenerative capacity [51]. Neurogenic drugs may be used to reverse or compensate deficits and impairments of neurological diseases and disorders, associated with the olfactory bulb, such as anosmia in AD, by stimulating neural progenitor and stem cells in the SVZ. Neurogenic drugs may also have a potential for regenerative medicine, to repair and restore degenerated or injured nerve pathways, and for the treatment of brain tumors. Further studies will be required to confirm and characterize the modulation of neurogenesis in neurological and neurodegenerative diseases and the activities of neurological drugs on adult neurogenesis, and to devise and develop more stringent and more specific assays that target specifically the NSCs of the adult brain.

Declaration of Interest

The author states no conflict of interest and has received no payment in preparation of this manuscript.

Acknowledgments

Reproduced with permission from Informa Healthcare: Taupin P. Neural stem cells as a tool for screening future neurodegenerative disorder treatments. Expert Opinion On Drug Discovery (2010) 5(10):921-925. Copyright 2010, Informa Healthcare (Informa UK Ltd).

Bibliography

[1]   Goldman SA. Adult neurogenesis: from canaries to the clinic. *J Neurobiol* 1998;36:267-86.

[2]   Taupin P. Adult neural stem cells, neurogenic niches and cellular therapy. *Stem Cell Rev* 2006;2:213-20.

[3]   Duan X, Kang E, Liu CY, et al. Development of neural stem cell in the adult brain. *Curr Opin Neurobiol* 2008;18:108-15.

[4]   Taupin P. Neurogenesis in the adult central nervous system. *C R Biol* 2006;329:465-75.

[5] Curtis MA, Penney EB, Pearson AG, et al. Increased cell proliferation and neurogenesis in the adult human Huntington's disease brain. *Proc Natl Acad Sci USA* 2003;100:9023-7.

[6] Jin K, Peel AL, Mao XO, et al. Increased hippocampal neurogenesis in Alzheimer's disease. *Proc Natl Acad Sci USA* 2004;101:343-7.

[7] Parent JM, Yu TW, Leibowitz RT, et al. Dentate granule cell neurogenesis is increased by seizures and contributes to aberrant network reorganization in the adult rat hippocampus. *J Neurosci* 1997;17:3727-38.

[8] Jin K, Galvan V, Xie L, et al. Enhanced neurogenesis in Alzheimer's disease transgenic (PDGF-APPSw,Ind) mice. *Proc Natl Acad Sci USA* 2004;101:13363-7.

[9] Feng R, Rampon C, Tang YP, et al. Deficient neurogenesis in forebrain-specific presenilin-1 knockout mice is associated with reduced clearance of hippocampal memory traces. Neuron 2001;32:911-26, Erratum in: *Neuron* 2002;33:313.

[10] Verret L, Jankowsky JL, Xu GM, et al. Alzheimer's-type amyloidosis in transgenic mice impairs survival of newborn neurons derived from adult hippocampal neurogenesis. *J Neurosci* 2007;27:6771-80.

[11] Rodriguez JJ, Jones VC, Tabuchi M, et al. *Impaired adult neurogenesis in the dentate gyrus of a triple transgenic mouse model of Alzheimer's disease.* PLoS ONE 2008;3:e2935.

[12] Donovan MH, Yazdani U, Norris RD, et al. Decreased adult hippocampal neurogenesis in the PDAPP mouse model of Alzheimer's disease. *J Comp Neurol* 2006;495:70-83.

[13] Reif A, Fritzen S, Finger M, et al. Neural stem cell proliferation is decreased in schizophrenia, but not in depression. *Mol Psychiatry* 2006;11:514-22.

[14] Taupin P. Adult neurogenesis pharmacology in neurological diseases and disorders. *Expert Rev Neurother* 2008;8:311-20.

[15] Duan X, Chang JH, Ge S, et al. Disrupted-In-Schizophrenia 1 regulates integration of newly generated neurons in the adult brain. *Cell* 2007;130:1146-58.

[16] Taupin P. Adult neurogenesis, neural stem cells and Alzheimer's disease: developments, limitations, problems and promises. *Curr Alzheimer Res* 2009;6:461-70.

[17] Jin K, Xie L, Mao XO, et al. Alzheimer's disease drugs promote neurogenesis. *Brain Res* 2006;1085:183-8.

[18] Malberg JE, Eisch AJ, Nestler EJ, et al. Chronic antidepressant treatment increases neurogenesis in adult rat hippocampus. *J Neurosci* 2000;20:9104-10.

[19] Banasr M, Soumier A, Hery M, et al. Agomelatine, a new antidepressant, induces regional changes in hippocampal neurogenesis. *Biol Psychiatry* 2006;59:1087-96.

[20] Perera TD, Coplan JD, Lisanby SH, et al. Antidepressant-induced neurogenesis in the hippocampus of adult nonhuman primates. *J Neurosci* 2007;27:4894-901.

[21] Boldrini M, Underwood MD, Hen R, et al. Antidepressants increase neural progenitor cells in the human hippocampus. *Neuropsychopharmacology* 2009;34:2376-89.

[22] Malberg JE, Duman RS. Cell proliferation in adult hippocampus is decreased by inescapable stress: reversal by fluoxetine treatment. *Neuropsychopharmacol* 2003;28:1562-71.

[23] Santarelli L, Saxe M, Gross C, et al. Requirement of hippocampal neurogenesis for the behavioral effects of antidepressants. *Science* 2003;310:805-9.

[24] Taupin P. Adult neurogenesis and drug therapy. *Cent Nerv Syst Agents Med Chem* 2008;8:198-202.

[25] Holick KA, Lee DC, Hen R, et al. Behavioral effects of chronic fluoxetine in BALB/cJ mice do not require adult hippocampal neurogenesis or the serotonin 1A receptor. *Neuropsychopharmacology*. 2008;33:406-17.

[26] Couillard-Despres S, Wuertinger C, Kandasamy M, et al. Ageing abolishes the effects of fluoxetine on neurogenesis. *Mol Psychiatry* 2009;14:856-64.

[27] Lucassen PJ, Stumpel MW, Wang Q, et al. Decreased numbers of progenitor cells but no response to antidepressant drugs in the hippocampus of elderly depressed patients. *Neuropharmacology* 2010;58:940-9.

[28] Taupin P. Neurogenic factors are target in depression. *Drug Discov Today Ther Strateg* 2008;5:157-60.

[29] Gould E, Beylin A, Tanapat P, et al. Learning enhances adult neurogenesis in the hippocampal formation. *Nat Neurosci* 1999;2:260-5.

[30] Shors TJ, Miesegaes G, Beylin A, et al. Neurogenesis in the adult is involved in the formation of trace memories. Nature 2001;410:372-6, Erratum in: *Nature* 2001;414:938.

[31] Taupin P. Neurogenesis and the effects of antidepressants. *Drug Target Insights* 2006;1:13-7.

[32] Reynolds BA, Weiss S. Generation of neurons and astrocytes from isolated cells of the adult mammalian central nervous system. *Science* 1992;255:1707-10.

[33] Gage FH, Coates PW, Palmer TD, et al. Survival and differentiation of adult neuronal progenitor cells transplanted to the adult brain. *Proc Natl Acad Sci USA* 1995;92:11879-83.

[34] Roy NS, Wang S, Jiang L, et al. In vitro neurogenesis by progenitor cells isolated from the adult human hippocampus. *Nat Med* 2000;6:271-7.

[35] Palmer TD, Schwartz PH, Taupin P, et al. Cell culture. Progenitor cells from human brain after death. *Nature* 2001;411:42-3.

[36] Taupin P. Nootropic agents stimulate neurogenesis. *Expert Opin Ther Pat* 2009;19:727-30.

[37] Taupin P. Fourteen compounds and their derivatives for the treatment of diseases and injuries characterized by reduced neurogenesis and neurodegeneration. *Expert Opin Ther Pat* 2009;19:541-7.

[38] Taupin P. Apigenin and related compounds stimulate adult neurogenesis. *Expert Opin Ther Pat* 2009;19:523-7.

[39] Miller MW, Nowakowski RS. Use of bromodeoxyuridineimmunohistochemistry to examine the proliferation, migration and time of origin of cells in the central nervous system. *Brain Res* 1998;457:44-52.

[40] Pereira AC, Huddleston DE, Brickman AM, et al. An in vivo correlate of exercise-induced neurogenesis in the adult dentate gyrus. *Proc Natl Acad Sci USA* 2007;104:5638-43.

[41] Taupin P. Magnetic resonance imaging for monitoring neurogenesis in the adult hippocampus. *Expert Opin Med Diagn* 2009;3:211-16.

[42] Reynolds BA, Rietze RL. Neural stem cells and neurospheres-re-evaluating the relationship. *Nat Methods* 2005;2:333-6.

[43] Chin VI, Taupin P, Sanga S, et al. Microfabricated platform for studying stem cell fates. *Biotechnol Bioeng* 2004;88:399-415.

[44] Crook JM, Kobayashi NR. Human stem cells for modeling neurological disorders: accelerating the drug discovery pipeline. *J Cell Biochem* 2008;105:1361-6.

[45] Kobayashi NR, Sui L, Tan PS, et al. Modelling disrupted-in-schizophrenia 1 loss of function in human neural progenitor cells: tools for molecular studies of human neurodevelopment and neuropsychiatric disorders. *Mol Psychiatry* 2010;15:672-5.

[46] Nowakowski RS, Hayes NL. Stem cells: the promises and pitfalls. *Neuropsychopharmacology* 2001;25:799-804.

[47] Taupin P. BrdU immunohistochemistry for studying adult neurogenesis: paradigms, pitfalls, limitations, and validation. *Brain Res Rev* 2007;53:198-214.

[48] Taupin P. Protocols for studying adult neurogenesis: insights and recent developments. *Regen Med* 2007;2:51-62.

[49] Taupin P. Characterization and isolation of synapses of newly generated neuronal cells of the adult hippocampus at early stages of neurogenesis. *J Neurodegener Regene* 2009;2:9-17.

[50] Taupin P. Neurogenic Drugs and compounds. *Recent Pat CNS Drug Discov* 2010;5:253-257.

[51] Taupin P. Aneuploidy and adult neurogenesis in Alzheimer's disease: therapeutic strategies. *Drug Discovery Today* 2010; In Press.

Chapter X

Neurogenic Drugs and Compounds[*]

Abstract

The advent of adult neurogenesis and neural stem cell (NSC) research opens new avenues and opportunities for treating neurological diseases and disorders, particularly for the discovery and development of novel drugs. Adult neurogenesis is modulated by a broad range of stimuli, physio- and pathological processes, trophic factors/cytokines and drugs, particularly drugs used for treating neurological diseases and disorders. Hence, adult neurogenesis is the target of drugs used for treating neurological diseases and disorders, such as Alzheimer's disease and depression, and the activities of neurological drugs may be mediated by adult NSCs. Although the contribution and mechanism of adult neurogenesis and newly generated neuronal cells of the adult brain in the activities of neurological drugs remain to be determined, new research is geared toward discovering and developing novel drugs that target specifically adult neurogenesis and the NSCs of the adult brain. Neurogenic drugs may reverse or compensate deficits and impairments associated with neurological diseases and disorders, particularly those associated with the hippocampus. They may have a potential for regenerative medicine and for the treatment of brain tumors. However, limitations in established models and protocols currently used in the drug discovery and development process of these drugs may hinder their potency and specificity. Here, we reviewed and discussed recent patents on neurogenic drugs and compounds, particularly nootropic agents and apigenin and related compounds.

Introduction

Neurogenesis occurs in the adult brain and neural stem cells (NSCs) reside in the adult central nervous system of mammals in various species, including in humans [1-4]. Neurogenesis occurs constitutively throughout adulthood primarily in two regions, the dentate

---

[*] Copyright notice. Reproduced with permission from Bentham Science Publishers, Ltd.: Taupin P. Neurogenic drugs and compounds. Recent Patents on CNS Drug Discovery (2010) 5(3):253-257. Copyright 2010, Bentham Science Publishers, Ltd.

.

gyrus (DG) of the hippocampus and the subventricular zone (SVZ) [5]. In the adult hippocampus, newly generated neuronal cells, generated in the subgranular zone, migrate to the granule cell layer, where they establish synaptic contacts with their target cells, in the CA3 region of the hippocampus [6,7]. The number of neuronal cells generated per day in the adult DG concerns a relatively small fraction of the nerve cells of the hippocampus, estimated at about 0.1% and 0.004% of the granule cell population in adult mice and macaque monkeys, respectively [8,9]. Neural progenitor and stem cells have been isolated and characterized *in vitro* from the adult brain of various mammalian species, including humans [10-14]. NSCs are the self-renewing multipotent cells that generate the main phenotypes of the nervous system. They are defined by five attributes: proliferation, self-renewal over an extended period of time, generation of a large number of differentiated progeny, regeneration of the tissue following injury and a flexibility of the use of these options. Neural progenitor cells are, as most broadly defined, any cells that do not fulfil all of the attributes of NSCs [15]. NSCs reside in specialized microenvironments in the adult brain or "niches" that control their developmental potential [16,17]. In the adult brain, newly generated neuronal cells would originate from a residual population of NSCs [18]. NSCs hold tremendous potential for cellular therapy and regenerative medicine, to treat and cure a broad range of neurological diseases and injuries, particularly neurodegenerative diseases, cerebral strokes and spinal cord injuries. To this aim, the stimulation of endogenous neural progenitor or stem cells of the adult brain and the transplantation of adult-derived neural progenitor and stem cells, are proposed to repair and restore the degenerated or injured nerve pathways. Johe et al. described a method for the transplantation of neural stem cells for the treatment of neurodegenerative diseases [19].

Neurogenesis is modulated in the adult mammalian brain, particularly in the hippocampus. It is modulated by a broad range of stimuli, physio- and pathological processes, trophic factors/cytokines and drugs. Among the factors and conditions that modulate adult neurogenesis in the hippocampus are environmental enrichment, learning and memory tasks, neurological diseases and disorders, such as Alzheimer's disease (AD) and epilepsy, insulin growth factor and drugs used for treating neurological diseases and disorders, particularly AD and depression [20-28]. This suggests that adult NSCs and newly generated neuronal cells of the adult brain may be involved in the physio- and pathology of the nervous system, as well as in drug therapy [29]. The involvement and contribution of adult neurogenesis to these processes remain to be elucidated and determined. The modulation of adult neurogenesis by environmental enrichment, by learning and memory tasks and in the brain of patients with neurological diseases and disorders would contribute to plasticity and regenerative attempts of the nervous system [30]. The modulation of adult neurogenesis by drugs used to treat AD and depression, like galantamine, memantine and fluoxetine [23, 27, 28], suggests that neural progenitor and stem cells of the adult brain may be the target of drugs used for the treatment neurological diseases and disorders [31]. Hence, adult neurogenesis and NSCs offer the new avenues and opportunities to discover and develop novel drugs for treating neurological diseases and disorders; drugs that target the NSCs of the adult brain or neurogenic drugs. Patent applications have been previously filed claiming the activities of drugs and compounds that target specifically the neural progenitor and stem cells of the adult brain and their therapeutic potential [15, 32]. A patent application has been filed that discloses a method for treating neurodegenerative diseases by the modulation of neurogenesis [33].

Recent patents on Compounds and Drugs Modulating Neurogenesis in the Adult Brain Nootropic Agents

Nootropic agents are substances that improve cognitive and mental functions [34]. Among them are the glutamate agonist AMPA (α-amino-3-hydroxyl-5-methyl-4-isoxazolepropionate), piracetam (2-oxo-l-pyrrolidineacetamide) and the analogue of piracetam, SGS-111. Barlow and collaborators have assessed the activities of these drugs on adult NSCs *in vitro* and *in vivo* [35]. The authors show that i) these compounds induce and stimulate the differentiation of human neural progenitor and stem cells, *in vitro*, into immature neuronal cells, immuno-positive for class III β-tubulin isotype, ii) AMPA promotes the neuronal differentiation of human-derived neural progenitor and stem cells, in presence of SGS-111, iii) PEPA (2-[2,6-difluoro-4-({2-[(phenylsulfonyl)amino]ethyl}thio) phenoxy]acetamide), an allosteric potentiator of AMPA receptor, promotes, in presence of AMPA, the differentiation of human-derived neural progenitor and stem cells into the neuronal pathway, iv) NBQX (2,3-dihydroxy-6-nitro-7-sulfamoyl-benzo[f]quinoxaline-2,3-dione), an antagonist of the AMPA receptor, inhibits the stimulation of neuronal differentiation of the human-derived neural progenitor and stem cells by AMPA and piracetam and v) SGS-111 increases the number of visits to the novel object, in rodents tested for their behavioural activity on the novel object recognition task. The novel object recognition task is a task in which animals are tested on their natural tendency to investigate a novel object rather than a familiar one, a test of object recognition memory [36].

This shows that SGS-111 elicit neurogenic activity *in vitro* and *in vivo*, that the neurogenic activity of AMPA is mediated through the AMPA receptors, that piracetam and

SGS-111 exerts some of their neurogenic effects *in vitro* through AMPA receptor activation and that SGS-111 acts as cognitive enhancer. The neurogenic activity of SGS-111 may contribute and play a role in its nootropic activity. However, this remains to be further evaluated and demonstrated. Barlow and collaborators filed a patent application in 2007 claiming the use of nootropic agents for their neurogenic activity and for the treatment of neurological diseases and injuries, by stimulating or increasing the generation of neuronal cells in the adult brain [37]. The publication number of the patent is: WO2007104035.

The Activity of 15 Compounds and their Derivatives

Kelleher Andersson assessed the activities of 15 compounds and their derivatives on adult NSCs *in vitro* [38]. The compounds: 4-(3-Cyano-6-ethoxy-quinoKn-2-yl)-[l,4]diazepane-l-carboxylic acid (2-fluoro-phenyl)-amide; 4-(3-Cyano-5,7-dimethyl-quinolin-2-yl)-[1,4]diazepane-1-carbothioic acid (2-methoxy-phenyl)-amide and 1-(2-Chloro-7,8-dimethyl-quinolin-3-yhnethyl)-1-(2-methoxy-ethyl)-3-(2-methoxy-phenyl)-urea stimulate the differentiation of adult human-derived neural progenitor and stem cells, into mature neuronal cells immuno-positive for Map-2, by 140%, 110% and 132%, respectively [38]. This shows that these compounds and their derivatives, a total of 15 compounds (compounds I to XV), elicit neurogenic activity *in vitro*.

Kelleher Andersson filed a patent application in 2007 claiming the use of the 15 compounds and their derivatives for the treatment of diseases and injuries particularly characterized by reduced neurogenesis and neuronal loss, including AD, depression, cerebral strokes and spinal cord injuries [39]. The publication number of the patent is: WO2007035722.

Kelleher Andersson described another method and composition to stimulate neurogenesis and thus can be used to treat neurodegenerative diseases [40].

Apigenin and Related Compounds

Apigenin and related compounds are derivatives used in food products. Hammerstone and collaborators assessed the activities of apigenin and related compounds on adult NSCs *in vitro* and *in vivo* [41]. These compounds promote the differentiation of adult-derived neural progenitor and stem cells in the neuronal pathway *in vitro*, in the absence of basic fibroblast growth factor. Administration of 25mg/kg apigenin promotes neurogenesis in the hippocampus of adult mice, when administered intraperitoneally (i.p.) or orally. Mice administered with 25mg/kg (i.p.) of apigenin perform significantly better in the Morris water maze task than control group [41]. The Morris water maze task is a task in which mice are tested for the speed to find a platform in a pool after being submitted to various treatments, a test of associative learning that require the hippocampus [42]. Mice administered with 25mg/kg (i.p.) of apigenin selected to receive voluntary running exercise have a significant higher number of new neuronal cells in the DG than mice of all other groups and perform significantly better in the Morris water maze task than the mice selected to receive voluntary running exercise without drug treatment and the control groups [41]. Voluntary running exercise has been previously described as enhancing neurogenesis in rodents [43]. This shows that apigenin increases neurogenesis in the hippocampus of adult mice. It increases learning and memory performances, with or without exercise, and exercise provides an additional benefit at low doses of apigenin. Apigenin may elicit its activity on adult neurogenesis through the induction and stimulation of neuronal differentiation. However, this remains to be further evaluated and demonstrated. Hammerstone and collaborators filed a patent application in 2008 claiming the use of apigenin and related compounds for stimulating adult neurogenesis and for the treatment of neurological diseases, disorders and injuries, by stimulating the generation of neuronal cells in the adult brain [44]. The publication number of the patent is: WO200814748.

Discussion

Nootropic, the 15 compounds and their derivatives (compounds I-XV) and apigenin and related compounds elicit neurogenic activities. These drugs and compounds may mediate some of their biological activities through their neurogenic activity.

The hippocampus is involved in numerous physio- and pathological processes, such as learning and memory, AD, depression and epilepsy [45-50]. Learning and memory tasks stimulate hippocampal neurogenesis in adult rodents [22]. Neurogenesis is enhanced in the adult hippocampus of animal models of epilepsy and of patients with AD [21, 23]. Hippocampal neurogenesis in the adult brain is required for the activity of anti-depressants, such as fluoxetine [51]. This suggests that adult neurogenesis and newly generated neuronal cells of the adult brain are involved in various physio- and pathological conditions and processes of the nervous system, particularly associated with the hippocampus [50-52]. As consequence, adult neurogenesis may be the target of drugs used for the treatment neurological diseases and disorders, particularly those associated with the hippocampus. The mechanisms and functions underlying the activities of neurological drugs on newly generated neuronal cells of the adult brain remain to be elucidated. Drugs may act directly or indirectly on NSCs and/or on newly generated neuronal cells of the adult brain. They may act via their pharmacological activities, on messenger signaling pathways, and/or via a neurogenic activity, by modulating neurogenesis and/or compensating for neuronal loss [53]. In support of this contention, AD and depression are associated with loss of nerve cells particularly in the hippocampus [46-50]. Drug treatments that stimulate neurogenesis in the adult hippocampus may therefore be beneficial for the treatment of AD and depression particularly, by modulating neurogenesis and/or compensating for the neuronal loss.

The mossy fibers (MF) are the axons of the dentate granule cells. They project to the CA3 regions of the adult hippocampus [54]. In the adult hippocampus, newly generated neuronal cells in the DG establish synaptic contacts with their target cells, in the CA3 region of the hippocampus, like mature granule cells [6,7]. The MF synapses represent a small fraction of the synapses of the adult hippocampus, less than 1% in mice [54]. Hence, the signals transmitted through the MF pathway, the link between the granule cells of the

DG and the pyramidal cells of the CA3 region of the hippocampus are subject to saturation [54]. The generation of nerve cells in the adult DG and the modulation of adult neurogenesis, in a saturated circuit, may therefore play a critical role in the signals transmitted to the CA3 region and in the physio- and pathology of the hippocampus [7]. Accordingly, drugs and compounds that modulate adult neurogenesis may reverse or compensate deficits and impairments associated with the hippocampus.

Hence, drugs that target specifically adult neurogenesis and NSCs, or neurogenic drugs, represent candidate drugs that are highly potent and highly specific for treating neurological diseases and disorders. They may be used for the treatment of neurological diseases and disorders to reverse or compensate deficits and impairments, particularly associated with the hippocampus, such as learning and memory deficits, AD, depression, epilepsy, schizophrenia and sleep disorders. They may also elicit potential for regenerative medicine, for the treatment of a broad range of neurological diseases and injuries, such as neurodegenerative diseases, cerebral strokes and traumatic brain and spinal cord injuries. They may also be used for the treatments of brain tumors.

Current and Future Developments

Adult neurogenesis and NSCs offer the new avenues and opportunities to discover and develop novel drugs that target specifically the NSCs of the adult brain, or neurogenic drugs, and that are highly potent and highly specific for treating neurological diseases and disorders. There are however currently limitations to the discovery and development of neurogenic drugs [55]. Firstly, the heterogeneity of the established protocols to isolate and propagate, *in vitro*, neural progenitor and stem cells from the adult brain is a factor limiting in the discovery and development process of potent and specific drugs [56, 57]. Secondly, there are limitations and pitfalls over the use of the paradigms and protocols used to study and quantify adult neurogenesis *in vivo*, particularly the bromodeoxyuridine labeling paradigm and the immunohistochemistry for markers of the cells cycle [58-61]. Both of which limits the potency and specificity of the identified and characterized drugs as targeting adult NSCs *in vitro* and *in vivo*, and therefore limits their therapeutic potential and applications. Future studies will aim at devising and developing assays that target specifically the NSCs of the adult brain *in vitro*, *ex vivo* and *in vivo*, to discover and develop novel neurogenic drugs that are more potent and more specific for treating neurological diseases and disorders [7].

Conflict of Interest

The author states no conflict of interest and has received no payment in preparation of this manuscript.

References

[1]   Eriksson PS, Perfilieva E, Bjork-Eriksson T, Alborn AM, Nordborg C, Peterson DA, et al. Neurogenesis in the adult human hippocampus. *Nat Med* 1998; 4(11); 1313-7.

[2]   Taupin P. Neurogenesis in the adult central nervous system. *C R Biol* 2006; 329(7): 465-75.

[3]   Duan X, Kang E, Liu CY, Ming GL, Song H. Development of neural stem cell in the adult brain. *Curr Opin Neurobiol* 2008; 18(1): 108-15.

[4]   Li Y, Mu Y, Gage FH. Development of neural circuits in the adult hippocampus. *Curr Top Dev Biol* 2009; 87: 149-74.

[5]   Taupin P, Gage FH. Adult neurogenesis and neural stem cells of the central nervous system in mammals. J *Neurosci Res* 2002; 69(6): 745-9.

[6]   Toni N, Teng EM, Bushong EA, Aimone JB, Zhao C, Consiglio A, et al. Synapse formation on neurons born in the adult hippocampus. *Nat Neurosci* 2007; 10(6): 727-34.

[7]   Taupin P. Characterization and isolation of synapses of newly generated neuronal cells of the adult hippocampus at early stages of neurogenesis. *J Neurodegener Regene* 2009; 2(1): 9-17.

[8]   Kornack DR, Rakic P. Continuation of neurogenesis in the hippocampus of the adult macaque monkey. *Proc Natl Acad Sci USA* 1999; 96(10): 5768-73.

[9]   Cameron HA, McKay RD. Adult neurogenesis produces a large pool of new granule cells in the dentate gyrus. *J Comp Neurol* 2001; 435(4): 406-17.

[10]   Reynolds BA, Weiss S. Generation of neurons and astrocytes from isolated cells of the adult mammalian central nervous system. *Science* 1992; 255(5052): 1707-10.

[11]   Gage FH, Coates PW, Palmer TD, Kuhn HG, Fisher LJ, Suhonen JO, et al. Survival and differentiation of adult neuronal progenitor cells transplanted to the adult brain. *Proc Natl Acad Sci USA* 1995; 92(25): 11879-83.

[12] Roy NS, Wang S, Jiang L, Kang J, Benraiss A, Harrison-Restelli C, et al. In vitro neurogenesis by progenitor cells isolated from the adult human hippocampus. *Nat Med* 2000; 6(3): 271-7.

[13] Taupin P, Ray J, Fischer WH, Suhr ST, Hakansson K, Grubb A, Gage FH. FGF-2-responsive neural stem cell proliferation requires CCg, a novel autocrine/paracrine cofactor. *Neuron* 2000; 28(2): 385-97.

[14] Palmer TD, Schwartz PH, Taupin P, Kaspar B, Stein SA, Gage FH. Cell culture. Progenitor cells from human brain after death. *Nature* 2001; 411(6833): 42-3.

[15] Taupin P. Therapeutic potential of adult neural stem cells. *Recent Pat CNS Drug Discov* 2006; 1(3): 299-303.

[16] Taupin P. Adult neural stem cells, neurogenic niches and cellular therapy. *Stem Cell Rev* 2006; 2(3): 213-20.

[17] Mitsiadis TA, Barrandon O, Rochat A, Barrandon Y, De Bari C. Stem cell niches in mammals. *Exp Cell Res* 2007; 313(16): 3377-85.

[18] Taupin P. Neural progenitor and stem cells in the adult Central Nervous System. *Ann Acad Med Singapore* 2006; 35(11): 814-817.

[19] Johe, K.K., Hazel, T.G. *Transplantation of human neural cells for treatment of neurodegenerative conditions*. US7691629 (2010).

[20] Kempermann G, Kuhn HG, Gage FH. More hippocampal neurons in adult mice living in an enriched environment. *Nature* 1997; 386(6624): 493-5.

[21] Parent JM, Yu TW, Leibowitz RT, Geschwind DH, Sloviter RS, Lowenstein DH. Dentate granule cell neurogenesis is increased by seizures and contributes to aberrant network reorganization in the adult rat hippocampus. *J Neurosci* 1997; 17(10): 3727-38.

[22] Gould E, Beylin A, Tanapat P, Reeves A, Shors TJ. Learning enhances adult neurogenesis in the hippocampal formation. *Nat Neurosci* 1999; 2(3): 260-5.

[23] Malberg JE, Eisch AJ, Nestler EJ, Duman RS. Chronic antidepressant treatment increases neurogenesis in adult rat hippocampus. *J Neurosci* 2000; 20(24): 9104-10.

[24] Jin K, Peel AL, Mao XO, Xie L, Cottrell BA, Henshall DC, et al. Increased hippocampal neurogenesis in Alzheimer's disease. *Proc Natl Acad Sci USA* 2004; 101(1): 343-7.

[25] Taupin P. Adult neurogenesis in the mammalian central nervous system: Functionality and potential clinical interest. *Med Sci Monit* 2005; 11(7): RA247-52.

[26] Banasr M, Soumier A, Hery M, Mocaër E, Daszuta A. Agomelatine, a new antidepressant, induces regional changes in hippocampal neurogenesis. *Biol Psychiatry* 2006; 59(11): 1087-96.

[27] Jin K, Xie L, Mao XO, Greenberg DA. Alzheimer's disease drugs promote neurogenesis. *Brain Res* 2006; 1085(1): 183-8.

[28] Perera TD, Coplan JD, Lisanby SH, Lipira CM, Arif M, Carpio C, et al. Antidepressant-induced neurogenesis in the hippocampus of adult nonhuman primates. *J Neurosci* 2007; 27(18): 4894-901.

[29] Taupin P. Adult neurogenesis pharmacology in neurological diseases and disorders. *Exp Rev Neurother* 2008; 8(2): 311-20.

[30]. Taupin P. Adult neurogenesis and neuroplasticity. *Restor Neurol Neurosci* 2006; 24(1): 9-15.

[31] Taupin P. Neurogenic factors are target in depression. *Drug Discov Today Ther Strateg* 2008; 5(3): 157-60.

[32] Taupin P. Therapeutic neuronal stem cells: Patents at the forefront. *Expert Opin Ther Pat* 2008; 18: 1107-10.

[33] Barlow, C., Carter, T.A., Morse, A., Treuner, K., Lorrain, K.I. *MCC-257 modulation of neurogenesis.* US20090239834 (2009).

[34] Malik R, Sangwan A, Saihgal R, Jindal DP, Piplani P. Towards better brain management: Nootropics. *Curr Med Chem* 2007; 14(2): 123-31.

[35] Barlow, C., Carter, T.A., Morse, A., Treuner, K., Lorrain, K.I., Gitnick, D., Pires, J.C. *Modulation of neurogenesis by nootropic agents.* WO2007104035 (2007).

[36] Ennaceur A, Meliani K. A new one-trial test for neurobiological studies of memory in rats. III. Spatial vs. non-spatial working memory. *Behav Brain Res* 1992; 51(1): 83-92.

[37] Taupin P. Nootropic agents stimulate neurogenesis. *Expert Opin Ther Pat* 2009; 19(5): 727-30.

[38] Kelleher Andersson, J. *Methods and compositions for stimulating neurogenesis and inhibiting neuronal degeneration.* WO2007035722 (2007).

[39] Taupin P. Fourteen compounds and their derivatives for the treatment of diseases and injuries characterized by reduced neurogenesis and neurodegeneration. *Expert Opin Ther Pat* 2009; 19(4): 541-7.

[40] Kelleher, A.J. *Methods and compositions for stimulating neurogenesis and inhibiting neuronal degeneration using isothiazolopyrimidinones.* EP2170340 (2010).

[41] Hammerstone, J.F. Jr., Kelm, M.A., Gage, F.H., van Praag, H. *Neurogenic compounds.* WO200814748 (2008).

[42] Morris RG, Garrud P, Rawlins JN, O'Keefe J. Place navigation impaired in rats with hippocampal lesions. *Nature* 1982; 297(5868): 681-3.

[43] van Praag H, Kempermann G, Gage FH. Running increases cell proliferation and neurogenesis in the adult mouse dentate gyrus. *Nat Neurosci* 1999; 2(3): 266-270.

[44] Taupin P. Apigenin and related compounds stimulate adult neurogenesis. *Expert Opin Ther Pat* 2009; 19(4): 523-7.

[45] Holmes GL, Ben-Ari Y. The neurobiology and consequences of epilepsy in the developing brain. *Pediatr Res* 2001; 49(3): 320-5.

[46] Burns A, Byrne EJ, Maurer K. Alzheimer's disease. *Lancet* 2002; 360(9327):163-5.

[47] Campbell S, Marriott M, Nahmias C, MacQueen GM. Lower hippocampal volume in patients suffering from depression: a metaanalysis. *Am J Psychiatry* 2004; 161(4): 598-607.

[48] Bielau H, Trübner K, Krell D, Agelink MW, Bernstein HG, Stauch R, et al. Volume deficits of subcortical nuclei in mood disorders. A postmortem study. *Eur Arch Psychiatry Clin Neurosci* 2005; 255(6): 401-12

[49] Taupin P. Neurogenesis and the Effects of Antidepressants. *Drug Target Insights* 2006; 1: 13-7.

[50] Taupin P. Adult neurogenesis, neural stem cells and Alzheimer's disease: Developments, limitations, problems and promises. *Curr Alzheimer Res* 2009; 6(6): 461-70.

[51] Santarelli L, Saxe M, Gross C, Surget A, Battaglia F, Dulawa S, et al. Requirement of hippocampal neurogenesis for the behavioural effects of antidepressants. *Science* 2003; 310(5634): 805-9.

[52] Shors TJ, Miesegaes G, Beylin A, Zhao M, Rydel T, Gould E. Neurogenesis in the adult is involved in the formation of trace memories. Nature 2001; 410(6826): 372-6. Erratum in: *Nature* 2001; 414(6866): 938.

[53] Taupin P. Adult neurogenesis and drug therapy. *Cent Nerv Syst. Agents Med Chem* 2008; 8: 198-202.

[54] Braitenberg V, Schüz A. Some anatomical comments on the hippocampus. In W Seifert, editor. Neurobiology of the hippocampus. *Academic Press* 21-37 (1983).

[55] Taupin P. Editorial. Adult neural stem cells from promise to treatment: The road ahead. *J Neurodegener Regene* 2008; 1: 7-8.

[56] Chin VI, Taupin P, Sanga S, Scheel J, Gage FH, Bhatia SN. Microfabricated platform for studying stem cell fates. *Biotechnol Bioeng* 2004; 88(3): 399-415.

[57] Reynolds BA, Rietze RL. Neural stem cells and neurospheres--re-evaluating the relationship. *Nat Methods* 2005; 2(5): 333-6.

[58] Nowakowski RS, Hayes NL. New neurons: Extraordinary evidence or extraordinary conclusion? *Science* 2000; 288(5467): 771.

[59] Rakic P. Adult neurogenesis in mammals: An identity crisis. *J Neurosci* 2002; 22(3): 614-8.

[60] Taupin P. BrdU Immunohistochemistry for Studying Adult Neurogenesis: Paradigms, pitfalls, limitations, and validation. *Brain Res Rev* 2007; 53(1): 198-214.

[61] Taupin P. Protocols for Studying Adult Neurogenesis: Insights and recent developments. *Regen Med* 2007; 2(1): 51-62.

Chapter XI

Very Small Embryonic-like Stem Cells for Regenerative Medicine[*]

Abstract

Background

The application is in the field of stem cells and regenerative medicine. Objective: It aims at identifying and characterising a population of pluripotent stem cells present in adult tissues.

Methods

Cells were isolated and purified using Fluorescence-Activated Cell Sorting and Direct ImageStream analysis from various adult and umbilical cord tissues of rodents and humans. Cells were propagated in the presence of trophic factors and feeder cell layers of C2C12 cells. Cells were characterised by electron microscopy and immunocytology.

Results

A population of cells that do not express a panleukocytic antigen CD45 and are negative for other markers of haematopoietic lineages were isolated and purified. The isolated cells elicit morphological features of embryonic stem cells (ESCs). They express

---

[*] Patent Details
Title: Methods for isolating very small embryonic-like stem cells
Assignee: University of Louisville Research Foundation, Inc. and Neostem, Inc.
Inventors: Zuba-Surma EK, Ratajczak M, Ratajczak J and Kucia M
Priority data: 24/09/2009
Filing date: 30/09/2009
Publication date: 08/04/2010
Publication no.: WO2010039241

.

markers of pluripotent stem cells, such as Nanog, Oct-4 and SSEA-1. On culturing on feeder cell layers, the isolated and purified cells generate embryoid body-like sphere. Conclusion: The identified and characterised cells elicit features of pluripotent stem cells and similarities with ESCs. They are termed very small embryonic-like stem cells (VSELs). The application claims the use of VSELs for cellular therapy and regenerative medicine.

Introduction

Stem cells are self-renewing cells that generate the differentiated phenotypes of the body [1,2]. Pluripotent stem cells are self-renewing cells that generate tissues of the three germ layers, neurectoderm, mesoderm and endoderm. Embryonic stem cells (ESCs) are the archetype of pluripotent stem cells [3]. They are derived from the inner cell mass of blastocysts of various species including primates, non-humans and humans [4,5]. Multipotent stem cells are self-renewing cells that generate the phenotypes of the tissue in which they reside. Multipotent stem cells have been isolated and characterised from various foetal and adult tissues, including liver, muscles, skin and blood. Over a decade ago, multipotent stem cells were isolated and characterised from the adult brain of rodents and human post-mortem tissues and biopsies [6,7]. It is now accepted that neurogenesis occurs in the adult brain and neural stem cells reside in the adult CNS of mammals, in various species, including humans [8-11].

A conventional dogma is that pluripotent stem cells are present in the embryo during development, whereas multipotent stem cells are present in foetal and adult tissues. Several reports have challenged the notion that multipotent stem cells generate differentiated phenotypes restricted to the tissues in which they reside. Among them, adult-derived neural progenitor and stem cells give rise to blood cells on transplantation into irradiated mice [12]. Adult bone marrow progenitor and stem cells and purified haematopoietic stem cells give rise to neurons and glia cells on transplantation [13,14]. These landmark studies and others revealed that adult-derived progenitor and stem cells might not be restricted to generate tissue specific cell types [15]. Whether adult stem cells are pluripotent or elicit a broader potential remain to be fully understood. There are also controversies over some of the studies, as some of the observations reported have been attributed to phenomena such as artefacts, contamination, transformation, transdifferentiation or cell fusion [16]. Niches are a specialised microenvironment that controls the developmental potential of stem cells [17]. It is proposed that the microenvironment underlies the broader potential of adult stem cells [16,17]. Despite these controversies and debates, the broader potential of adult stem cells opens new avenues and opportunities for cellular therapy.

Because of their potential to generate the main phenotypes of the body, ESCs represent a promising model for cellular therapy. However, there are ethical and political constraints associated with the use of human ESCs for research and therapy. The identification and characterisation of pluripotent adult stem cells would represent a model of choice for cellular therapy, without the debates and controversies associated with either the broader potential of adult stem cells or the ethical and political concerns over the use of human ESCs for research and therapy. The application claims the isolation and characterisation of pluripotent stem cells from various adult tissues, including bone marrow, peripheral blood and spleen, and from cord blood tissues. The application may be used for regenerative medicine for the treatment of a broad range of diseases and injuries, ranging from diabetes, heart diseases and muscle repair to neurological diseases and injuries, including neurodegenerative diseases and spinal cord injuries.

Chemistry

The application reports a method for: i) isolating and purifying a population of cells that do not express a panleukocytic antigen CD45 and are negative for other haematopoietic lineage markers, such as $CD34^+/CD45^-Lin^-$ or $Sca-1^+/CD45^-Lin^-$ cells and ii) generating embryoid body-like sphere *in vitro*, from the isolated and purified cells. Cells that do not express a panleukocytic antigen CD45 and are negative for other haematopoietic lineage markers, such as $CD45^-Lin^-$ cells, were isolated and purified by Fluorescence-Activated Cell Sorting and Direct Image Stream analysis from the non-haematopoietic compartment of various adult tissues, including bone marrow, peripheral blood and spleen, and from cord blood tissues of mice and humans [18-20]. Embryoid body-like sphere formation from the isolated and purified cells were induced in the presence of trophic factors, such as EGF and fibroblast growth factor-2, or by co-culturing the cells on feeder layers of C2C12 cells.

Biology and Action

Isolated and purified cells were identified and characterised by electron microscopy. On the ultrastructural level, they elicit, like ESCs, a small size - with an average diameter of 3.6 mm - a large nucleus, a narrow rim of cytoplasm surrounding the nucleus and open-type chromatin or euchromatin [21]. Immunocytological and RT-PCR studies reveal that the isolated and purified cells express *in vitro* markers of pluripotent stem cells, particularly Nanog, Oct-4 and SSEA-1 [22]. When plated over feeder layers of C2C12 murine sarcoma cells, a proportion, 5 - 10%, of the isolated and purified cells form spheres with similar morphology to embryoid bodies generally observed when culturing ESCs *in vitro*. Cells of the embryoid body-like structure express markers of pluripotent stem cells, such as CXCR4, SSEA-1 and Oct-4 [22]. The isolated and purified cells that elicit properties of pluripotent stem cells *in vitro* and features of ESCs are termed very small embryonic-like stem cells (VSELs).

Expert Opinion

VSELs are a population of cells isolated and purified from various adult tissues and cord blood tissues that elicit a phenotype of pluripotent cells *in vitro*. A fraction of the VSELs cultured *in vitro*, in the presence of feeder layers, generates embryoid body-like structures and shares similar ultrastructural and immunological features with ESCs. VSELs correspond to a rare population of cells in adult tissues, estimated at 0.01% of the mononuclear cells in the bone marrow [23]. VSELs represent an alternative source of pluripotent stem cells, present in adult tissues, for cellular therapy and regenerative medicine.

VSELs were originally identified and characterised from the bone marrow of adult mice and the umbilical cord blood of humans [18-20]. Since then, VSELs have been isolated and purified from various adult tissues, including foetal liver, spleen and thymus in mice and humans [24,25]. VSELs identified and characterised from bone marrow tissues give rise to haematopoietic stem cells, mesenchymal stem cells and endothelial progenitor cells [24,25]. It is proposed that VSELs contribute to tissue homeostasis and regeneration of tissues after injuries [26]. VSELs represent a rare population of primitive stem cells that are deposited during early gastrulation in developing tissues and organs, such as the bone marrow [23]

Because of their potential to generate the main phenotypes of the body, VSELs represent a promising and alternative model to ESCs for cellular therapy and regenerative medicine. The use of ESCs for therapy is primarily limited by ethical and political concerns and constraints associated with their derivation from human embryos [27]. The use of ESCs for therapy is also limited by the difficulties in generating cell lines of ESCs for autologous transplantations or a sufficient number of cells lines for matching human leukocyte antigens for allogeneic transplantations [3]. VSELs are isolated and purified from various adult tissues and from umbilical cord tissues, thereby, providing an easily accessible source of tissues for therapy and for autologous transplantation, without the ethical and political constraints and limitations over the use of human embryonic tissue for therapy. VSELs represent a model of pluripotent stem cells of choice for cellular therapy and regenerative medicine. There are, however, limitations to the use of VSELs for therapy. Among them, because VSELs share characteristics with ESCs, they may elicit tumorigenic risks. More studies need to be conducted to further characterise the properties of VSELs and their potential for therapy before VSELs are brought to therapy.

Declaration of Interest

The author states no conflict of interest and has received no payment in preparation of this manuscript.

Acknowledgments

Reproduced with permission from Informa Healthcare: Taupin P. Very small embryonic-like stem cells for regenerative medicine: WO2010039241. Expert Opinion on Therapeutic Patents (2010) 20(8):1103-1106. Copyright 2010, Informa Healthcare (Informa UK Ltd).

References

Papers of special note have been highlighted as either of interest (*) or of considerable interest (**) to readers.

[1] Potten CS, Loeffler M. Stem cells: attributes, cycles, spirals, pitfalls and uncertainties. Lessons for and from the crypt. *Development* 1990;110:1001-20.

[2] Taupin P. Therapeutic potential of adult neural stem cells. *Recent Pat CNS Drug Discov* 2006;1:299-303.

[3] Taupin P. Derivation of embryonic stem cells for cellular therapy: challenges and new strategies. *Med Sci Monit* 2006;12:RA75-8.

[4] Thomson JA, Kalishman J, Golos TG, et al. Isolation of a primate embryonic stem cell line. *Proc Natl Acad Sci USA* 1995;92:7844-8.

[5] Thomson JA, Itskovitz-Eldor J, Shapiro SS, et al. Embryonic stem cell lines derived from human blastocysts. Science 1998;282:1145-7. Erratum in: *Science* 1998;282:1827.

[6] Reynolds BA, Weiss S. Generation of neurons and astrocytes from isolated cells of the adult mammalian central nervous system. *Science* 1992;255:1707-10.

**   Original report of the isolation and characterisation of neural progenitor and stem cells from the adult brain of mammals. Neural progenitor and stem cells are cultured as neurospheres.

[7] Palmer TD, Schwartz PH, Taupin P, et al. Cell culture. Progenitor cells from human brain after death. *Nature* 2001;411:42-3.

*   First isolation and chracterisation of neural progenitor and stem cells from human post-mortem tissues and biopsies.

[8] Eriksson PS, Perfilieva E, Bjork-Eriksson T, et al. Neurogenesis in the adult human hippocampus. *Nat Med* 1998;4:1313-17.

*   First evidence of adult neurogenesis in the hippocampus of human brains.

[9] Taupin P, Gage FH. Adult neurogenesis and neural stem cells of the central nervous system in mammals. *J Neurosci Res* 2002;69:745-9.

[10] Curtis MA, Kam M, Nannmark U, et al. Human neuroblasts migrate to the olfactory bulb via a lateral ventricular extension. *Science* 2007;315:1243-9.

[11] Duan X, Kang E, Liu CY, et al. Development of neural stem cell in the adult brain. *Curr Opin Neurobiol* 2008;18:108-15.

[12] Bjornson CR, Rietze RL, Reynolds BA, et al. Turning brain into blood: a hematopoietic fate adopted by adult neural stem cells in vivo. *Science* 1999;283:534-7.

[13] Brazelton TR, Rossi FM, Keshet GI, et al. From marrow to brain: expression of neuronal phenotypes in adult mice. *Science* 2000;290:1775-9.

[14] Mezey E, Chandross KJ, Harta G, et al. Turning blood into brain: cells bearing neuronal antigens generated in vivo from bone marrow. *Science* 2000;290:1779-82.

[15] D'Amour D'Amour KA, Gage FH. Are somatic stem cells pluripotent or lineage-restricted? *Nat Med* 2002;8:213-14.

[16] Taupin P. Adult neural stem cells, neurogenic niches and cellular therapy. *Stem Cell Rev* 2006;2:213-19.

[17] Mitsiadis TA, Barrandon O, Rochat A, et al. Stem cell niches in mammals. *Exp Cell Res* 2007;313:3377-85.

[18] Kucia M, Reca R, Jala VR, et al. Bone marrow as a home of heterogenous populations of nonhematopoietic stem cells. *Leukemia* 2005;19:1118-27.

[19] Kucia M, Halasa M, Wysoczynski M, et al. Morphological and molecular characterization of novel population of CXCR4(+) SSEA-4(+) Oct-4(+) very small embryonic-like cells purified from human cord blood-preliminary report. *Leukemia* 2007;21:297-303.

[20] Zuba-Surma EK, Kucia M, Dawn B, et al. Bone marrow-derived pluripotent very small embryonic-like stem cells (VSELs) are mobilized after acute myocardial infarction. *J Mol Cell Cardiol* 2008;44:865-73.

[21] Zuba-Surma EK, Kucia M, Abdel-Latif A, et al. Morphological characterization of Very Small Embryonic-Like stem cells (VSELs) by Image Stream system analysis. *J Cell Mol Med* 2008;12:292-303.

[22] Kucia M, Reca R, Campbell F.R, et al. A population of very small embryonic-like (VSELs) CXCR4(+) SSEA-1(+)Oct-4+ stem cells identified in adult bone marrow. *Leukemia* 2006;20:857-69.

[23] Ratajczak MZ, Zuba-Surma EK, Wysoczynski M, et al. Very small embryonic-like stem cells: characterization, developmental origin, and biological significance. *Exp Hematol* 2008;36:742-51.

[24] Ratajczak MZ, Machalinski B, Wojakowski W, et al. A hypothesis for an embryonic origin of pluripotent Oct-4 stem cells in adult bone marrow and other tissues. *Leukemia.* 2007;21:860-7.

[25] Ratajczak MZ, Zuba-Surma EK, Wysoczynski M, et al. Hunt for pluripotent stem cell and regenerative medicine search for almighty cell. *J Autoimmun* 2008;30:151-62.

[26] Kucia M, Zhang YP, Reca R, et al. Cells enriched in markers of neural tissue-committed stem cells reside in the bone marrow and are mobilized into the peripheral blood following stroke. *Leukemia* 2006;20:18-28.

[27] Taupin P. Stem cells engineering for cell-based therapy. *J Neural Eng* 2007;4:R59-63.

Chapter XII

Transplantation of Cord Blood Stem Cells for Treating Hematologic Diseases and Strategies to Improve Engraftment

Executive Summary

- Umbilical cord blood (CB) offers an alternative source of hematopoietic stem cells for the treatment of malignant and nonmalignant hematologic diseases.
- Umbilical CB is used for pediatric and adult transplants, but is associated with high rate of mortality and morbidity, particularly in adults.
- Various strategies are being developed and considered to improve CB transplantation, among them are double CB transplantation and improving the homing and engraftment capabilities of CB stem cells.
- Administration of double doses of CB improves the rate of success of transplantation, but the conditions are still suboptimal.
- *Ex vivo* fucosylation of CB stem cells prior transplantation provides a novel strategy for improving homing and engraftment to the bone marrow, but it remains to be confirmed and validated. Other strategy for improving homing and engraftment consists of using Notch-mediated expanded CB progenitor cells *ex vivo*.
- The expansion and propagation of CB stem cells *in vitro* provides an alternative strategy for treating hematologic diseases, as well as for regenerative medicine, but conditions for expansion and growth of the cells remain to be established.

Abstract

Umbilical cord blood (CB) offers an alternative source of hematopoietic stem cells for the treatment of malignant and nonmalignant hematologic diseases. Umbilical CB has high levels of repopulating hematopoietic stem cells and is depleted of immune cells. It elicits low cell dose, delayed and poor engraftment to the bone marrow. Umbilical CB is used for pediatric transplants, and also in adults. CB transplantation is associated with high rate of mortality and morbidity, particularly in adults. To improve the success rate, patients are treated with a double CB dose. However, such a strategy limits the availability of CB transplants for patients, and the conditions are still suboptimal. Novel avenues are being devised and considered, among them the expansion and propagation of CB stem cells *in vitro* and the improvement of homing and engraftment of CB stem cells to the bone marrow. Such strategies would overcome the low cell dose in CB units, by improving the delay and engraftment of CB stem cells to the bone marrow. Therefore, it would reduce the risk of early infections, improve the rate of success of CB transplantation and make CB transplantation available to more patients. Umbilical CB offers a promising model for cellular therapy and regenerative medicine.

Introduction

Umbilical cord blood (CB) offers an alternative source of hematopoietic stem cells (HSCs) to treat patients with malignant and nonmalignant hematologic diseases, such as leukemia, lymphoma, myeloma, Fanconi anemia, myelodysplasia and sickle cell anemia [1]. Umbilical CB contains a low cell dose, and the first transplantation CB was performed in children with Fanconi anemia, by Gluckman and collaborators at the hospital Saint Louis in Paris in 1989 [2]. Since then, CB transplantations have been performed with success in children, but also in adults. However, low cell dose, graft failure, poor engraftment in the bone marrow (BM) and delay in engraftment and in immune reconstitution lead to significant morbidity and mortality, particularly in adults.

The rate of morbidity and mortality after CB transplants remains high in adults, with 47% of patients dying within 100 days of the unrelated transplant [3]. To improve the rate of success of CB transplantation, double doses of CB units are being infused into patients. However, this limits the availability of CB for therapy, conditions are still suboptimal, and it does not address the main limitations of CB for the treatment of hematologic diseases. CB is considered a standard source of HSCs for pediatric transplants, and the transplantation of HSCs from CB is a viable alternative even in adults, as demonstrated by the number of adult patient transplants exceeding transplants in child patients in the last 2–3 years [4-7].

Umbilical CB contains 3–6-times more repopulating hematopoietic progenitor and stem cells than the BM and mobilized peripheral blood (MPB) [8]. It is depleted of immune cells, particularly T lymphocytes and has decreased natural killer cell activity, reduced alloproliferative, allostimulatory and allocytolytic capacity of mononuclear cells, and a lower frequency of alloreactive cytotoxic T lymphocyte precursors in CB mononuclear cells [9,10]. This allows for greater disparity of HLA antigens when matching donors to recipients than with BM and MPB. Currently, worldwide donor registries include over 14 million donors, including 8 million Americans, and CB inventory represents only a small fraction of them.

The registry of potential BM donors meets the needs of an estimated 60% of Caucasians in the USA, and only 5–15% of minorities. The chance that siblings will be a match is only 25%. Hence, umbilical CB provides an alternative model for unrelated allogeneic transplantation of HSCs and for potentially treating more patients, particularly minorities who are underrepresented in BM registries. Novel strategies are being devised and considered to address the main limitations of umbilical CB for transplantation and are necessary to take full advantage of its potential for cellular therapy and regenerative medicine [11]. Among them, four strategies are being primarily reviewed and discussed in the manuscript: the direct delivery of umbilical CB to the BM, the transplantation of a double unit of CB, the fucosylation of selectin glycoprotein ligands *ex vivo*, and the expansion and propagation of CB stem cells *in vitro*.

HSCs and Cord Blood Stem Cells

The BM is primary the source of HSCs in the adult body. HSCs reside in the extravascular space of the endosteum region and in periarterial sites of the BM primarily, but also that of other organs, from which they give rise to the differentiated lineages of the blood and immune systems [12]. Hematopoietic progenitor and stem cells, identified and characterized as populations highly enriched in $CD34^+$ and $CD34^+$ $CD38^{-/low}$ cells in various species, including rodents and humans, reconstitute the pool of HSCs of the BM after in irradiation. Owing to their potential to generate the main phenotypes of the blood and immune systems, HSCs represent a model of choice for treating a broad range of hematopoietic diseases. Populations of $CD34^+$ hematopoietic progenitor and stem cells, capable of repopulating irradiated BM after transplantation, have been identified and characterized in umbilical CB [13,14]. The umbilical CB contains 3–6 times more repopulating hematopoietic progenitor and stem cells than the BM and MPB [8]. Hence, the umbilical CB demonstrates a greater potential to reconstitute the recipient BM than BM and MPB.

Umbilical CB is depleted of immune cells, particularly of T lymphocytes. It also contains a high proportion of 'naïve' T cells that express the $CD45RA^+/$ $CD45RO^-$, $CD62L^+$ phenotype. The CB produces increased amounts of IL-10, an anti-inflammatory cytokine, and expresses little cytotoxic activity. The CB, in contrast to BM and MPB, elicits low immunogenicity. This allows for greater the disparity of HLA antigens when matching donors to recipients with CB, compared to BM and MPB, and potentially permits treatment of more patients [15].

Selectins and the Homing of HSCs

Hematopoietic stem cells migrate to their niches in the BM, a process referred as homing [12]. The homing contributes to the replenishment and maintenance of the pool of hematopoietic progenitor and stem cells in the BM, and other tissues, and to the recruitment and mobilization of HSCs during injuries, particularly during immune responses and stress-induced recruitment of leukocytes. During development, this process is involved in the seeding of fetal HSCs to the BM, which involves the rolling and arresting of hematopoietic progenitor and stem cells through the blood vessels and across the endothelial vasculature, and complex molecular and cellular interactions.

P- and E-selectins and Selectin Glycoprotein Ligands

P- and E-selectins are membrane bound C-type lectins involved in the homing of HSCs to the BM. They are expressed on endothelial cells and BM vessels in mice and humans (Figure 1) [16-19]. P- and E-selectins bind ligands that are cell-surface proteo-O-glycan conjugated ligands, or selectin glycoprotein ligands (SGLs). SGLs are expressed on various cell types, particularly CD34+ hematopoietic progenitor and stem cells of the BM, particularly in mice and humans (Figure 1). P-SGL-1 is the best characterized P-selectin ligand. It is a mucin expressed on CD34+ cells and on leukocytes [20-23]. P- and E-selectins elicit differential binding affinity with P-SGL-1.

Selectin glycoprotein ligands have a characteristic N-terminal glycan determinant; a N-terminal glycan capped with a sialylated Lewis x (sLex) and a site for fucosylation (NeuAca2-3Galb1-4[Fuca1-3]GlcNAcb1-R). The enzymes alpha1–3 fucosyltransferase (FT)VI and FTVII are responsible for alpha1–3 FT activity [24-28]. These enzymes are present on the cell surfaces of various cell types, particularly hematopoietic cells of the BM of mice and humans, where they fucosylate their substrates. SGLs on CD34+ cells of the BM elicit N-terminal glycan determinants with an alpha 2–3-linked sialic acid and an alpha1–3-linked fucose. The N-terminal glycan determinant of SGLs corresponds to the binding site of hematopoietic cells to P- and E-selectins (Figure 1) [20,23]. The site for fucosylation is most likely to occur at a core 2 O-glycan linked to a threonine in the N-terminal binding site for P-selectin on SGLs [21,23]. The residues of the binding site of SGLs to P- and E-selectins include fucose, galactose, sialic acid and sulphated tyrosines [29-31]. P-SGL-1 that are capped with sLex and that are sulphated bind with strong affinity to P- and E-selectins [30]. Hence, post-translational modifications, particularly fucosylation, of SGLs on hematopoietic cells and HSCs, underlie their binding to P- and E-selectins.

Homing of Hematopoietic Progenitor and Stem Cells of the BM and CB

CD34$^+$ hematopoietic progenitor and stem cells isolated and purified from human BM or MPB and administered intravenously, in irradiated nonobese diabetic/severe combined immune deficiency (NOD/SCID) mice, home to the BM of those mice. Their rolling activities on microvessels of and homing to the BM are diminished after injection of blocking monoclonal antibodies to P-selectin or to P-SGL-1. Their homing capabilities are also impaired in irradiated NOD/SCID mice deficient for P- and E-selectins [22]. By contrast, CD34$^+$ hematopoietic progenitor and stem cells isolated and purified from human CB elicit poor rolling activities on microvessels of and poor homing capabilities to the BM, after transplantation into irradiated NOD/SCID mice [22]. Hence, HSCs of the BM and CB demonstrate different capabilities of homing to the BM. CD34$^+$ hematopoietic progenitor and stem cells of the BM and MPB roll on endothelial cells and BM vessels and home to the BM, a process mediated by the interaction of SGLs with selectins, in contrast to their CB counterpart. HSCs of the BM bind to P- and E-selectins on endothelial cells and BM vessels for rolling and homing to the BM in mice and humans. P-SGL-1 underlies the tethering of leukocytes to E-selectin in flow studies *in vitro* and the tethering and rolling of leukocytes to, and on, P-selectin *in vivo* [32]. The interaction SGLs with selectins also plays an important role in the homing of leukocytes to lymphoid tissues and their recruitment to sites of inflammation [18,20,21,23,33].

Like human CD34$^+$ hematopoietic progenitor and stem cells of the BM, human CB CD34$^+$ cells express P-SGL-1 on their surface. As opposed to BM CD34$^+$ cells, most, approximately 75%, of CB CD34$^+$CD38$^{-/low}$ cells lack the sLex and site for fucosylation of the N-glycan determinant of SGLs and do not bind to P- and E-selectins. Hence, SGLs of hematopoietic progenitor and stem cells of the CB express a form of P-SGL-1 that does not bind to P-and E-selectins [22]. It is proposed that the inability of SGLs of CB hematopoietic progenitor and stem cells to bind P- and E-selectins underlies the diminished rolling and homing activity of the cells on BM vessels and to the BM in NOD/SCID mice [22]. The inability of SGLs of CB hematopoietic progenitor and stem cells to bind to P- and E-selectins originate from the low or absent expression of the N-glycan determinant on hematopoietic progenitor and stem cells of the CB (Figure 1) [34,35]. This low or absent expression of the N-glycan determinant – a post-translational event – particularly the fucosylation, may originate from insufficient levels of FTVI to physiologically fucosylate the SGLs on their surface.

Overall, the interaction of SGLs with selectins plays an important role in the homing of HSCs and leukocytes. The N-glycan determinant, the sLex and the site for fucosylation on SGLs is critical for the rolling and homing of HSCs on endothelial cells and BM vessels and to the BM.

Other factors are involved in the process of migration on endothelial cells and homing of HSCs to the BM. These include CD44, chemokines, integrins, lymphocyte function-associated antigen 1, P- and E-selectins, stem cell factor (SCF), stromal-derived factor 1, vascular cell adhesion molecule-1, very late antigen 4/5 and their respective ligands or receptors [17-19,33,36,37].

Transplantation of Cord Blood Stem Cells for the Treatment of Hematologic Diseases

The CB contains 3–6-times more repopulating hematopoietic progenitor and stem cells than the BM and MPB, providing a promising source of transplant for the treatment of hematologic diseases. However, CB transplants are associated with low cell count, graft failure and delayed engraftment and immune reconstitution leading to significant morbidity and mortality, particularly in adults. Transplantation-related mortality (TRM) following unrelated CB transplantation is primarily due to infections related to slow engraftment and immune-incompetence.

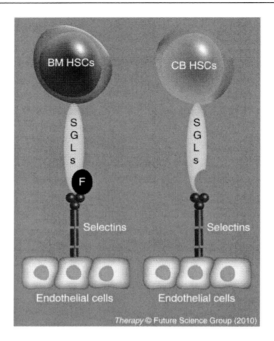

Figure 1. Selectins and selectin glycoprotein ligands on endothelial cells and on hematopoietic stem cells of the bone marrow and cord blood. P- and E-Selectins are membrane bound C-type lectins involved in the homing of HSCs. They are expressed on endothelial cells and vessels of the BM. SGLs are expressed on CD34$^+$ hematopoietic progenitor and stem cells of the BM and CB. SGLs elicit a characteristic N-terminal glycan determinant; a N-terminal glycan capped with a sialylated Lewis x and a site for fucosylation. SGLs on HSCs of the BM, but not of the CB, have N-terminal glycan determinants with a alpha1-3-linked fucose (F). The N-terminal glycan determinant of SGLs corresponds to the binding site of HSCs to P- and E-selectins. SGLs for which the N-terminal glycan determinant is not fucosylated have a defect in binding to P- and E-selectins. HSCs of the BM and CB elicit different capabilities of homing to the BM. CD34$^+$ hematopoietic progenitor and stem cells of the BM roll on endothelial cells and BM vessels and home to the BM, a process mediated by the interaction of SGLs-selectins, in contrast to their CB counterpart. The defect in fucosylation of SGLs on the surface of CB HSCs underlies their poor capabilities of homing to the BM. Hence, post-translational modifications, particularly fucosylation, of SGLs on HSCs underlie their binding to P- and E-selectins and their homing capabilities to the BM.
BM: Bone marrow; CB: Cord blood; F: Fucose; HSC: Hematopoietic stem cell; SGL: Selectin glycoprotein ligand.

Total Nucleated Cell Count and Age of Patients

Cord blood has a low total nucleated cell count and a low number of CD34$^+$ cells. The rate of success of unrelated-CB transplantation is positively correlated with the nucleated cell dose and the number of CD34$^+$ cells of the CB transplanted per kilogram of body weight of the recipient and with the younger age of the patient [38-40]. Higher total nucleated cell count, number of CD34+ cells in the graft and younger age of the patients correlate positively with improved engraftment, survival of the graft and outcome for the patient [3,41]. A 20% TRM after 100 days was reported for children with acute myeloid leukemia following unrelated CB transplantation with a collected nucleated cell dose higher than 5.2 x 10^7/kg [42]. The rate of success of unrelated-CB transplantation for treating hematologic diseases is reported to be higher in children than in adult patients [40]. The transplantation of CB in children still has delays in engraftment and in immune reconstitution, despite receiving sufficient nucleated cell doses [43-47]. Hence, even in children, the transplantation of CB is still suboptimal. Owing to the low nucleated cell dose, unrelated CB transplantation is considered a standard procedure for the treatment of hematologic diseases in children, particularly for children with very poor-prognosis acute myeloid leukemia and who lack an HLA-identical sibling [1,4,42,48,49].

In adults, the rate of mortality of patients with hematologic diseases who are treated with unrelated, matched, CB transplants is as high as 47%, and the rate of disease-free survival is 26% in the first 100 days after myeloablative transplantations [3]. After 3 years, the rate of leukemia-free survival is 23% for adult patients treated with unrelated, matched, CB transplants; it is 33% for patients treated with unrelated matched BM transplants and 19% for unrelated single antigen mismatched BM transplant [50,51]. In nonmyeloablative regimen, a 26% unrelated, matched, CB TRM was reported at 3 years [52]. While most studies reveal that, for unrelated transplantation, BM has a higher rate of success in adult patients than CB, others report a TRM rate of 9% for adults with hematologic malignancies following unrelated CB transplantation [53]. Hence, nonmyeloablative conditioning favors CB transplantation as a strategy for treating patients with hematologic diseases, particularly for older ones, and unrelated CB transplantation could be as effective as unrelated BM or MPB transplantation for treating adult patients.

Early Infections and Delayed Engraftment

As chemotherapy and radiation treatments to kill the cancer cells suppress patient immune systems, the patients are at risks of early infections. After chemotherapy and radiation treatment, impaired recipient thymopoiesis and lack of transferred memory cells contribute to the delayed T cell recovery. This results in an increased risk of opportunistic infections. This is a major risk for patients undergoing HSC transplant. Unrelated CB transplant is associated with delayed engraftment and, therefore, with delayed reconstitution of the patients' immune system and with higher risks of early infections than BM and MPB transplants [38,54,55]. Hence, early infection is a major risk for patients undergoing CB transplantation and is one of the reasons for the lower rate of success of CB transplantation. Patients treated with CB transplants for hematologic diseases face months of recovery and treatments to ensure a successful transplantation therapy.

The delayed engraftment of CB HSCs in patients after transplants reveals that CB cells have poor homing and engraftment capabilities to the BM after intravenous infusion, compared to BM and MBP transplants. In addition, the fact that T lymphocytes of the CB show decreased expression of two enzymes that contribute to eradicating viral infections - granzyme and perforin - is a contributing factor to risk of early infections, particularly viral infections, in patients treated with a CB transplant [56,57]. Both of these factors contribute to the higher risks of early infections in patients treated with CB transplants.

Graft-versus-Host Disease

Graft-versus-host disease (GVHD) is the immunological reaction and associated damages that occur when transplanting immunologically competent cells into a host whose immune system is compromised. The degree of severity of GVHD is related to the HLA disparity between the donor and the recipient, with the severity enhanced with increased HLA disparity. It ranges from mild to fatal [58]. Mild forms of GVHD can also beneficial to the patients, particularly for cancer patients (e.g. leukemia patients). In mild forms of GVHD, the graft-derived lymphocytes attack the cancer cells, increasing the chance of successful therapy for the patients, a phenomenon referred as graft-versus tumor effect (e.g. graft-versus-leukemia effect). The transplantation of allogeneic CB has a low risk of severe GVHD, particularly lower risks of grade II, III or IV acute GVHD than after unrelated BM transplantation [38,51,54,55]. The reasons for the low risk of severe GVHD for CB transplants are two-fold; firstly the CB is depleted of immune cells and secondly it produces increased amounts of IL-10, an anti-inflammatory cytokine, and little cytotoxic activity [15]. The increased production of the anti-inflammatory cytokine IL-10 and low cytotoxic activity may down modulate GVHD after CB transplant [59-61].

On the one hand, because allogeneic CB transplantation allows for greater HLA disparity and has a lower risk of severe GVHD, it is appropriate for a broader range of patients than BM or MPB transplantations. On the other hand,as allogeneic CB transplantation has a low risk of GVHD, it is more suited for the treatment of patients with nonmalignant hematologic diseases, for whom GVHD risk must be minimized and for whom there is no need for a graft-versus-tumor effect, than for patients with malignant diseases such as leukemia [62-64]. In addition, patients with nonmalignant hematologic diseases have a lower risk of relapse, and are less likely to be in need of post-transplant therapies. Therefore, allogeneic CB transplantation is particularly suited for a broad range of patients with nonmalignant hematologic diseases, particularly children. Similarly, the autologous transplantation of BM is more suited for the treatment of patients with nonmalignant hematologic diseases [65].

Overall, unrelated CB transplantation is promising for the treatment of hematologic diseases, particularly for children and adults with acute leukemia who lack a HLA-matched BM donor. Despite the CB having a higher potential to reconstitute the recipients' BM, there are still limitations to the use of CB for therapy for the treatment of hematologic diseases, beside the low nucleated cell dose in the CB. The main limitations of CB for transplantation are the delayed in engraftment and immune reconstitution leading to significant morbidity and mortality, particularly in adults. CB transplantation is more suited for the treatment of nonmalignant hematologic diseases for a broad range of patients, particularly children. Strategies aimed at improving the nucleated cell dose, homing and engraftment of CB must be devised and developed to improve the rate of success of CB transplantation and to reduce the risk of early infections and the mortality and morbidity rate after CB transplantation, particularly in adult.

Strategies to Improve the Outcome of CB Transplantation for the Treatment of Hematologic Diseases

Several strategies are being devised and proposed to improve the outcome of CB transplantation for the treatment of hematologic diseases. Among them are the direct delivery of CB stem cells to the BM, the increase of doses or units of CB transplanted, the improvement of the engraftment and homing of CB stem cells to the BM and the expansion and propagation of CB stem cells *in vitro* to generate cell lines for transplantation.

Direct Delivery of Cord Blood Stem Cells to the Bone Marrow

To overcome the poor engraftment and homing capabilities of CB stem cells to the BM, a strategy has been proposed to directly transplant umbilical CB into the BM cavities. Studies report mixed results and benefits for the patients [66,67]. Further investigations are required to prove the benefits of a strategy that is more invasive for the patients than the intravenous infusion of CB stem cells.

Transplantation of Double Cord Blood Units

To overcome the low nucleated cell dose present in CB, it is proposed to transplant either pooled or sequential multiple units of umbilical CB [54,68-70]. The use of multiple CB units for allogeneic transplantation requires matching of the various donors to the recipient HLA antigens, as well as the various donors to each other, a difficult and less probable task as the number of units increases. The transplanted units must be closely HLA-matched to the recipients to reduce the risk of GVHD. They must be closely HLA-matched to each other to reduce the risk of immunoreactivity among them or graft-versus-graft effect that would prevent engraftment of the units. Henceforth, the use of two CB units is considered as the standard for multiple CB unit transplantation. Double CB units achieve a nucleated cell dose of 0.23×10^8 nucleated cells/kg [54]. They are generally composed of a matched and a partially matched CB unit to the recipient HLA antigens.

Double CB unit transplantation has been applied successfully to improve the outcome of CB transplantation in children and in adults in need of HSC transplant. Successful therapies with double CB unit transplantation have been reported with no graft failures and 54% disease-free survival at the 3 years mark in myeloablative transplantations [71]. Double CB unit transplantation improves the outcome of the transplantation in humans [72-74]. It improves myeloid and platelet engraftment rates, but not the time to engraftment and does not trigger immunologic rejection in patients [68]. Cases of chronic GVHD have been reported [75]. Conflicting data have been reported on the contribution of each CB unit to the transplant. Some studies report that only one unit contributes to long-term hematopoiesis, while others report that both CB units contribute to hematopoiesis, with the unit eliciting a higher nucleated cell and CD34$^+$ cell dose being associated with cord predominance in the transplant [72,73,75-77]. The failure of one unit to engraft results from the immune rejection mediated by effector CD8$^+$ T cells that develop after CB transplantation [73]. Despite only one unit engrafting in most patients, double CB unit transplantation improves the outcome of the transplantation by increasing the probability of one/the most viable CB unit engrafting [74].

Double CB unit transplantation increases the nucleated cell count of the transplant, improves engraftment of the cells and immune reconstitution in patients. It is associated with an improved rate of success of CB transplantation [78-80]. Nonetheless, the engraftment is still suboptimal. Double CB unit transplantation is still associated with delayed engraftment and a higher rate of engraftment failure than BM and MPB transplantations. Several strategies have been devised and used successfully to circumvent problems associated with the engraftment in double CB transplantation. Among them are the use of a reduced-intensity conditioning regimen of fludarabine, melphalan and antithymocyte globulin that leads to a 14% TRM after 100 days [81], and the use of specific antibodies, such as rituximab [82]. Reduced-intensity or nonmyeloablative regimens use lower doses of pretransplant chemotherapy drugs and/or radiation than the traditional high dose, myeloablative regimens, reducing the toxicity of these treatments. Rituximab is a monoclonal antibody against the protein CD20, a phosphoprotein expressed on the surface of B cells. It is used in transplants involving incompatible blood groups. Hence, double CB unit transplantation represents a promising strategy for the treatment of hematologic diseases in children and in adults. It is particularly suited for patients for whom a perfectly single matched unit is not available, and may reduce the risk of relapse in patients treated for hematologic malignancies owing to higher graft-versus-tumor effect than with single CB unit transplantation.

Fucosylation of Selectin Glycoprotein Ligands Ex Vivo

To overcome the poor engraftment capabilities of CB stem cells to the BM, it is proposed to fucosylate *ex vivo* the SGLs expressed on CB cells, prior transplantation. CB CD34+ hematopoietic progenitor and stem cells express forms of SGLs that lack proper N-glycan determinant, the sLex and the site for fucosylation. The lack of proper N-glycan determinant of SGLs on the surface of HSCs results in the inability of the SGLs to bind to P- and E-selectins, and poor rolling and homing capabilities of CB HSCs on BM vessels and to the BM [22]. The fucosylation of the N-glycan determinant of SGLs has been reported to be critical for the homing and rolling activities of HSCs *in vivo*. Rolling and homing on blood and BM vessels and to the BM are key steps for therapies involving the transplantation of HSCs [12]. It is proposed that improved homing capabilities of CB HSCs would improve their engraftment to the BM. *Ex vivo* fucosylation, by FTVI, of SGLs in the surface of CB HSCs would restore the binding properties of SGLs and the homing and rolling potential of CB HSCs to the BM. Therefore, *ex vivo* fucosylation of SGLs expressed on CB cells would improve their engraftment to the BM. As a consequence, it would reduce the delayed engraftment and reduce the risk of early infections associated with CB transplants, thereby improving the rate of success of CB transplantation.

The treatment of human CB CD34[+] hematopoietic progenitor and stem cells *ex vivo*, by FTVI in presence of GDP fucose increases the yield of fucosylation of sLex determinants on the surface of the cells, particularly on P-SGL-1 (Figure 2). It results in improved binding of the cells to fluid-phase P- and E-selectins and improves cell rolling on P- and E-selectins under flow *in vitro* [83]. It enhances the homing of the cells to and their engraftment into the BM, through more effective rolling interactions of CD34+ cells with P- and E-selectins in BM vessels, in irradiated NOD/SCID mice after infusion [83]. Hence, the fucosylation of CB CD34[+] hematopoietic progenitor and stem cells *ex vivo*, by FTVI, improves the homing of CB HSCS to and their engraftment in the BM [83].

A blocking antibody to the P- and E-selectin-binding region of P-SGL-1 does not inhibit the binding of CB CD34+ cells to fluid-phase P-selectin, after fucosylation *ex vivo* [83]. This reveals that surface fucosylation creates additional binding sites for P- and E-selectin on other regions of PSGL-1 or on other glycoproteins or glycolipids. It further reveals that CB HSCs may not necessarily roll on P- and E-selectins, after their surface fucosylation; they may roll on other glycoproteins or glycolipids. In addition, surface fucosylation of CB cells does not adversely affect their ability to repopulate the BM after homing.

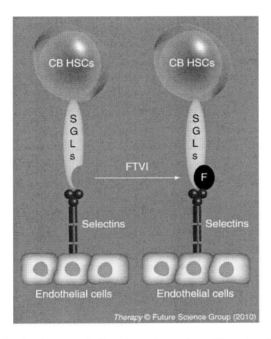

Figure 2. Fucosylation of selectin glycoprotein ligands on the surface of hematopoietic stem cells of the cord blood *ex vivo*. HSCs of the CB elicit a defect in binding to P- and E-selectins and poor homing capabilities to the bone marrow. The defect in fucosylation of SGLs on the surface of HSCs of the CB underlies their inability to bind to P- and E-selectins and their poor capabilities of homing to the bone marrow. The enzyme alpha1-3 FTVI is responsible for alpha1-3 fucosyltransferase activity. The defect in fucosylation of SGLs on the surface of CB HSCs may originate from insufficient levels of FTVI to physiologically fucosylate the SGLs on their surface. The treatment of human CB CD34$^+$ hematopoietic progenitor and stem cells *ex vivo* by FTVI in the presence of guanosine diphosphate fucose increases the yield of fucosylation of the N-glycan determinant of SGLs on the surface of the HSCs (F). *Ex vivo* fucosylation of SGLs by FTVI in the surface of CB HSCs would restore the binding properties of SGLs and the homing and rolling potential of CB HSCs to the bone marrow. Surface fucosylation of CB stem cells would improve their engraftment to the bone marrow. As a consequence, it would reduce the delayed engraftment and reduce the risk of early infections associated with CB transplants, thereby improving the rate of success of CB transplantation.
CB: Cord blood, FTVI: Fucosyltransferase VI; HSC: Hematopoietic stem cell; SGL: glycoprotein ligand.

Hence, the surface fucosylation of CB stem cells has important consequences for therapeutic applications involving CB transplants for treating hematologic diseases. The force-fucosylation of the SGLs, and other glycoprotein or glycolipid sites expressed on the surface of human CB cells, is proposed to improve the homing of CB HSCs to the BM and their engraftment to the BM. It is a simple and efficient procedure performed *ex vivo* prior to transplantation. It involves a 30 min incubation, at 37°C, of the CB cells with FTVI. Short-term biochemical treatment with exogenous FTVI and GDP fucose only transiently increases fucosylated glycans on CB cells, which decline as glycoproteins and glycolipids turn over and as cells divide. Owing to the fact that the increased fucosylation is transient, it is less likely to affect the long-term functions of HSCs and accessory cells after they enter the BM of conditioned recipients [83]. It would improve homing of CB HSCs to the BM and their engraftment in the BM. However, forced fucosylation of CB HSCs might improve rolling on selectins, but not increase entry into the BM if the cells also lack integrins, chemokine receptors or other molecules essential for homing [84]. Many factors, including SCF, fetal liver tyrosine kinase 3-ligand, erythropoietin, granulocyte colony-stimulating factor (G-CSF) and IL-11, are involved in the osteoblastic niche and in the interaction between the niche and the stem cells [85]. The modulation of these factors may affect the homing and engraftment of CB stem cells to the BM, and particularly the rolling on selectins and entry into the BM. In addition, *ex-vivo* manipulations on the graft are hampered by difficulties, such as stem cell loss and dendritic cell activation, and are extremely expensive if performed under good manufacturing practice-grade conditions. Hence, forced fucosylation of CB HSCs represents an alternative strategy for improving engraftment of CB stem cells to the BM. However, it remains to be further confirmed and validated, particularly in humans, before being brought to therapy.

Expansion and Propagation of Cord Blood Stem Cells In Vitro

Another strategy to overcome the low nucleated cell dose present in CB is to expand and propagate CB stem cells *in vitro*, to generate populations of CB stem and progenitor cells for transplantation. Stem cells are self-renewing multipotent cells that generate a large number of differentiated progenies though a transient amplifying population [86]. Three strategies have been proposed and are being considered for the expansion and propagation of CB stem cells *in vitro*.

The first strategy is the expansion and propagation of progenitor and stem cells from CB *in vitro*, or liquid culture. Progenitor and stem cells are isolated from umbilical CB and cultured *in vitro*, in the presence of growth factors and cytokines [5,87,88]. Several protocols and cocktails of growth factors/cytokines have been reported for propagating CB-derived progenitor and stem cells *in vitro*. Among the latter are [71,87]:

- SCF, IL-3, IL-6 and G-CSF
- SCF, thrombopoietin (TPO) and G-CSF
- Fetal liver tyrosine kinase-3 ligand, SCF, IL-3, IL-6, IL-11 and G-CSF.

Delta-1, a membrane-bound ligand of the Notch receptor, induces a 100-fold increase in the number of human $CD34^+$ $CD38^-$ CB cells and promotes their lymphoid differentiation *in vitro* [89]. The cytokine pleiotrophin also promotes the expansion of repopulating populations of human CB, $CD34^+$ $CD38^-$ Lin^- cells, *in vitro* and in vivo. As well as its use *in vitro* to promote the expansion and propagation of human CB stem cells, pleiotrophin may be used to promote hematopoiesis *in vivo* [90]. Generally, CB-derived progenitor and stem cells expand and propagate more rapidly and generate larger number of progenies *in vitro* than their BM counterpart. The second strategy involves the co-culture of progenitor and stem cells from the CB with mesenchymal stromal cells *in vitro* or stromal co-culture. The microenvironment or niche controls the developmental potential of stem cells [91]. Mesenchymal cells from the marrow stroma elicit immuno-modulatory activity on and promote the engraftment of CB $CD34^+$ cells when co-administered in NOD-SCID mice [71,92,93]. CB progenitor and stem cells co-cultured with mesenchymal stromal cells, in presence of fetal bovine serum and a growth factor cocktail (such as SCF, thrombopoietin and G-CSF) promote the growth and expansion of CB-derived progenitor and stem cells by 10–20 fold and of $CD34^+$ cells by 16–37 fold [71,94]. The third strategy involves the culture of progenitor and stem cells from the CB *in vitro* in bioreactors, or continuous perfusion culture systems.

The *in vitro* expansion and propagation of CB stem cells may benefit not only the transplantation of CB for the treatment of hematologic and immune diseases. This is achieved by generating and expanding CB stem cells in an unlimited fashion, thereby overcoming the low nucleated cell count present in CB - the main limiting factor in CB transplantation. It may also benefit the use of CB stem cells for regenerative medicine and gene therapy, for the treatment of a broad range of diseases and injuries [95,96]. With this aim in mind, it is important to note the ability of CB stem cells to generate and differentiate into other phenotypes, including the neuronal lineages, to produce neurotropic factors/cytokines and to modulate immune and inflammatory reactions that may contribute to extend their potential for regenerative medicine, particularly for the treatment of neurological diseases and disorders [97]. One of the main advantages of expanding CB stem cells *in vitro* is the availability of the generated stem cells for the recipients for post-transplant therapies. In one schema, it is proposed to transplant an un-manipulated CB unit to the patient and expand the same unit for later use [98-102]. The main limitations regarding the expansion and propagation of CB stem cells for therapeutic use are: the risk of altering the developmental and therapeutic potential of the cells, particularly stem cell loss and dendritic cell activation, the fact that optimal culture conditions remain to be established, and the high cost associated with generating cell lines under good manufacturing practice-grade conditions [103-105].

Other strategies are also being considered to improve engraftment of CB stem cells to the BM, such as the *ex-vivo* graft engineering to improving T cell recovery, pharmacologic interventions to preserve thymopoiesis, the reduction of the toxicity of the conditioning regimens and the transplantation of two populations of stem cells, as well as other methods of improving homing [106-108]. Delaney and collaborators recently reported recently the development of a Notch-mediated expansion of human $CD34^+$ CB progenitor cells *ex vivo* [109]. Cells were cultured for 17–21 days on immobilized engineered Notch ligand in the presence of cytokines. Notch-mediated expansion CB progenitor cells resulted in over a 100-fold increase in the absolute number of stem/progenitor cells *ex vivo* and in the rapid engraftment of stem cells to the BM of humans in clinical trial [109]. These strategies are at different stages of therapeutic applications, from basic research to advanced phases of clinical studies. Hence, several strategies are being devised and considered, and are promising to improve the engraftment of CB stem cells to the BM. In all, CB is considered a standard source of HSCs for pediatric transplants, but its use is not limited to children. More than 80% of CB transplants are performed in adults with malignancies, and results in nonmalignant disorders have been improved by the use of reduced-intensity conditioning and double CB transplant.

Conclusion

Umbilical CB is enriched in repopulating HSCs, is depleted of immune cells and is easily accessible. It provides a model choice for treating hematologic and BM diseases. CB transplant is considered a standard procedure for the treatment of hematologic diseases in children. It is more suited for the treatment of nonmalignant hematologic diseases for a broad range of patients, including adults. There are, however, limitations to the use of umbilical CB for transplantation: low cell dose, delayed engraftment and early infections, particularly. Current strategies to improve the rate of success of CB transplantation, particularly in adults, involve the infusion of double CB doses. However, this limits the availability of CB units for therapy and the engraftment is still suboptimal. Future strategies to improve the rate of success of CB transplantation, particularly in adult patients, involve the forced fucosylation of CB stem cells *ex vivo*, the expansion and propagation of CB stem cells *in vitro*, reduced-intensity conditioning and the use of Notch-mediated expanded CB progenitor cells *ex vivo*. Forced fucosylation of CB stem cells *ex vivo* and Notch-mediated expanded CB progenitor cells *ex vivo* are being considered to improve the homing and engraftment capabilities of CB stem cells to the BM, whereas the expansion and propagation of CB stem cells *in vitro* are aimed at providing cell lines for cellular therapy and regenerative medicine. These strategies will give the opportunity to treat more patients. Strategies aiming at improving the homing and engraftment capabilities of the CB stem cells to the BM may also be applied to other types of stem cells, such as embryonic stem cells, induced pluripotent stem cells, mesenchymal stem cells, neural stem cells and very small embryonic-like stem cells, to improve their engraftment and therapeutic potential, particularly when administered intravenously [110-112]. Future investigations will aim at validating the novel technologies that will not only take advantage of the full potential of umbilical CB for therapy, but will also enhance it.

Future Perspectives

In 5–10 years, CB stem cell therapy will be the model of choice of the treatment of malignant and nonmalignant hematologic diseases. Improvement in engraftment and immune reconstitution after CB transplantation will lead to more successful treatments not only in children, but also in adults. CB stem cell therapy will also be a model of choice for regenerative medicine.

Financial and Competing Interests Disclosure

The author has no relevant affiliations or financial involvement with any organization or entity with a financial interest in or financial conflict with the subject natter or materials discussed in the manuscript. This includes employment, consultancies, honoraria, stock ownership or options, expert testimony, grants or parents received or pending, or royalties.

No writing assistance was utilized in the production of this manuscript.

Acknowledgments

Reproduced from Therapy (2010) 7(6), 703-715 with permission of Future Medicine Ltd.

References

Papers of special note have been highlighted as either of interest (*) or of considerable interest (**) to readers.

[1] Wagner JE, Gluckman E: Umbilical cord blood transplantation: the first 20 years. *Semin. Hematol.* 47(1), 3-12 (2010).

[2] Gluckman E, Broxmeyer HA, Auerbach AD, *et al.*: Hematopoietic reconstitution in a patient with Fanconi's anemia by means of umbilicalcord blood from an HLA-identical sibling. *N Engl. J Med.* 321(17), 1174-1178 (1989).

** First successful transplantation cord blood stem cells, performed in children with Fanconi anemia.

[3] Long GD, Laughlin M, Madan B, *et al.*: Unrelated umbilical cord blood transplantation in adult patients. *Biol. Blood Marrow Transplant.* 9(12), 772-780 (2009).

* The rate of morbidity and mortality after cord blood transplants remains high in adults, with 47% of patients dying within 100 days of the unrelated transplant.

[4] Rocha V, Cornish J, Sievers EL, *et al.*: Comparison of outcomes of unrelated bone marrow and umbilical cord blood transplants in children with acute leukemia. *Blood.* 97(10), 2962-2971 (2001).

[5] Ballen K, Becker PS, Greiner D, *et al.*: Effect of ex vivo cytokine treatment on human cord blood engraftment in NOD-scid mice. *Br. J Haematol.* 108(3), 629-640 (2000).

[6] Rodrigues CA, Sanz G, Brunstein CG, et al.: Analysis of risk factors for outcomes after unrelated cord blood transplantation in adults with lymphoid malignancies: a study by the Eurocord-Netcord and lymphoma working party of the European group for blood and marrow transplantation. J Clin Oncol. 27(2): 256-263 (2009). Erratum in: J Clin Oncol. 27(11): 1923 (2009).

[7] Eapen M, Rocha V, Sanz G, et al.: Effect of graft source on unrelated donor haemopoietic stem-cell transplantation in adults with acute leukaemia: a retrospective analysis. Lancet Oncol. 11(7): 653-660 (2010).

[8] Wang JC, Doedens M, Dick JE: Primitive human hematopoietic cells are enriched in cord blood compared with adult bone marrow or mobilized peripheral blood as measured by the quantitative in vivo SCID-repopulating cell assay. *Blood.* 89(11), 3919-3924 (1997).

* Umbilical cord blood contains 3–6 times more repopulating hematopoietic progenitor and stem cells than the bone marrow and mobilized peripheral blood.

[9] Keever CA, Abu-Hajir M, Graf W, *et al.*: Characterization of the alloreactivity and anti-leukemia reactivity of cord blood mononuclear cells. *Bone Marrow Transplant.* 15(3): 407-419 (1995).

[10] Wang XN, Sviland L, Ademokun AJ, *et al.*: Cellular alloreactivity of human cord blood cells detected by T-cell frequency analysis and a human skin explant model. *Transplantation.* 66(7): 903-909 (1998).

[11] Rocha V, Broxmeyer HE. New approaches for improving engraftment after cord blood transplantation. *Biol Blood Marrow Transplant.* 16(1 Suppl): S126-132 (2010).

[12] Lapidot T, Dar A, Kollet O: How do stem cells find their way home? *Blood.* 106(6), 1901-1910 (2005).

[13] Broxmeyer HE, Hangoc G, Cooper S, *et al.*: Growth characteristics and expansion of human umbilical cord blood and estimation of its potential for transplantation in adults. *Proc. Natl. Acad. Sci. U S A* 89(9), 4109-4113 (1992).

[14] Kurtzberg J, Laughlin M, Graham ML, *et al.*: Placental blood as a source of hematopoietic stem cells for transplantation into unrelated recipients. *N Engl. J Med.* 335(3), 157-166 (1996).

[15] Cohen Y, Nagler A: Umbilical cord blood transplantation: how, when and for whom? *Blood Rev.* 18(3), 167-179 (2004).

[16] Schweitzer KM, Drager AM, Van der Valk P, *et al.*: Constitutive expression of E-selectin and vascular cell adhesion molecule-1 on endothelial cells of hematopoietic tissues. *Am. J Pathol.* 148(1), 165-175 (1996).

[17] Frenette PS, Subbarao S, Mazo IB, *et al.*: Endothelial selectins and vascular cell adhesion molecule-1 promote hematopoietic progenitor homing to bone marrow. *Proc. Natl. Acad. Sci. U S A* 95(24), 14423-14428 (1998).

[18] Mazo IB, Gutierrez-Ramos JC, Frenette PS, *et al.*: Hematopoietic progenitor cell rolling in bone marrow microvessels: parallel contributions by endothelial selectins and vascular cell adhesion molecule 1. *J Exp. Med.* 188(5), 465-474 (1998).

[19] Katayama Y, Hidalgo A, Furie BC, *et al.*: PSGL-1 participates in E-selectin-mediated progenitor homing to bone marrow: evidence for cooperation between E-selectin ligands and alpha 4 integrin. *Blood.* 102(6), 2060-2067 (2003).

[20] Vestweber D, Blanks JE.: Mechanisms that regulate the function of the selectins and their ligands. *Physiol. Rev.* 79(1), 181-213 (1999).

[21] McEver RP: Adhesive interactions of leukocytes, platelets, and the vessel wall during hemostasis and inflammation. *Thromb. Haemost.* 86(3), 746-756 (2001).

[22] Hidalgo A, Weiss LA, Frenette PS: Functional selectin ligands mediating human CD34+ cell interactions with bone marrow endothelium are enhanced postnatally. *J Clin. Invest.* 110(4), 559-569 (2002).

[23] McEver RP: Selectins: lectins that initiate cell adhesion under flow. *Curr. Opin. Cell. Biol.* 14(5), 581-586 (2002).

[24] Maly P, Thall AD, Petryniak B, *et al.*: The alpha (1,3)Fucosyltransferase Fuc-TVII controls leukocyte trafficking through an essential role in L-, E-, and Pselectin ligand biosynthesis. *Cell.* 86(4), 643-653 (1996).

[25] Blander JM, Visintin I, Janeway CA Jr, *et al.*: Alpha(1,3)-fucosyltransferase VII and alpha(2,3)-sialyltransferase IV are up-regulated in activated CD4 T cells and maintained after their differentiation into Th1 and migration into inflammatory sites. *J Immunol.* 163(7), 3746-3752 (1999).

[26] Lim YC, Henault L, Wagers AJ, *et al.*: Expression of functional selectin ligands on Th cells is differentially regulated by IL-12 and IL-4. *J Immunol.* 162(6), 3193-3201 (1999).

[27] Weninger W, Ulfman LH, Cheng G, *et al.*: Specialized contributions by alpha(1,3)-fucosyltransferase-IV and FucT-VII during leukocyte rolling in dermal microvessels. *Immunity.* 12(6), 665-676 (2000).

[28] Bengtson P, Lundblad A, Larson G, *et al.*: Polymorphonuclear leukocytes from individuals carrying the G329A mutation in the 1,3-fucosyltransferase VII gene (FUT7) roll on E- and P-selectins. *J Immunol.* 169(7), 3940-3946 (2002).

[29] Leppainen A, Mehta P, Ouyang YB, *et al.*: A novel glycosulfopeptide binds to P-selectin and inhibits leukocyte adhesion to P-selectin. *J Biol. Chem.* 274(35), 24838-24848 (1999).

[30] Somers WS, Tang J, Shaw GD, *et al.*: Insights into the molecular basis of leukocyte tethering and rolling revealed by structures of P- and E-selectin bound to SLe(X) and PSGL-1. *Cell.* 103(3), 467-479 (2000).

[31] Leppainen A, Yago T, Otto VI, *et al.*: Model glycosulfopeptides from P-selectin glycoprotein ligand-1 require tyrosine sulfation and a core 2-branched O-glycan to bind to L-selectin. *J Biol. Chem.* 278(29), 26391–26400 (2003).

[32] Yang J, Hirata T, Croce K, *et al.*: Targeted gene disruption demonstrates that P-selectin glycoprotein ligand 1 (PSGL-1) is required for P-selectinmediated but not E-selectin-mediated neutrophil rolling and migration. *J Exp. Med.* 190(12), 1769-1782 (1999).

[33] Papayannopoulou T, Priestley GV, Nakamoto B, *et al.*: Molecular pathways in bone marrow homing: dominant role of alpha(4)beta(1) over beta(2)-integrins and selectins. *Blood.* 98(8), 2403- 2411 (2001).

[34] Fuhlbrigge RC, Kieffer JD, Armerding D, *et al.*: Cutaneous lymphocyte antigen is a specialized form of PSGL-1 expressed on skin-homing T cells. *Nature.* 389(6654), 978-981 (1997).

[35] Wagers AJ, Waters CM, Stoolman LM, *et al.*: Interleukin 12 and interleukin 4 control cell adhesion to endothelial selectins through opposite effects on alpha1,3-fucosyltransferase VII gene expression. *J Exp. Med.* 188(12), 2225-2231 (1998).

[36] Wright DE, Bowman EP, Wagers AJ, *et al.*: Hematopoietic stem cells are uniquely selective in their migratory response to chemokines. *J Exp. Med.* 195(9), 1145-1154 (2002).

[37] Naiyer AJ, Jo DY, Ahn J, *et al.*: Stromal derived factor-1-induced chemokinesis of cord blood CD34(+) cells (long-term culture-initiating cells) through endothelial cells is mediated by E-selectin. *Blood.* 94(12), 4011-4019 (1999).

[38] Rubinstein P, Carrier C, Scaradavou A, *et al.*: Outcomes among 562 recipients of placental-blood transplants from unrelated donors. *N Engl. J Med.* 339(22), 1565-1577 (1998).

[39] Migliaccio AR, Adamson JW, Stevens CE, *et al.*: Cell dose and speed of engraftment in placental/umbilical cord blood transplantation: graft progenitor cell content is a better predictor than nucleated cell quantity. *Blood.* 96(8), 2717-2722 (2000).

[40] Laughlin MJ, Barker J, Bambach B, *et al.*: Hematopoietic engraftment and survival in adult recipients of umbilical-cord blood from unrelated donors. *N Engl. J Med.* 344(24), 1815-1822 (2001).

[41] Gluckman E, Rocha V, Arcese W, *et al.*: Factors associated with outcomes of unrelated cord blood transplant: guidelines for donor choice. *Exp. Hematol.* 32(4), 397-407 (2004).

[42] Michel G, Rocha V, Chevret S, *et al.*: Unrelated cord blood transplantation for childhood acute myeloid leukemia: a Eurocord Group analysis. *Blood.* 102(13), 4290-4297 (2003).

[43] Thomson BG, Robertson KA, Gowan D, *et al.*: Analysis of engraftment, graft-versus-host disease, and immune recovery following unrelated donor cord blood transplantation. *Blood.* 96(8), 2703-2711 (2000).

[44] Sawczyn KK, Quinones R, Malcolm J, *et al.*: Cord blood transplant in childhood ALL. *Pediatr. Blood Cancer.* 45(7), 964-970 (2005).

[45] Martin PL, Carter SL, Kernan NA, *et al.*: Results of the cord blood transplantation study (COBLT): outcomes of unrelated donor umbilical cord blood transplantation in pediatric patients with lysosomal and peroxisomal storage diseases. *Biol. Blood Marrow Transplant.* 12(2), 184-194 (2006).

[46] Szabolcs P, Niedzwiecki D: Immune reconstitution after unrelated cord blood transplantation. *Cytotherapy.* 9(2), 111-122 (2007).

[47] Kurtzberg J, Prasad VK, Carter SL, *et al.*: Results of the Cord Blood Transplantation Study (COBLT): clinical outcomes of unrelated donor umbilical cord blood transplantation in pediatric patients with hematologic malignancies. *Blood.* 112(10), 4318-4327 (2008).

[48] Ballen K: Challenges in umbilical cord blood stem cell banking for stem cell reviews and reports. *Stem Cell Rev.* 6(1), 8-14 (2010).

[49] Ljungman P, Bregni M, Brune M, *et al.*: Allogeneic and autologous transplantation for haematological diseases, solid tumours and immune disorders: current practice in Europe 2009. *Bone Marrow Transplant.* 45(2): 219-234 (2010).

[50] Laughlin MJ, Eapen M, Rubinstein P, *et al.*: Outcomes after transplantation of cord blood or bone marrow from unrelated donors in adults with leukemia. *N Engl. J Med.* 351(22), 2265-2275 (2004).

[51] Rocha, V, Labopin, M, Sanz, G, *et al.*: Transplants of umbilical cord blood or bone marrow from unrelated donors in adults with acute leukemia. *N Engl. J Med.* 351(22), 2276-2285 (2004).

[52] Brunstein CG, Barker JN, Weisdorf DJ, *et al.*: Umbilical cord blood transplantation after nonmyeloablative conditioning: impact on transplantation outcomes in 110 adults with hematologic disease. *Blood.* 110(8), 3064-3070 (2007).

[53] Takahashi S, Ooi J, Tomonari A, *et al.*: Comparative single-institute analysis of cord blood transplantation from unrelated donors with bone marrow or peripheral blood stem-cell transplants from related donors in adult patients with hematologic malignancies after myeloablative conditioning regimen. *Blood.* 109(3), 1322-1330 (2007).

[54] Barker JN, Wagner JE: Umbilical cord blood transplantation: current practice and future innovations. *Crit. Rev. Oncol. Hematol.* 48(1), 35-43 (2003).

* The transplantation of allogeneic umbilical cord blood has a low risk of severe graft-versus-host disease.

[55] Grewal SS, Barker JN, Davies SM, *et al.*: Unrelated donor hematopoietic cell transplantation: marrow or umbilical cord blood? *Blood.* 101(11), 4233-4244 (2003).

[56] Berthou, C, Legros-Maida, S, Soulie, A, *et al.*: Cord blood T lymphocytes lack constitutive perforin expression in contrast to adult peripheral blood T lymphocytes. *Blood.* 85(6), 1540-1546 (1995).

[57] Choy JC: Granzymes and perforin in solid organ transplant rejection. *Cell Death Differ.* 17(4), 567-576 (2010).

[58] Taupin P: OTI-010 Osiris Therapeutics/JCR Pharmaceuticals. *Curr. Opin. Investig. Drugs.* 7(5), 473-481 (2006).

[59] Vaziri, H, Dragowska, W, Allsopp, R. C, *et al.*: Evidence for a mitotic clock in human hematopoeitic stem cells: loss of telomeric DNA with age. *Proc. Natl. Acad. Sci. U S A.* 91(21), 9857-9860 (1994).

[60] Kim YJ, Brutkiewicz PR, Broxmeyer HE: Role of 4-1BB (CD137) in the functional activation of cord blood CD28-CD8+ T cells. *Blood.* 100(9), 3253-3260 (2002).

[61] Szabolcs P, Park KD, Reese M, *et al.*: Coexistant naïve phenotype and higher cycling rate of cord blood T cells compared to adult peripheral blood. *Exp. Hematol.* 31(8), 708-714 (2003).

[62] Staba SL, Escolar ML, Poe M, *et al.*: Cord-blood transplants fromunrelated donors in patients with Hurler's syndrome. *N Engl. J Med.* 350(19), 1960-1969 (2004).

[63] Escolar ML, Poe MD, Provenzale JM, *et al.*: Transplantation of umbilical-cord blood in babies with infantile Krabbe's disease. *N Engl. J Med.* 352(20), 2069-2081 (2005).

[64] Kobayashi, R, Ariga, T, Nonoyama, S, *et al.*: Outcome in patients with Wiskott-Aldrich syndrome following stem cell transplantation: an analysis of 57 patients in Japan. *Br. J Haematol.* 135(3), 362-366 (2006).

[65] Gale KB: Backtracking leukemia to birth: identification of clonotypic gene fusion sequences in neonatal blood spots. *Proc. Natl. Acad. Sci. U S A.* 94(25), 13950-13954 (1997).

[66] Frassoni F, Gualandi F, Podesta M, *et al.*: Direct intrabone transplant of unrelated cord-blood cells in acute leukaemia: a phase I/II study. *Lancet Oncol.* 9(9), 831-839 (2008).

[67] Brunstein CG, Barker JN, Weisdorf DJ, *et al.*: Intra-BM injection to enhance engraftment after myeloablative umbilical cord blood transplantation with two partially HLA-matched units. *Bone Marrow Transplant.* 43(12), 935-940 (2009).

[68] Weinreb S, Delgado JC, Clavijo OP, *et al.*: Transplantation of unrelated cord blood cells. *Bone Marrow Transplant.* 22(2), 193-196 (1998).

[69] Fernandez MN, Regidor C, Cabrera R, *et al.*: Cord blood transplants: early recovery of neutrophils from co-transplanted sibling haploidentical progenitor cells and lack of engraftment of cultured cord blood cells, as ascertained by analysis of DNA polymorphisms. *Bone Marrow Transplant.* 28(4), 355-363 (2001).

[70] De Lima M, St John LS, Wieder ED, *et al.*: Double-chimaerism after transplantation of two human leucocyte antigen mismatched, unrelated cord blood units. *Br. J Haematol.* 119(3), 773-776 (2002).

[71] Kelly SS, Parmar S, De Lima M, *et al.*: Overcoming the barriers to umbilical cord blood transplantation. *Cytotherapy.* 12(2), 121-130 (2010).

[72] Bradstock K, Hertzberg M, Kerridge I, *et al.*: Single versus double unrelated umbilical cord blood units for allogeneic transplantation in adults with advanced haematological malignancies: a retrospective comparison of outcomes. *Intern. Med. J.* 39(11), 744-751 (2009).

[73] Gutman JA, Turtle CJ, Manley TJ, *et al.*: Single-unit dominance after double-unit umbilical cord blood transplantation coincides with a specific CD8+ T-cell response against the nonengrafted unit. *Blood.* 115(4), 757-765 (2010).

[74] Scaradavou A, Smith KM, Hawke R, *et al.*: Cord blood units with low CD34+ cell viability have a low probability of engraftment after double unit transplantation. *Biol. Blood Marrow Transplant.* 16(4), 500-508 (2010).

[75] Barker JN, Weisdorf DJ, Wagner JE: Creation of a double chimera after the transplantation of umbilical-cord blood from two partially matched unrelated donors. *N Engl. J Med.* 344(24), 1870-1871 (2001).

[76] Wang FR, Huang XJ, Zhang YC, *et al.*: Successful transplantation of double unit umbilical-cord blood from unrelated donors in high risk leukemia with a long follow-up. *Chin. Med. J (Engl).* 118(9), 772-776 (2005).

[77] Delaney M, Cutler CS, Haspel RL, *et al.*: High-resolution HLA matching in doubleumbilical cord blood reduced-intensity transplantation in adults. *Transfusion.* 49(5), 995-1002 (2009).

[78] Broxmeyer HE, Douglas GW, Hangoc G, *et al.*: Human umbilical cord blood as a potential source of transplantable hematopoietic stem/progenitor cells. *Proc. Natl. Acad. Sci. U S A.* 86(10), 3828-3832 (1989).

[79] Majhail NS, Weisdorf DJ, Wagner JE, *et al.*: Comparable results of umbilical cord blood and HLA-matched sibling donor hematopoietic stem cell transplantation after reduced-intensity preparative regimen for advanced Hodgkin lymphoma. *Blood.* 107(9), 3804-3807 (2006).

[80] Ballen KK, Barker JN, Stewart SK, *et al.*: Collection and preservation of cord blood for personal use. *Biol. Blood Marrow Transplant.* 14(3), 356-363 (2008).

[81] Ballen KK, Spitzer TR, Yeap BY, *et al.*: Double unrelated reduced-intensity umbilical cord blood transplantation in adults. *Biol. Blood Marrow Transplant.* 13(1), 82-89 (2007).

[82] Blaes AH, Cao Q, Wagner JE, *et al.*: Monitoring and preemptive rituximab therapy for Epstein-Barr virus reactivation after antithymocyte globulin containing nonmyeloablative conditioning for umbilical cord blood transplantation. Biol. Blood Marrow Transplant 16(2), 287-291 (2010).

[83] Xia L, McDaniel JM, Yago T, *et al.*: Surface fucosylation of human cord blood cells augments binding to P-selectin and E-selectin and enhances engraftment in bone marrow. *Blood.* 104(10), 3091-3096 (2004).

** The treatment of human cord blood CD34$^+$ hematopoietic progenitor and stem cells *ex vivo*, by fucosyltransferase VI in presence of guanosine diphosphate fucose, enhances the homing of the cells to and their engraftment in the BM, in irradiated nonobese diabetic/severe combined immunodeficiency mice after infusion.

[84] Hidalgo A, Frenette PS: Enforced fucosylation of neonatal CD34+ cells generates selectin ligands that enhance the initial interactions with microvessels but not homing to bone marrow. *Blood.* 105(2), 567-575 (2005).

** Forced fucosylation of cord blood hematopoietic stem cells might improve rolling on selectins, but not increase entry into the bone marrow.

[85] Gonzalez S, Amat L, Azqueta C, *et al.*: Factors modulating circulation of hematopoietic progenitor cells in cord blood and neonates. *Cytotherapy.* 11(1), 35-42 (2009).

[86] Taupin P: Therapeutic potential of adult neural stem cells. *Recent Pat. CNS Drug. Discov.* 1(3), 299-303 (2006).

[87] Purdy MH, Hogan CJ, Hami L, *et al.*: Large volume ex vivo expansion of CD34-positive hematopoietic progenitor cells for transplantation. *J Hematother*. 4(6), 515-525 (1995).

[88] Piacibello W, Sanavio F, Severino A, *et al.*: Engraftment in nonobese diabetic severe combined immunodeficient mice of human CD34(+) cord blood cells after ex vivo expansion: evidence for the amplification and self-renewal of repopulating stem cells. *Blood*. 93(11), 3736-3749 (1999).

[89] Ohishi K, Varnum-Finney B, Bernstein ID: Delta-1 enhances marrow and thymus repopulating ability of human CD34(+)CD38(-) cord blood cells. *J. Clin. Invest*. 110(8), 1165-1174 (2002).

** Delta-1, a membrane-bound ligand of the Notch receptor, induces a 100-fold increase in the number of human $CD34^+$ $CD38^-$ cord blood cells and promotes their lymphoid differentiation *in vitro*.

[90] Himburg HA, Muramoto GG, Daher P, *et al.*: Pleiotrophin regulates the expansion and regeneration of hematopoietic stem cells. *Nat. Med*. 16(4), 475-482 (2010).

[91] Taupin P: Adult neural stem cells, neurogenic niches and cellular therapy. *Stem Cell Rev*. 2(3), 213-219 (2006).

[92] Noort WA, Kruisselbrink AB, in't Anker PS, *et al.*: Mesenchymal stem cells promote engraftment of human umbilical cord blodderived CD34(+) cells in NOD/SCID mice. *Exp. Hematol*. 30(8), 870-878 (2002).

[93] in't Anker PS, Noort WA, Kruisselbrink AB, *et al.*: Nonexpanded primary lung and bone marrow-derived mesenchymal cells promote the engraftment of umbilical cord blood-derived CD34(+) cells in NOD/SCID mice. *Exp. Hematol*. 31(10), 881-889 (2003).

[94] McNiece I, Harrington J, Turney J, *et al.*: Ex vivo expansion of cord blood mononuclear cells on mesenchymal stem cells. *Cytotherapy*. 6(4), 311-317 (2004).

[95] Boissel L, Tuncer HH, Betancur M, *et al.*: Umbilical cord mesenchymal stem cells increase expansion of cord blood natural killer cells. *Biol. Blood Marrow Transplant*. 14(9), 1031-1038 (2008).

[96] Mazur MA, Davis CC, Szabolcs P: Ex vivo expansion and Th1/Tc1 maturation of umbilical cord blood T cells by CD3/CD28 costimulation. *Biol. Blood Marrow Transplant*. 14(10), 1190-1196 (2008).

[97] Park DH, Borlongan CV, Willing AE, *et al.*: Human umbilical cord blood cell grafts for brain ischemia. *Cell Transplant*. 18(9), 985-998 (2009).

[98] Pecora AL, Stiff P, Jennis A, *et al.*: Prompt and durable engraftment in two older adult patients with high risk chronic myelogenous leukemia (CML) using ex vivo expanded and unmanipulated unrelated umbilical cord blood. *Bone Marrow Transplant*. 25(7), 797-799 (2000).

[99] Pecora AL, Stiff P, LeMaistre CF, *et al.*: A phase II trial evaluating the safety and effectiveness of the AastromReplicell system for augmentation of low-dose blood stem cell transplantation. *Bone Marrow Transplant*. 28(3), 295-303 (2001).

[100] Shpall EJ, Quinones R, Giller R, *et al.*: Transplantation of ex vivo expanded cord blood. *Biol. Blood Marrow Transplant*. 8(7), 368-376 (2002).

[101] Jaroscak J, Goltry K, Smith A, *et al.*: Augmentation of umbilical cord blood (UCB) transplantation with ex vivo-expanded UCB cells: results of a phase 1 trial using the AastromReplicell System. *Blood*. 101(12), 5061-5067 (2003).

[102] de Lima M, McMannis J, Gee A, *et al.*: Transplantation of ex vivo expanded cord blood cells using the copper chelator tetraethylenepentamine: a phase I/II clinical trial. *Bone Marrow Transplant.* 41(9), 771-778 (2008).

[103] Williams DA: Ex vivo expansion of hematopoietic stem and progenitor cells: robbing Peter to pay Paul? *Blood.* 81(12), 3169-3172 (1993).

[104] Holyoake TL, Alcorn MJ, Richmond L, *et al.*: CD34 positive PBPC expanded ex vivo may not provide durable engraftment following myeloablative chemoradiotherapy regimens. *Bone Marrow Transplant.* 19(11), 1095-1101 (1997).

[105] McNiece IK, Almeida-Porada G, Shpall EJ, *et al.*: Ex vivo expanded cord blood cells provide rapid engraftment in fetal sheep but lack long-term engrafting potential. *Exp. Hematol.* 30(6), 612-616 (2002).

[106] Goldstein G, Toren A, Nagler A: Transplantation and other uses of human umbilical cord blood and stem cells. *Curr. Pharm. Des.* 13(13), 1363-1373 (2007).

[107] Escalon MP, Komanduri KV: Cord blood transplantation: evolving strategies to improve engraftment and immune reconstitution. *Curr. Opin. Oncol.* 22(2), 122-129 (2010).

[108] Taupin P: Transplantation of two populations of stem cells to improve engraftment: WO2008060932. *Expert Opin. Ther. Pat.* 20(9), 1259-1263 (2010).

[109] Delaney C, Heimfeld S, Brashem-Stein C, *et al.* Notch-mediated expansion of human cord blood progenitor cells capable of rapid myeloid reconstitution. *Nat Med.* 16(2): 232-236 (2010).

** Notch-mediated expanded cord blood progenitor cells for improving homing and engraftment to the bone marrow show promising results *ex vivo* and in clinical trial.

[110] Taupin P: VSELs; Very small embryonic-like stem cells for regenerative medicine: WO2010039241. *Expert Opin. Ther. Pat.* 20(8), 1103-1106 (2010).

[111] Taupin P: Ex vivo fucosylation to improve the engraftment capability and therapeutic potential of human cord blood stem cells. *Drug Discov. Today.* 15(17/18), 698-699 (2010).

[112] Taupin P: Ex vivo fucosylation of stem cells to improve engraftment: WO2004094619. *Expert Opin. Ther. Pat.* 20(9), 1265-1269 (2010).

Chapter XIII

Transplantation of Two Populations of Stem Cells to Improve Engraftment[*]

Abstract

Background

The application is in the field of haematopoietic stem cells (HSCs) and cellular therapy. Objective: It aims at improving the outcome and rate of success of HSC transplantation for treating patients with haematologic diseases, primarily following allogeneic transplantation

Methods

The patients are administered two intravenous infusions of cord blood (CB) tissue between a 2 and 24 h interval

Results

Patients who receive a first infusion of CB stem cells, followed by a second infusion within a 24 h interval, elicit a better outcome and rate of success of CB transplantation than patients receiving only one injection or two injections in whom the second injection was administered several days or weeks following the first one. The double infusion of

---

[*] Patent details:
Title: Methods for improved engraftment following stem cell transplantation
Assignee: Aldagen, Inc.
Inventor: Balber AE
Priority data: 08/11/2006
Filing date: 08/11/2007
Publication date: 22/05/2008
Publication no.: WO2008060932

CB tissue, within a 24 h interval, accelerates the time to neutrophil and platelet engraftment and immune reconstitution following myeloablative therapy.

Conclusion

The application claims the transplantation of at least two populations of HSCs, separated by an interval of time between 2 and 24 h, to improve the outcome of HSC transplantation for the treatment of haematologic diseases. The procedure may be extended to other types of stem cells for treating a broad range of diseases and injuries.

Introduction

Haematopoietic stem cells (HSCs) are the self-renewing multipotent cells that generate the cell lineages of the blood and immune systems. The bone marrow (BM) is the main source of HSCs in the body. HSCs are also present in mobilised peripheral blood (MPB) and in umbilical cord blood (CB) tissues [1,2]. BM transplants have been used for treating a broad range of malignant and non-malignant haematologic diseases [3]. Allogeneic transplants are the most common form of transplantation for the treatment of haematologic diseases, particularly leukaemia. They are chosen from human leukocyte antigen (HLA)-compatible donors, preferably from a related donor, a sibling or parent (allowing single-locus mismatched donor), or from an unrelated donor (fully matched donor). In related-heterologous transplantation, the tissue originates from an identical twin, or syngeneic transplantation, or from a matched sibling or a mismatched family or relative member, or allogeneic transplantation. In unrelated-heterologous allogeneic transplantation, the tissue originates from an unrelated individual. Tissues for unrelated-allogeneic BM transplantations originate from banks which lack donors and are not highly populated.

CB tissues elicit a high level of repopulating HSCs and represent an alternative source of tissue for HSC transplantation [4]. CB tissues are also easily accessible and CB banks are more populated than the BM and MPB registries. In addition, CB tissues are depleted of immune cells, particularly T lymphocytes, allowing for greater disparity of HLA compatibility when matching donors--recipients in allogeneic transplantation than with BM and MPB tissues. The depletion in immune cells of the CB results also in low risk of severe graft-versus-host disease (GVHD) in patients treated with CB transplants. GVHD is the immunological reaction and associated damage that occur when transplanting immunologically competent cells into a host whose immune system is compromised [5]. CB transplantations for the treatment of haematologic diseases have been performed successfully in children and in adults [6,7]. The rate of success of CB transplantation is correlated with the nucleated cell dose and the age of the patients [8]. The higher the nucleated cell dose in the transplant and the younger the patient, the higher the rate of success of CB transplantation [9]. However, CB transplantation remains characterised by a high rate of morbidity and mortality, particularly in adults. The rate of mortality of patients with haematologic diseases treated with CB transplants is as high as 47% of patients dying prior to the 100 days mark after allogeneic transplantation [10]. Low cell doses, delayed engraftment, poor engraftment and early infections are the main limitations of the outcome of CB transplants for treating haematologic diseases, particularly in adults, but also in children [11,12].

With the aim of improving the outcome of CB transplantation for treating haematologic diseases, several approaches are being developed and considered; among them, the transplantation of multiple units of CB tissue, the expansion and propagation of CB stem cells *in vitro* and the fucosylation of CB stem cells *ex vivo* [13-17]. The transplantation of double units of CB tissue improves the outcome of CB transplantation, but does not shorten the time to neutrophil or platelet engraftment, the two criteria defining engraftment. In addition, the conditions of transplantation are still suboptimal. Optimal culture conditions for the expansion and propagation of CB stem cells *in vitro* for use in transplantation remain to be established and the fucosylation of CB stem cells *ex vivo* to improve the outcome of CB transplantation remains to be confirmed and validated [18-20].

The application claims the transplantation of two preparations or populations of CB stem cells to improve the outcome of HSC transplantation for treating patients with haematologic diseases, such as the two transplantations that are performed by intravenous infusion between a 2 and 24 h interval. The application may be used primarily for allogeneic transplantation of HSCs from CB tissues, but also from other sources such as the BM and MPB, to treat patients with haematologic diseases. It may also be used for the transplantation of other types of stem cells, such as liver stem cells, mesenchymal stem cells and neural stem cells, when administered intravenously to improve the treatment of a variety of diseases and injuries, ranging from liver diseases, diabetes and heart diseases to neurological diseases and injuries, including neurodegenerative diseases and spinal cord injuries.

Methods

Transplant

The transplant consists of two preparations or populations of CB stem cells for allogeneic transplantation in patients in need of HSC transplants. The two populations of cells from the donor and host are matched for HLA compatibility (fully or partially matched) to minimise the risk of graft rejection. The cells originate from one or several donors matched for HLA compatibility with the host. The cells of the two populations may originate from different source of HSCs, for example, CB, BM and/or MPB. Each population of cells may be composed of a different ratio of different source of HSCs. The number of nucleated cells for each population depends on the composition of the first cell population, such as: i) if the first cell population contains a sufficient number of cells to facilitate release of the second or supplemental cell population from the liver and/or lungs after its administration, the second cell population may contain fewer stem cells, ii) if the second cell population contains a sufficient number of stem cells to engraft, the first cell population may not need to be abundant and iii) the first and second cell populations may be optimised to promote engraftments of stem cells in the BM. The first cell population may contain 1×10^5 to 1×10^6 cells/kg body weight or in a combination of the first and second cell populations. Cells are prepared in buffers such as neutral buffered saline or phosphate buffered saline.

Transplantation

The two populations of CB stem cells are administered intravenously in patients by infusion, injection or transfusion. The two populations of cells may be administered by different routes. The second or supplemental population of cells are administered between 2 and 24 h following the first population.

Biology and Action

The intravenous infusion of two preparations or populations of CB stem cells, within a 24 h interval, accelerates haematopoiesis and improves the outcome of CB transplantation in patients with haematologic diseases after allogeneic transplantation. Specifically, the intravenous infusion of two populations of CB stem cells, between a 2 and 24 h interval, shortens the time to neutrophil and platelet engraftment.

The mechanism underlying the improvement of CB transplantation when two populations of CB stem cells are administered intravenously between a 2 and 24 h interval remains to be determined.

The reticuloendothelial system (RES) consists of macrophages of the BM, liver, lungs and spleen. It provides the body with a variety of immunological defences and responses, such as protection against infection, neoplasia surveillance and recognition of foreign antigens. The recognition of foreign antigens by the RES plays a role in the capacity of the recipient to reject allogeneic tissues and organ transplants [21]. The RES also plays a role in the flow of transplanted tissue through the microvasculature of the lungs. When tissues are administered intravenously, by injection, infusion or transfusion, they flow through the pulmonary circulation to the lungs, where they are retarded by the microvasculature in the area around the alveoli (where the pulmonary venous capillaries join the pulmonary arterioles). The alveoli are lined up with pulmonary macrophages of the RES. These macrophages remove particulate material and dying cells present in grafted tissues. Hence, the RES of the lungs contributes to slow the flow of grafted tissue in the body. It results in delaying the process of engraftment when the tissue is administered intravenously.

It is proposed that the intravenous infusion of the first preparation or population of CB stem cells suppresses the activity of the RES. Thereby, it permits the second population to be less prone to recognition of foreign antigens by the macrophages of the RES and to travel through the blood to the BM, being less retarded by the microvasculature in the area around the alveoli. In this process, the first population of transplanted cells hides or 'masks' the endothelium from the cells in the second population that expresses similar ligands, whereas the second population of cells benefits from the suppression of the RES when administered within 24 h of the first one; this is achieved by reducing the capacity of the host to reject the transplanted tissues in allogeneic transplantation and the capacity of the lung to delay the flow of grafted tissue administered intravenously. As a result, the second population of cells elicits a higher survival rate and is free to leave the liver and lungs, to travel through the blood to the BM, and successfully engraft in the BM when both populations of cells are administered intravenously.

The intravenous infusion of two preparations or populations of CB stem cells, within a 24 h interval, results in a better engraftment and improves the outcome of CB transplantation in patients with haematologic diseases, particularly after allogeneic transplantation.

Expert Opinion

The intravenous infusion of two populations of CB stem cells, between a 2 and 24 h interval, accelerates haematopoiesis and improves the outcome of CB transplantation in patients with haematologic diseases after allogeneic transplantation. The intravenous infusion of two populations of CB stem cells, within a 24 h interval, shortens the time to neutrophil and platelet engraftment, thereby, reducing the delay in engraftment and the risk of early infections.

The time to absolute neutrophil count (ANC) recovery and to platelet engraftment is a major indicator of successful engraftment of HSCs to the BM. Delay in time to neutrophil and/or platelet engraftment reduces the overall probability of engraftment and reduces the rate of success of HSC transplantation. The intravenous infusion of two populations of

HSCs, several days or weeks after the first transplantation, does not improve the outcome of HSC transplantation, when compared to subjects receiving only one infusion of cells after allogeneic transplantation [22,23]. When the second transplantation is performed days or weeks after the first one, the activity of the RES is restored in the host. Other strategies have been devised and proposed to decrease the time to neutrophil and/or platelet engraftment. Among them, fucosylation of CB tissue *ex vivo*, prior to transplantation, reduces the delay in engraftment CB tissues in the BM and the risk of early infections, in rodents [17]. This latter strategy remains to be confirmed and validated, particularly in humans [19,20]. Hence, the intravenous infusion of two populations of CB stem cells, within a 24 h interval, facilitates the engraftment by decreasing time to ANC recovery and platelet engraftment, resulting in overall improvement of engraftment of CB HSCs to the BM after allogeneic transplantation. Engraftment after HSC transplantation is a major predictor of successful transplantation. Thereby, the intravenous infusion of two populations of CB stem cells, between a 2 and 24 h interval, provides a promising strategy to improve the rate of success of CB transplants after allogeneic transplantation. It may also benefit autologous transplantation. The intravenous infusion of two populations of CB stem cells, within a 24 h interval, may be also be used for other sources of HSCs, such as BM HSCs and MPB HSCs, including HSCs expanded and propagated *in vitro*, for the treatment of haematologic diseases to improve the rate of success of HSC transplantation. It may also be applied to other types of stem cells, including liver stem cells, pancreatic stem cells, and neuronal stem cells, when administered intravenously to improve the treatment of a variety of diseases and injuries, ranging from liver diseases, diabetes and heart diseases to neurological diseases and injuries, brain tumours and MS [24-28].

Declaration of Interest

The author states no conflict of interest and has received no payment in preparation of this manuscript.

Acknowledgments

Reproduced with permission from Informa Healthcare: Taupin P. Transplantation of two populations of stem cells to improve engraftment: WO2008060932. Expert Opinion on Therapeutic Patents (2010) 20(9):1259-1263. Copyright 2010, Informa Healthcare (Informa UK Ltd).

Bibliography

Papers of special note have been highlighted as either of interest (*) or of considerable interest (**) to readers.

[1] Kurtzberg J, Laughlin M, Graham ML, et al. Placental blood as a source of hemat opoietic stem cells for transplantation into unrelated recipients. *N Engl J Med* 1996;335:157-66.

[2] Cohen Y, Nagler A. Umbilical cord blood transplantation: how, when and for whom? *Blood Rev* 2004;18:167-79.

[3] Thomas ED. History, current results, and research in marrow transplantation. *Perspect Biol Med* 1995;38:230-7.

[4] Wang JC, Doedens M, Dick JE. Primitive human hematopoietic cells are enriched in cord blood compared with adult bone marrow or mobilized peripheral blood as measured by the quantitative in vivo SCID-repopulating cell assay. *Blood* 1997;89:3919-24.

[5] Taupin P. OTI-010 Osiris Therapeutics/JCR Pharmaceuticals. *Curr Opin Investig Drugs* 2006;7:473-81.

[6] Rocha V, Labopin M, Sanz G, et al. Transplants of umbilical cord blood or bone marrow from unrelated donors in adults with acute leukemia. *N Engl J Med* 2004;351:2276-85.

[7] Takahashi S, Iseki T, Ooi J, et al. Single-institute comparative analysis of unrelated bone marrow transplantation and cord blood transplantation for adult patients with hematologic malignancies. *Blood* 2004;104:3813-20.

[8] Gluckman E, Rocha V, Arcese W, et al. Factors associated with outcomes of unrelated cord blood transplant: guidelines for donor choice. *Exp Hematol* 2004;32:397-407.

[9] Laughlin MJ, Barker J, Bambach B, et al. Hematopoietic engraftment and survival in adult recipients of umbilical-cord blood from unrelated donors. *N Engl J Med* 2001;344:1815-22.

[10] Long GD, Laughlin M, Madan B, et al. Unrelated umbilical cord blood transplantation in adult patients. *Biol Blood Marrow Transplant* 2003;9:772-80.

* The rate of mortality of patients with haematologic diseases treated with CB transplants is as high as 47% of patients dying prior to the 100 days mark after transplant.

[11] Szabolcs P, Niedzwiecki D. Immune reconstitution after unrelated cord blood transplantation. *Cytotherapy* 2007;9:111-22.

[12] Kurtzberg J, Prasad VK, Carter SL, et al. Results of the Cord Blood Transplantation Study (COBLT): clinical outcomes of unrelated donor umbilical cord blood transplantation in pediatric patients with hematologic malignancies. *Blood* 2008;112:4318-27.

[13] De Lima M, St John LS, Wieder ED, et al. Double-chimaerism after transplantation of two human leucocyte antigen mismatched, unrelated cord blood units. *Br J Haematol* 2002;119:773-6.

* The transplantation of double units of CB tissue improves the outcome of CB transplantation.

[14] Barker JN, Wagner JE. Umbilical cord blood transplantation: current practice and future innovations. *Crit Rev Oncol Hematol* 2003;48:35-43.

[15] Piacibello W, Sanavio F, Severino A, et al. Engraftment in nonobese diabetic severe combined immunodeficient mice of human CD34(+) cord blood cells after ex vivo expansion: evidence for the amplification and self-renewal of repopulating stem cells. *Blood* 1999;93:3736-49.

[16] Ballen K, Becker PS, Greiner D, et al. Effect of ex vivo cytokine treatment on human cord blood engraftment in NOD-scid mice. *Br J Haematol* 2000;108:629-40.

[17] Xia L, McDaniel JM, Yago T, et al. Surface fucosylation of human cord blood cells augments binding to P-selectin and E-selectin and enhances engraftment in bone marrow. *Blood* 2004;104:3091-6.

[18] McNiece IK, Almeida-Porada G, Shpall EJ, et al. Ex vivo expanded cord blood cells provide rapid engraftment in fetal sheep but lack long-term engrafting potential. *Exp Hematol* 2002;30:612-6.

* Optimal culture conditions for the expansion and propagation of CB stem cells *in vitro* for use in transplantation remain to be established.

[19] Hidalgo A, Frenette PS. Enforced fucosylation of neonatal CD34+ cells generates selectin ligands that enhance the initial interactions with microvessels but not homing to bone marrow. *Blood* 2005;105:567-75.

[20] Taupin P. Ex vivo fucosylation to improve the engraftment capability and therapeutic potential of human cord blood stem cells. *Drug Discov Today* 2010; In press.

[21] Brouwer A, Knook DL. The reticuloendothelial system and aging: a review. *Mech Ageing Dev* 1983;21:205-28.

[22] Shpall EJ, Quinones R, Giller R, et al. Transplantation of ex vivo expanded cord blood. *Biol Blood Marrow Transplant* 2002;8:368-76.

** The intravenous infusion of two populations of HSCs, several days or weeks after the first transplantation, does not improve the outcome of HSC transplantation when compared to subjects receiving only one infusion of cells.

[23] Fernandez MN, Regidor C, Cabrera R, et al. Unrelated umbilical cord blood transplants in adults: early recovery of neutrophils by supportive co-transplantation of a low

number of highly purified peripheral blood CD34+ cells from an HLA-haploidentical donor. *Exp Hematol* 2003;31:535-44.

[24] Brown AB, Yang W, Schmidt NO, et al. Intravascular delivery of neural stem cell lines to target intracranial and extracranial tumors of neural and non-neural origin. *Hum Gene Ther* 2003;14:1777-85.

[25] Pluchino S, Quattrini A, Brambilla E, et al. Injection of adult neurospheres induces recovery in a chronic model of multiple sclerosis. *Nature* 2003;422:688-94.

[26] Taupin P. The therapeutic potential of adult neural stem cells. *Curr Opin Mol Ther* 2006;8:225-31.

[27] Rice CM, Mallam EA, Whone AL, et al. Safety and feasibility of autologous bonemarrow cellular therapy in relapsing-progressive multiple sclerosis. *Clin Pharmacol Ther 2010;* In press.

[28] Wang J, Zhang S, Rabinovich B, et al. Human CD34+ cells in experimental myocardial infarction. Long-term survival, sustained functional improvement, and mechanism of action. *Circ Res 2010;* In press.

Chapter XIV

Ex Vivo Fucosylation of Stem Cells to Improve Engraftment[*]

Abstract

Background

The application is in the field of haematopoietic stem cell (HSC) and umbilical cord blood (CB) transplantation.

Objective

It aims at determining an enzymatic procedure to improve the engraftment of CB stem cells to the bone marrow (BM) as well as the rate of success of CB transplantation.

Methods

Human CB stem cells were treated with $\alpha 1$ - 3 fucosyltransferase VI (FTVI) for 30 min *ex vivo* prior to transplantation. Human CB stem cells were administered intravenously in irradiated nonobese diabetic/severe combined immune deficiency (NOD/SCID) mice.

---

[*] Patent details
Title: Haematopoietic stem cells treated by *in vitro* fucosylation and methods of use
Assignee: Oklahoma Medical Research Foundation
Inventors: Xia L and McEver RP
Filing date: 30/01/2004
Publication date: 21/10/2004
Publication no.: WO2004094619

Results

Treatment of CB stem cells with FTVI improves their engraftment in the BM of NOD/SCID mice.

Conclusion

Treatment of CB stem cells with FTVI, *ex vivo* prior to transplantation, may reduce the delay of engraftment of CB stem cells to the BM and the risk of early infections associated with CB transplants, particularly in adults. It may improve the outcome and rate of success of CB transplantation. The application claims the use of fucosyltransferase for improving the engraftment of CB HSCs to the BM for the treatment of haematologic diseases. The procedure may be used to improve the engraftment of HSCs from other sources and other types of stem cells, on transplantation, particularly when administered intravenously.

Introduction

Haematopoietic stem cells (HSCs) are the self-renewing multipotent cells that generate the main phenotypes of the blood and immune system. The transplantation of HSCs is used to treat patients with malignant and non-malignant haematologic and bone marrow (BM) diseases, such as leukaemia, lymphoma, myeloma, Fanconi anemia, myelodysplasia and thalassemia [1]. Three sources of tissues are available for HSC transplantation to treat patients with haematopoietic diseases: adult BM, mobilised peripheral blood (MPB) and umbilical cord blood (CB) [2,3]. The shortage of human leukocyte antigen (HLA)-matched donors is the main limitation of BM and MPB registries for HSC allogeneic transplantation.

CB tissues elicit a higher potential to reconstitute the recipient BM than BM and MPB transplants. This is because they contain three to six times more repopulating haematopoietic progenitor and stem cells than the BM and MPB [4].

CB tissues are depleted of immune cells, particularly of T lymphocytes. The depletion in immune cells of the CB results in low risk of severe graft-versus-host disease (GVHD) in patients treated with CB transplants. GVHD is the immunological reaction that occurs when immunologically competent cells are transplanted into a host whose immune system is compromised [5]. The depletion in immune cells of the CB allows for greater disparity of HLA compatibility when matching donors-recipients with CB tissues compared to BM and MPB tissues. As a result, it permits to treat potentially more patients, particularly minority groups, who are mostly under-represented in registries. The rate of success of CB transplantation is correlated with the nucleated cell dose and the age of the patients; the higher the nucleated cell dose in the transplant and the younger the age of the patient, the higher the rate of success of CB transplantation [6,7]. CB tissues are characterised by low nucleated cell doses and are considered a standard source of tissue for paediatric transplants of HSCs [8,9]. CB transplantations for the treatment of haematologic diseases have been performed successfully in children and in adults [10,11]. However, CB transplantation is characterised by a high rate of morbidity and mortality, particularly in adults. The rate of mortality of patients with haematologic diseases treated with CB transplants is as high as 47% of patients dying prior to the 100 days mark after transplant [12]. Low cell doses, graft failure, delayed engraftment, poor engraftment and early infections are the main limitations of the outcome of CB transplants for treating haematologic diseases, particularly in adults, but also in children [13,14].

With the aim of improving the outcome of CB transplantation for treating haematologic diseases, several approaches are being devised and considered; among them, the transplantation of multiple units of CB tissue and the expansion and propagation of CB stem cells *in vitro* [15-17]. The transplantation of double units of CB tissue improves the outcome of CB transplantation, but does not shorten the delay of engraftment. In addition, the conditions of transplantation are still suboptimal. Optimal culture conditions for the expansion and propagation of CB stem cells *in vitro* for use in transplantation remain to be established [18,19].

The application claims the fucosylation of CB stem cells *ex vivo* to improve the delayed and poor engraftment of CB stem cells to the BM and the outcome of CB transplantation for treating patients with haematologic diseases [20]. The application may be used to improve the engraftment of other sources of HSCs, such as HSCs of the BM and MPB, for transplantation to treat patients with haematologic diseases. It may also be used to improve the engraftment of other types of stem cells, such as embryonic stem cells, liver stem cells, mesenchymal stem cells and neural stem cells, for cellular therapy.

Biology and Action

In Vivo and In Vitro Studies

Human umbilical CB tissues were obtained from full-term vaginal deliveries. Populations of $CD34^+$ and $CD34^+$ $CD^{38-/low}$ haematopoietic progenitor and stem cells were isolated and purified from the CB tissues by fluorescence activated cell sorting. Isolated and purified cells were incubated with fucosyltransferase VI (FTVI) and GDP fucose for 30 min *ex vivo* prior to transplantation. Cells were washed and administered by intravenous injections in nonobese diabetic/severe combined immune deficiency (NOD/SCID) mice at a dose of 0.01×10^8 nucleated cells/kg of body weight. Cells were assayed on P- and E-selectin binding assays *in vitro*.

Fucosyltransferases

At least five different types of fucosyltransferase have been identified and characterized in humans (FTIII – VII) [21]. They fucosylate their substrates when GDP fucose is present. FTVI and FTVII elicit $\alpha 1$ - 3 fucosyltransferase activity [22,23]. The enzymes are present on the cell surface of various cell types.

Treatment of human CB $CD34^+$ and $CD34^+$ $CD^{38-/low}$ haematopoietic progenitor and stem cells, by FTVI, enhanced the binding of the cells to fluid-phase P- and E-selectins and improved cell rolling on P- and E-selectins under flow *in vitro*. The irradiated NOD/SCID mice that were administered with fucosylated CB CD34$^+$ cells elicit two to threefold more CD45$^+$ human derived haematopoietic cells in their BM and MPB than mice that received sham-treated CB HSCs, as revealed by flow cytometry studies.

The treatment of human CB CD34+ haematopoietic progenitor and stem cells *ex vivo*, by FTVI, increases the yield of fucosylation of the N-glycan determinants on the surface of the cells. It results in enhanced binding of CB HSCs to fluid-phase P- and E-selectins and improved cell rolling on P- and E-selectins under flow *in vitro*, and in improved rolling of the CB HSCs on P- and E-selectins on the surface of endothelial cells and in the homing of the cells to the BM *in vivo* [20].

Expert Opinion

The fucosylation of human CB haematopoietic progenitor and stem cells *ex vivo*, by FTVI, enhances the binding of the treated cells to P- and E-selectins *in vitro*. It improves their homing and engraftment to the BM *in vivo* after intravenous transplantation in irradiated NOD/SCID mice [20]. Homing is the process of migration of stem cells to their niches, the microenvironment that controls their developmental potential [24]. The migration of HSCs to their niches in the BM contributes to the replenishment and maintenance of their pool in the tissue, as well as their recruitment and mobilisation during injuries [25]. It involves the rolling of the haematopoietic progenitor and stem cells through the blood vessels and across the endothelial vasculature, and complex molecular and cellular interactions involving particularly P- and E-selectins. The process of homing of HSCs to the BM is a key factor for therapies involving the transplantation of HSCs when administered intravenously. Transplanted cells use the same physiological path to reconstitute, regenerate and repair the pool of HSCs of the patients.

P- and E-selectins are membrane bound C-type lectins expressed on endothelial cells and BM vessels and involved in the homing of HSCs to the BM [26]. They bind to ligands, selectin glycoprotein ligands (SGLs), which are cell-surface proteoglycan conjugated ligands. HSCs express SGLs on their surface [27,28]. SGLs elicit a characteristic N-terminal glycan determinant: an N-terminal glycan capped with a sialylated Lewis x (sLex) and a site for fucosylation. The N-terminal glycan determinant of SGLs corresponds to the binding site of haematopoietic cells to P- and E-selectins [29].

In contrast to human BM CD34+ haematopoietic progenitor and stem cells, human CB CD34$^+$ cells elicit poor rolling activities on endothelial cells and BM microvessels and poor homing and engraftment capabilities to the BM after intravenous transplantation in irradiated NOD/SCID mice [30]. In contrast to human BM CD34+ haematopoietic progenitor and stem cells, human CB CD34+ cells express forms of SGLs that lack proper N-glycan determinant, sLex and the site for fucosylation. Hence, human BM CD34+ haematopoietic progenitor and stem cells home and engraft efficiently to the BM of irradiated NOD/SCID mice through their rolling and binding interactions with P- and E-selectins on endothelial cells and in BM vessels, in contrast to human CB CD34$^+$ cells. The lack of proper N-glycan determinant of SGLs, sLex and the site for fucosylation on the surface of human CB CD34+ haematopoietic progenitor and stem cells underlies their poor homing and engraftment capabilities in the BM of irradiated NOD/SCID mice, and defect of the binding of SGLs to P- and E-selectins [30].

The fucosylation of human CB haematopoietic progenitor and stem cells *ex vivo*, by FTVI, improves their homing and engraftment to the BM *in vivo* after intravenous transplantation in irradiated NOD/SCID mice. The improvement of the homing and engraftment to the BM of the human CB HSCs fucosylated *ex vivo* results from more effective rolling interactions of the SGLs of treated cells with P- and E-selectins on endothelial cells and in BM vessels of the host, through the restoration of the binding properties of SGLs and of other sites on CB cells by the fucosylation [20]. Delayed and poor engraftments are major limitations for the outcome of CB transplants for treating haematologic diseases [13,14]. Improved engraftment optimises the cell dose required for successful CB transplantation therapy as well as reduces the risks of early infections in patients, thereby, improving the outcome of CB transplantation, particularly in adults, but also in children. It is proposed to fucosylate CB tissue *ex vivo*, prior to transplantation, to improve the rate of success of CB transplantation for treating patients with haematologic diseases. *Ex vivo* fucosylation may be used to improve the engraftment of other sources of HSCs, such as HSCs of the BM and MPB, to treat patients with haematologic diseases. It may also be applied to improve the engraftment of other types of stem cells, such as embryonic stem cells, liver stem cells, mesenchymal stem cells and neural stem cells, particularly when administered intravenously to improve the treatment of a variety of diseases and injuries, ranging from liver diseases, diabetes and heart diseases to neurological diseases and injuries, including neurodegenerative diseases and spinal cord injuries [31-35]. However, the therapeutic potential of *ex vivo* fucosylation of stem cells, including of CB stem cells, remains to be confirmed and validated [29,36].

Declaration of Interest

The author states no conflict of interest and has received no payment in preparation of this manuscript.

Acknowledgments

Reproduced with permission from Informa Healthcare: Taupin P. *Ex vivo* fucosylation of stem cells to improve engraftment: WO2004094619. Expert Opinion on Therapeutic Patents (2010) 20(9):1265-1269. Copyright 2010, Informa Healthcare (Informa UK Ltd).

Bibliography

Papers of special note have been highlighted as either of interest (*) or of considerable interest (**) to readers.

[1]   Thomas ED. History, current results, and research in marrow transplantation. *Perspect Biol Med* 1995;38:230-7.

[2] Kurtzberg J, Laughlin M, Graham ML, et al. Placental blood as a source of hematopoietic stem cells for transplantation into unrelated recipients. *N Engl J Med* 1996;335:157-66.

[3] Cohen Y, Nagler A. Umbilical cord blood transplantation: how, when and for whom? *Blood Rev* 2004;18:167-79.

[4] Wang JC, Doedens M, Dick JE. Primitive human hematopoietic cells are enriched in cord blood compared with adult bone marrow or mobilized peripheral blood as measured by the quantitative in vivo SCID-repopulating cell assay. *Blood* 1997;89:3919-24.

* CB tissues contain three to six times more repopulating haematopoietic progenitor and stem cells than BM and MPB.

[5] Taupin P. OTI-010 Osiris Therapeutics/JCR Pharmaceuticals. *Curr Opin Investig Drugs* 2006;7:473-81.

[6] Gluckman E, Rocha V, Arcese W, et al. Factors associated with outcomes of unrelated cord blood transplant: guidelines for donor choice. *Exp Hematol* 2004;32:397-407.

[7] Laughlin MJ, Barker J, Bambach B, et al. Hematopoietic engraftment and survival in adult recipients of umbilical-cord blood from unrelated donors. *N Engl J Med* 2001;344:1815-22.

[8] Rocha V, Cornish J, Sievers EL, et al. Comparison of outcomes of unrelated bone marrow and umbilical cord blood transplants in children with acute leukemia. *Blood* 2001;97:2962-71.

[9] Ballen K, Becker PS, Greiner D, et al. Effect of ex vivo cytokine treatment on human cord blood engraftment in NOD-scid mice. *Br J Haematol* 2000;108:629-40.

[10] Rocha V, Labopin M, Sanz G, et al. Transplants of umbilical cord blood or bone marrow from unrelated donors in adults with acute leukemia. *N Engl J Med* 2004;351:2276-85.

[11] Takahashi S, Iseki T, Ooi J, et al. Single-institute comparative analysis of unrelated bone marrow transplantation and cord blood transplantation for adult patients with hematologic malignancies. *Blood* 2004;104:3813-20.

[12] Long GD, Laughlin M, Madan B, et al. Unrelated umbilical cord blood transplantation in adult patients. *Biol Blood Marrow Transplant* 2003;9:772-80.

* The rate of mortality of patients with haematologic diseases treated with CB transplants is as high as 47% of patients dying prior to the 100 days mark after transplant.

[13] Szabolcs P, Niedzwiecki D. Immune reconstitution after unrelated cord blood transplantation. *Cytotherapy* 2007;9:111-22.

[14] Kurtzberg J, Prasad VK, Carter SL, et al. Results of the Cord Blood Transplantation Study (COBLT): clinical outcomes of unrelated donor umbilical cord blood transplantation in pediatric patients with hematologic malignancies. *Blood* 2008;112:4318-27.

[15] De Lima M, St John LS, Wieder ED, et al. Double-chimaerism after transplantation of two human leucocyte antigen mismatched, unrelated cord blood units. *Br J Haematol* 2002;119:773-6.

* The transplantation of double units of CB tissue improves the outcome of CB transplantation.

[16] Piacibello W, Sanavio F, Severino A, et al. Engraftment in nonobese diabetic severe combined immunodeficient mice of human CD34(+) cord blood cells after ex vivo

expansion: evidence for the amplification and self-renewal of repopulating stem cells. *Blood* 1999;93:3736-49.

[17]   Ballen K, Becker PS, Greiner D, et al. Effect of ex vivo cytokine treatment on human cord blood engraftment in NOD-scid mice. *Br J Haematol* 2000;108:629-40.

[18]   McNiece IK, Almeida-Porada G, Shpall EJ, et al. Ex vivo expanded cord blood cells provide rapid engraftment in fetal sheep but lack long-term engrafting potential. *Exp Hematol* 2002;30:612-6.

[19]   Barker JN, Wagner JE. Umbilical cord blood transplantation: current practice and future innovations. *Crit Rev Oncol Hematol* 2003;48:35-43.

[20]   Xia L, McDaniel JM, Yago T, et al. Surface fucosylation of human cord blood cells augments binding to P-selectin and E-selectin and enhances engraftment in bone marrow. *Blood* 2004;104:3091-6.

**   The fucosylation of human CB haematopoietic progenitor and stem cells ex vivo, by FTVI, improves their homing and engraftment to the BM in vivo, after intravenous transplantation in irradiated NOD/SCID mice.

[21]   Miyoshi E, Moriwaki K, Nakagawa T. Biological function of fucosylation in cancer biology. *J Biochem* 2008;143:725-9.

[22]   Weninger W, Ulfman LH, Cheng G, et al. Specializedcontributions by α (1,3)-fucosyltransferase-IV and FucT-VII during leukocyte rolling in dermal microvessels. *Immunity 2000;12:665-76.*

[23]   Bengtson P, Lundblad A, Larson G, et al. Polymorphonuclear leukocytes from individuals carrying the G329A mutation in the 1,3-fucosyltransferase VII gene (FUT7) roll on E- and P-selectins. *J Immunol* 2002;169:3940-6.

[24]   Taupin P. Adult neural stem cells, neurogenic niches and cellular therapy. *Stem Cell Rev* 2006;2:213-19.

[25]   Lymperi S, Ferraro F, Scadden DT. The HSC niche concept has turned 31. Has our knowledge matured? *Ann NY Acad Sci* 2010;1192:12-8.

[26]   Mazo IB, Gutierrez-Ramos JC, Frenette PS, et al. Hematopoietic progenitor cell rolling in bone marrow microvessels: parallel contributions by endothelial selectins and vascular cell adhesion molecule. *J Exp Med* 1998;188:465-74.

[27]   Katayama Y, Hidalgo A, Furie BC, et al. PSGL-1 participates in E-selectin-mediated progenitor homing to bone marrow: evidence for cooperation between E-selectin ligands and alpha 4 integrin. *Blood* 2003;102:2060-7.

[28]   McEver RP. Selectins: lectins that initiate cell adhesion under flow. *Curr Opin Cell Biol* 2002;14:581-6.

[29]   Hidalgo A, Frenette PS. Enforced fucosylation of neonatal CD34+ cells generates selectin ligands that enhance the initial interactions with microvessels but not homing to bone marrow. *Blood* 2005;105:567-75.

**   Forced fucosylation of CB HSCs might improve rolling on selectins but not increase entry into the BM.

[30]   Hidalgo A, Weiss LA, Frenette PS. Functional selectin ligands mediating human CD34+ cell interactions with bone marrow endothelium are enhanced postnatally. *J Clin Invest* 2002;110:559-69.

**   In contrast to human BM CD34+ haematopoietic progenitor and stem cells, human CB CD34+ cells elicit poor rolling activities on endothelial cells and BM microvessels and poor homing and engraftment capabilities to the BM, after intravenous transplantation in irradiated NOD/SCID mice.

[31] Brown AB, Yang W, Schmidt NO, et al. Intravascular delivery of neural stem cell lines to target intracranial and extracranial tumors of neural and non-neural origin. *Hum Gene Ther* 2003;14:1777-85.

[32] Pluchino S, Quattrini A, Brambilla E, et al. Injection of adult neurospheres induces recovery in a chronic model of multiple sclerosis. *Nature* 2003;422:688-94.

[33] Taupin P. The therapeutic potential of adult neural stem cells. *Curr Opin Mol Ther* 2006;8:225-31.

[34] Rice CM, Mallam EA, Whone AL, et al. Safety and feasibility of autologous bone marrow cellular therapy in relapsing-progressive multiple sclerosis. *Clin Pharmacol Ther 2010;* In press.

[35] Wang J, Zhang S, Rabinovich B, et al. Human CD34+ Cells in experimental myocardial infarction. Long-term survival, sustained functional improvement, and mechanism of action. *Circ Res* 2010; In press.

[36] Taupin P. Ex vivo fucosylation to improve the engraftment capability and therapeutic potential of human cord blood stem cells. *Drug Discov* Today 2010;15:698-699..

Chapter XV

Thirteen Compounds Promoting Oligodendrocyte Progenitor Cell Differentiation and Remyelination for Treating Multiple Sclerosis

Abstract

Background

The application is in the field of cellular therapy and neural repair

Objective

It aims at identifying and characterizing compounds and molecules that promote the differentiation of oligodendrocyte progenitor cells and remyelination of the nervous system.

Methods

Library of compounds and molecules were screened on a series of assays specifically designed and developed to assess the activity and potency of compounds and molecules on the differentiation of oligodendrocyte progenitor cells and on remyelination of nerve cells in in vitro and in vivo models, such as cultures of neural progenitor and stem cells, cerebellar organotypic cultures, the zebrafish and the cuprizone-mediated demyelination mouse models.

Results

In all, 13 compounds were identified and characterized, after a secondary screening, for inducing the differentiation of oligodendrocyte progenitor cells and for promoting myelination and remyelination in vitro and in vivo.

Conclusion

The 13 compounds, promoting the differentiation of oligodendrocyte progenitor cells and myelination of nerve cells, may be used for the treatment of multiple sclerosis (MS) and other myelin-related disorders. The application claims the use of the compounds to promote the differentiation of oligodendrocyte progenitor cells and endogenous remyelination for the treatment of demyelinating diseases alone or in combination with other agents and drugs, such as immunomodulatory, immunosuppressive, neuroprotective and neuroregenerative agents.

Introduction

MS is an autoimmune and inflammatory disease of the central nervous system (CNS). It is a complex neurological disease characterized by chronic inflammatory demyelination, axonal injuries and neurodegeneration in the CNS – the hallmarks of the disease – causing neurological disabilities [1]. The onset of the disease occurs usually in young adults and the life expectancy of patients with MS is 5 – 10 years lower than that of unaffected individuals. It is the most common form of demyelinating disease and myelin-related disorder which includes acquired disorders, such as transverse myelitis, chronic inflammatory demyelinating polyneuropathy and Guillain-Barre syndrome, and genetic inherited disorders, such as leukodystrophies. MS affects 2.5 million individuals worldwide, including 300,000 in the North America. There is currently no cure for MS [2].

As a result of autoimmune and inflammatory attacks, the oligodendrocytes of the CNS are destroyed in individuals with MS [3]. Oligodendrocytes are generated during development from a common glial progenitor cells. A population of oligodendrocyte progenitor cells remains throughout adulthood and plays a role in regenerating the myelin in the damaged and injured CNS. Oligodendrocyte progenitor cells are characterized by molecular markers, such as the platelet-derived growth factor (PDGF)-alpha receptor, the NG2 chondroitin sulfate proteoglycan and the ganglioside GD3. Immature/premyelinating oligodendrocytes are characterized by the molecular marker O4. Mature oligodendrocytes are characterized by molecular markers, such as the proteolipid protein (PLP), the myelin basic protein (MBP) and the myelin oligodendrocyte glycoprotein (MOG). The destruction of oligodendrocytes in MS leads to demyelination and scarring and to nerve damages, including axonal injuries and neuronal cell death, in the CNS. In MS, the demyelination affects the saltatory conduction, which speeds axonal electric impulse, causing MS-associated symptoms and increasing disabilities [4]. In individuals with MS, the population of oligodendrocyte progenitor cells in the adult CNS fails to repair and compensate for the myelin loss, leading to MS symptoms and pathology.

MS and myelin-related disorders are complex multifactorial diseases [3]. Treatment and cure for the diseases involve the development of compounds and drugs and a combination of therapies targeting the various aspects of the diseases, such as axonal degeneration, demyelination, immunomodulation, inflammation and neurodegeneration [5-9]. The application aims at identifying and characterizing compounds and molecules that promote the differentiation of oligodendrocyte progenitor cells and remyelination of nerve cells of the CNS for developing treatments and cures for MS and myelin-related disorders.

Chemistry and Synthesis

Seven classes of compounds have been identified and characterized for promoting the differentiation of oligodendrocyte progenitor cells and remyelination of nerve cells.

Compounds selected from the following general structures as in Figure 1, wherein R1, R2, R3, R4, R5, R6 and R7 consist of a hydrogen, alky, alkenyl, alkynyl, aryl, alkaryl, aralkyl, halohydroxyl, alkoxy, alkenyloxy, alkynyloxy, aryloxy, acyloxy alkoxycarbonyl, aryloxycarbonyl, halocarbonyl, alkylcarbonato, arylcarbonato, carboxy, carboxylato, carbamoyl, amino, substituted amino, alkylamido, arylamido, imino, alkylimino, arylimino, nitro and nitroso.

Compounds selected from the groups as given in Figure 2A, B.

The activities of these compounds have been identified and characterized by primary and secondary screenings on a series of assays in vitro and in vivo, specifically designed and developed.

Biology and Action

Culture of Oligodendrocyte Progenitor Cells

Oligodendrocyte progenitor cells were generated from fetal-derived neurospheres. The neurospheres were prepared and propagated from the cerebrum of 14.5 day embryos of wild-type mice and of PLP-enhanced green fluorescence protein (PLP-EGFP) transgenic mice in the presence of 10 ng/ml EGF, as previously described [10-13]. The generation and differentiation of oligodendrocyte progenitor cells from neurospheres was performed in the presence of 10 ng/ml PDGF and basic fibroblast growth factor (bFGF) for 24 h. Oligodendrocyte progenitor cells were further differentiated to mature oligodendrocytes in the presence of 1 ng/ml PDGF and bFGF. Differentiation of oligodendrocytes was scored under a phase contrast microscope using a 1 - 4 scale, such as 1 and 2: bipolar to tripolar cells, 3: cells with more than three processes and 4: cells showing numerous processes and membranous structures. Differentiation of oligodendrocytes was also assessed by immunocytology and confocal microscopy and by western blot analysis for PLP and MBP.

Cerebellar Organotypic Cultures and Lysolecithin Demyelination

Using 400 μm thick sections, postnatal day 4 - 7 cerebellar of wild-type mice or EGFP transgenic mice were prepared using a Leica VTlOOOS vibratome. The sections were maintained for 4 - 10 days before applying 0.5 mg/ml lysolecithin (r-monoacyl-L-3-glyccrylphosphorylcholine) for 17 h to induce demyelination. Demyelination and remyelination were assessed and monitored by GFP fluorescence and immunohistology for myelin-axonal proteins and confocal microscopy. Increased fluorescence in treated cerebellar organotypic cultures, after lysolecithin treatment was indicative of oligodendrocyte maturation and was quantified under the microscope.

Zebrafish Model

Transgenic-PLP-EGFP zebrafish were raised and maintained, as previously described [13]. Zebrafish embryos were processed for histology by standard procedures.

Cuprizone-mediated Demyelination Mouse Model

Mice were prepared and treated with cuprizone, as previously described [14]. The mice brains were prepared and processed for histology and immunohistochemistry by standard procedures. Compounds were administered by intraperiteonal injection.

Other Assays

Cellular toxicity was assessed by MTT assay, immunocytochemistry and western blot analysis for markers, such as 5-bromodeoxyuridine (a marker of DNA synthesis [15]), PLP, MBP, MOG and b-tubulin (a marker of immature neuronal cells). Black and gold staining of brain tissue was to detect total myelin. There was mass spectrometry detection of compounds in blood plasma and brain homogenates of mice.

Drug Screenings

Primary Screening

A library of 13,920 small molecules was screened (drug-like organic molecules with molecular mass in a range of 250 - 550 kDa dissolved in DMSO at a concentration of 5 mg/ml or 10 mM, Chembridge library) in cultured oligodendrocyte progenitor cells, in a 96-well plate (high-throughput screening). Cells were scored for oligodendrocyte progenitor cell differentiation and maturation in the presence of compounds.

Secondary Screening

Selected compounds from the primary screening were characterized for their activity on the differentiation of oligodendrocyte progenitor cells and on the remyelination of nerve cells on cerebellar organotypic cultures after lysolecithin treatment, Zebrafish model and the cuprizone-mediated demyelination mouse model.

In all, 0.01% of the compounds and molecules screened on the primary screening assay promote the differentiation and maturation of oligodendrocyte progenitor cells in vitro, 87.2% have no apparent effect and 12.8% induce cell death. The secondary screening leads to the identification and characterization of 13 compounds that promote the differentiation of oligodendrocyte progenitor cells and the remyelination of the nervous system in cerebellar organotypic cultures and in Zebrafish and mouse models. Among them, two lead compounds, A (C20 H24 N2 O4 S) and B (C12 H8 F2 N2 04 S), and a third one, as a result of database search for structural analogs and experimental functional analysis, A-7 (C21 H26 N2 O2), were identified and selected for in-depth studies and characterization. These compounds elicit dose-dependent activities in promoting the differentiation of oligodendrocyte progenitor cells and the remyelination of the nervous system. They elicit activities at concentrations ranging from 0.01 to 0.1 μM.

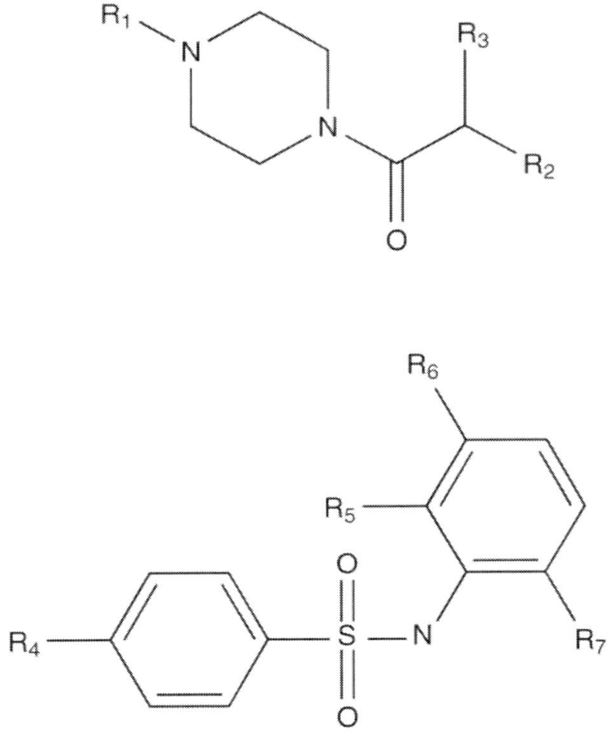

Figure 1. Compounds wherein R1, R2, R3, R4, R5, R6 and R7 consist of a hydrogen, alky, alkenyl, alkynyl, aryl, alkaryl, aralkyl, halo hydroxyl, alkoxy, alkenyloxy, alkynyloxy, aryloxy, acyloxy alkoxycarbonyl, aryloxycarbonyl, halocarbonyl, alkylcarbonato, arylcarbonato, carboxy, carboxylato, carbamoyl, amino, substituted amino, alkylamido, arylamido, imino, alkylimino, arylimino, nitro, nitroso.

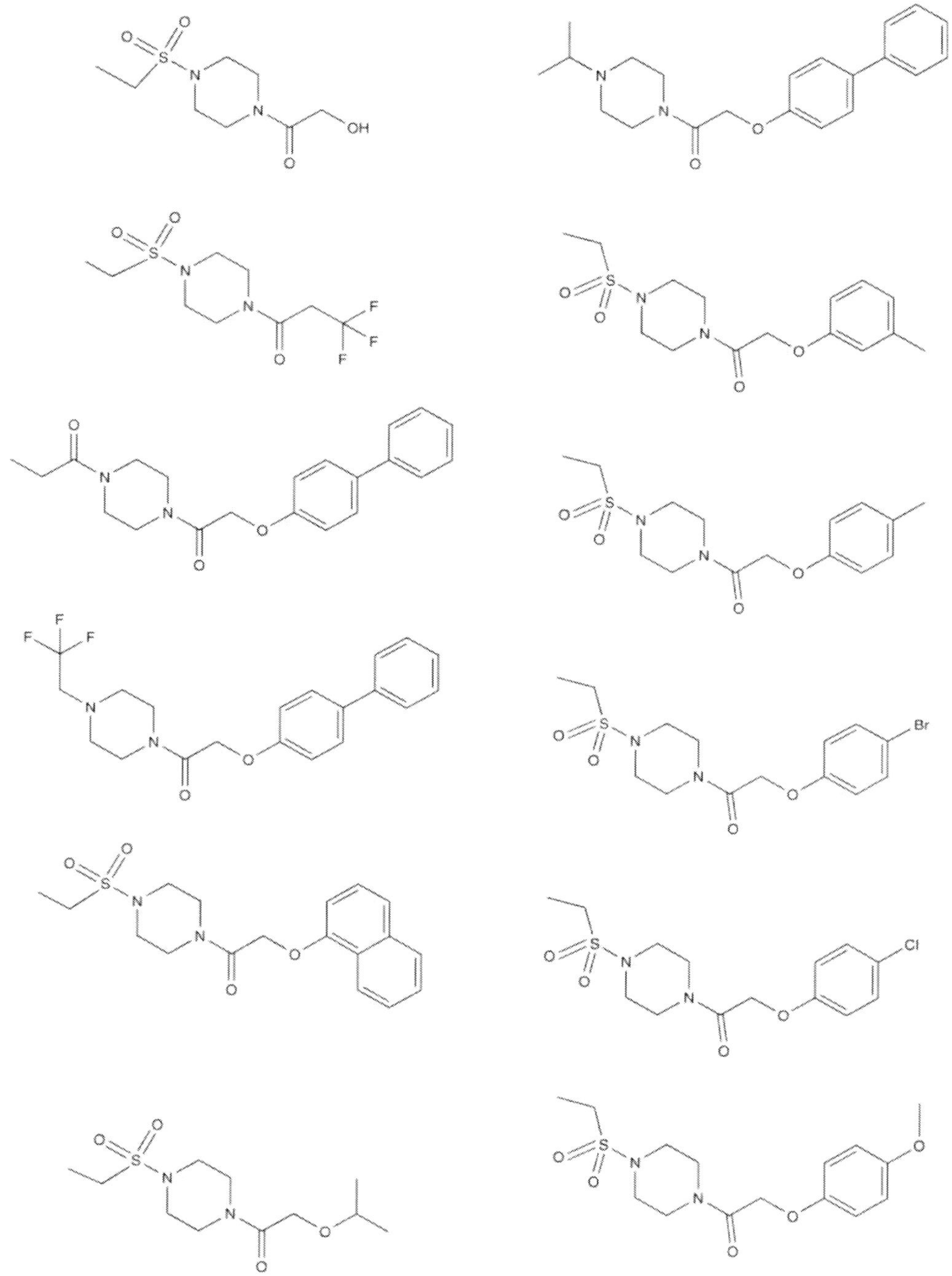

Figure 2. (Continued)

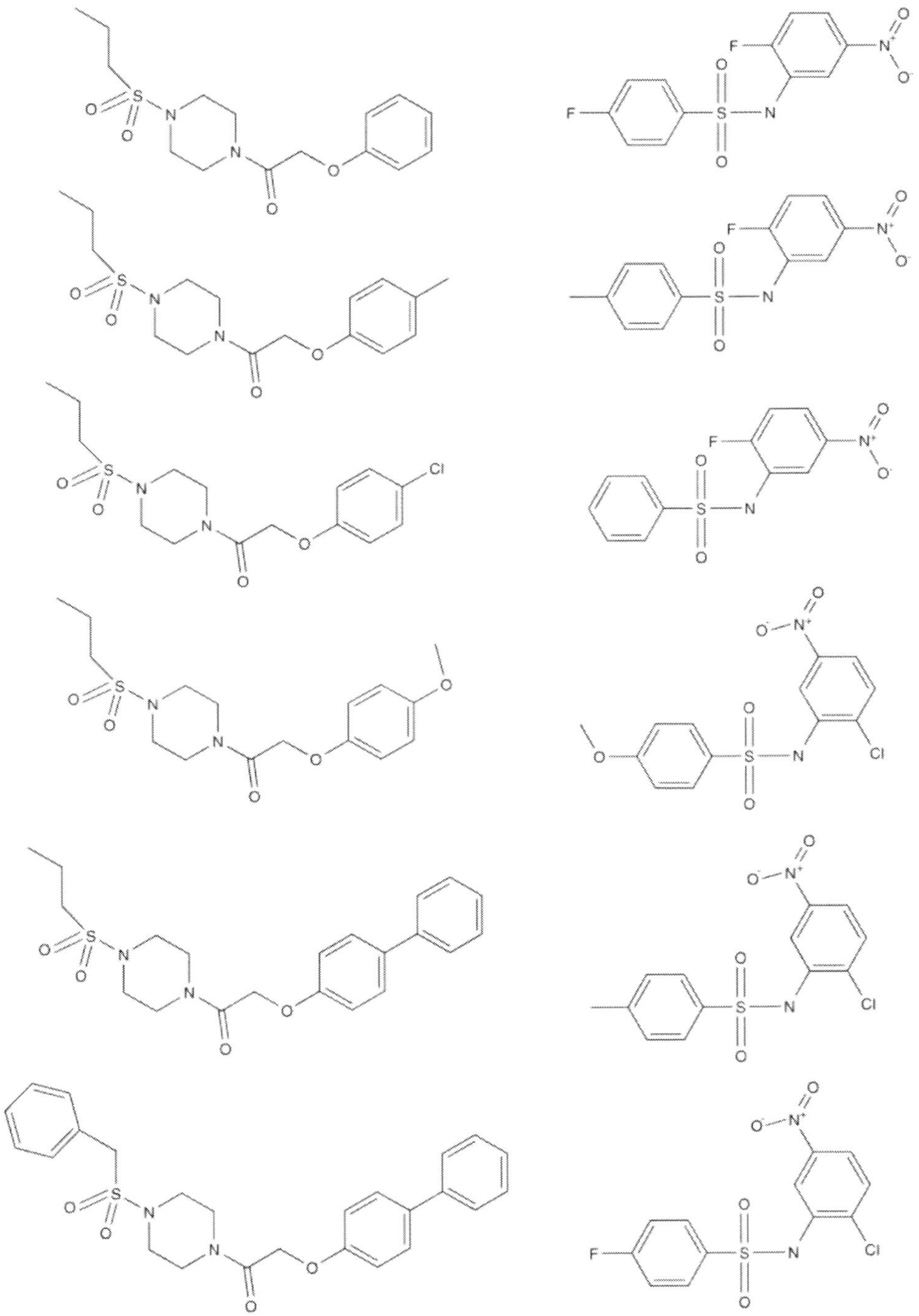

Figure 2. A. and B. Generic formula of compounds from patent WO2010054307.

Expert Opinion

The application claims the identification and characterization of 13 compounds and molecules after screening on multiple in vitro and in vivo assays – such as neural progenitor and stem cells in vitro, cerebellar organotypic cultures and zebrafish and mouse models in vivo – that promote the differentiation of oligodendrocyte progenitor cells and induce endogenous remyelination of nerve cells. Particularly, the application reports three compounds that have been identified and characterized in depth, compounds A, B and A-7. The characterization that compounds A and A-7 are present in the blood plasma and in the brain homogenates of mice, as shown by mass spectrometry studies, and that they induce the proliferation of oligodendrocyte progenitor cells in the brain of mice indicates that the compounds cross the blood-brain barrier (BBB) and mediate remyelination in vivo by promoting the proliferation and differentiation of oligodendrocyte progenitor cells. The activities of the compounds have been identified and characterized as being mediated through the protein kinase B, a second messenger involved in oligodendrocyte progenitor cell differentiation in vitro and in vivo. This shows that the multi-pronged strategy reported in the application allows identifying and discovering, with a high degree of confidence, compounds and molecules that target oligodendrocyte progenitor cells in vitro and in vivo and that the identified and characterized compounds and molecules promote the differentiation of oligodendrocyte progenitor cells and induce endogenous remyelination of nerve cells. The identified and characterized compounds and molecules represent new candidate drugs for treating MS and myelin-related disorders.

MS is a complex multifactorial disease and there is a need to discover and develop new drugs and treatments for the disease. To this endeavor, discovering and developing drugs and compounds that promote oligodendrocyte progenitor cell differentiation and remyelination of the CNS offer new opportunities and perspectives to target an aspect of the disease for treating MS and myelin-related disorders that have not been addressed thoroughly before. MS is an autoimmune and inflammatory disease and approaches to treat MS primarily focus on developing anti-inflammatory and neuroprotective treatments. The population of oligodendrocyte progenitor cells that remains in the CNS throughout adulthood represents a target for compounds and drugs aiming at repairing and restoring the myelin sheath and, therefore, to discover and develop new drugs and treatments for MS and other myelin-related disorders. Alternatively, oligodendrocyte progenitor cells or mature oligodendrocytes may be transplanted to repair and restore the myelin sheath [16]. However, this latter strategy would require multiple transplantation sites, limiting its effectiveness and clinical applicability. Hence, the compounds reported in the patent application may lead to new drugs and therapies for MS and myelin-related disorders.

However, further studies remain to be conducted before these compounds and molecules be brought to clinical trials and therapy. Among them, the characterization of their activities and potencies in other animal models of MS and related-myelin disorders, such as the experimental allergic encephalitis model, and in human models of neural progenitor and stem cells and of oligodendrocyte progenitor cells in vitro [17,18]. In the application, the compounds and molecules have been identified and characterized in a fetal-derived model of neural progenitor and stem cells. Because the onset of the disease occurs usually in young adults, it would be relevant to study and characterize the activity and potency of the compounds on neural progenitor and stem cells and on oligodendrocyte progenitor cells from the adult brain isolated and characterized in vitro. Neurogenesis occurs in the adult brain and neural progenitor and stem cells have been identified and characterized from the adult CNS, including from human biopsies and post mortem tissues [10,19-21]. The stimulation of endogenous neural progenitor or stem cells and the transplantation of adult-derived neural progenitor and stem cells are considered for repairing and restoring the degenerated or injured nerve pathways. Hence, adult-derived neural progenitor and stem cells offer new avenues and opportunities for the treatment of MS and myelin-related disorders, as well as to discover and develop novel drugs and compounds for treating neurological diseases and disorders, particularly MS [22-27].

In all, drugs and compounds that promote the differentiation of endogenous oligodendrocyte progenitor cells and induce the remyelination of nerve cells offer new opportunities for treating MS and myelin-related disorders. MS is a multifactorial disease and oligodendrocyte progenitor cell differentiation agents are mandated not only to promote remyelination, but also to treat and cure MS and myelin-related disorders. They may be used alone or in combination with other drugs, such as anti-inflammatory, immunemodulatory, neuro-protective and neuro-regenerative treatments. Future investigations will be needed to bring these compounds to clinical trials and therapy. Among them, the cytotoxicity, metabolism and pharmacokinetic of the drugs, the investigations in other preclinical models and the testing of the activities and potencies of the compounds on human-derived and on adult-derived oligodendrocyte progenitor cells will need to be addressed. Future directions will involve characterizing the potential of adult neurogenesis and neural stem cells for treating MS and other myelin-related disorders.

Declaration of Interest

P Taupin declares no conflict of interest and has received no payment in preparation of this manuscript.

Acknowledgments

Reproduced with permission from Informa Healthcare: Taupin P. Thirteen compounds promoting oligodendrocyte progenitor cell differentiation and remyelination for treating multiple sclerosis: WO2010054307. Expert Opinion on Therapeutic Patents (2010) 20(12):1767-1773. Copyright 2010, Informa Healthcare (Informa UK Ltd).

Bibliography

Papers of special note have been highlighted as either of interest (*) or of considerable interest (**) to readers.

[1]   Giuliani F, Yong VW. Immune-mediated neurodegeneration and neuroprotection in MS. *Int MS J* 2003;10:122-30.

[2]   Yong VW. Prospects for neuroprotection in multiple sclerosis. *Front Biosci* 2004;9:864-72.

[3]   Dhib-Jalbut S, Arnold DL, Cleveland DW, et al. Neurodegeneration and neuroprotection in multiple sclerosis and other neurodegenerative diseases. *J Neuroimmunol* 2006;176:198-215.

[4]   Glass CK, Saijo K, Winner B, et al. Mechanisms underlying inflammation in neurodegeneration. *Cell* 2010;140:918-34.

[5]   Aharoni R, Arnon R. Linkage between immunomodulation, neuroprotection and neurogenesis. *Drug News Perspect* 2009;22:301-12.

[6]   Aktas O, Kieseier B, Hartung HP. Neuroprotection, regeneration and immunomodulation: broadening the therapeutic repertoire in multiple sclerosis. *Trends Neurosci* 2010;33:140-52.

[7]   Mangas A, Covenas R, Geffard M. New drug therapies for multiple sclerosis. *Curr Opin Neurol* 2010;23:287-92.

[8]   Saijo K, Crotti A, Glass CK. Nuclear receptors, inflammation, and neurodegenerative diseases. *Adv Immunol* 2010;106:21-59.

[9]   Van der Walt A, Butzkueven H, Kolbe S, et al. Neuroprotection in multiple sclerosis: a therapeutic challenge for the next decade. *Pharmacol Ther* 2010;126:82-93.

[10]   Reynolds BA, Weiss S. Generation of neurons and astrocytes from isolated cells of the adult mammalian central nervous system. *Science* 1992;255:1707-10.

**   The first report of the isolation and characterization of populations of neural progenitor and stem cells from the adult brain *in vitro*. Neural progenitor and stem cells expand *in vitro*, as neurospheres, in the presence of 20 ng/ml EGF.

[11]   Reynolds BA, Tetzlaff W, Weiss S. A multipotent EGF-responsive striatal embryonic progenitor cell produces neurons and astrocytes. *J Neurosci* 1992;12:4565-74.

[12]   Weiss S, Reynolds B. *Novel growth factor-responsive progenitor cells which can be proliferated in vitro*. WO1993001275; 1993

**   Patent WO1993001275 lays the ground for the protection of the intellectual property for the preparation and use of neural progenitor and stem cells *in vitro*, *ex vivo* and *in vivo*.

[13]   Yoshida M, Macklin WB. Oligodendrocyte development and myelination in GFP-transgenic zebrafish. J Neurosci Res 2005;81:1-8.

[14]   Wu QZ, Yang Q, Cate HS, Kemper D, Binder M, et al. MRI identification of the rostral-caudal pattern of pathology within the corpus callosum in the cuprizone mouse model. *J Magn Reson Imaging* 2008;27:446-53.

[15]   Taupin P. BrdU Immunohistochemistry for Studying Adult Neurogenesis: paradigms, pitfalls, limitations, and validation. *Brain Res Rev* 2007;53:198-214.

*   BrdU is a thymidine analog used for birth dating and monitoring cell proliferation. BrdU is not a marker of cell proliferation and neurogenesis, but a marker of DNA synthesis.

[16]   Weiss S, Reynolds BA, Hammang JP. *Remyelination using neural stem cells*. EP0664832B1; 2002.

[17]   Yong VW, Giuliani F, Xue M, et al. Experimental models of neuroprotection relevant to multiple sclerosis. *Neurology* 2007;68:S32-7.

[18] De Santi L, Annunziata P, Sessa E, et al. Brain-derived neurotrophic factor and TrkB receptor in experimental autoimmune encephalomyelitis and multiple sclerosis. *J Neurol Sci* 2009;287:17-26.

[19] Palmer TD, Schwartz PH, Taupin P, et al. Cell culture. Progenitor cells from human brain after death. *Nature* 2001;411:42-3.

[20] Taupin P, Gage FH. Adult neurogenesis and neural stem cells of the central nervous system in mammals. *J Neurosci Res* 2002;69:745-9.

[21] Duan X, Kang E, Liu CY, et al. Development of neural stem cell in the adult brain. *Curr Opin Neurobiol* 2008;18:108-15.

[22] Taupin P. The therapeutic potential of adult neural stem cells. *Curr Opin Mol Ther* 2006;8:225-31.

[23] Taupin P. Nootropic agents stimulate neurogenesis. *Expert Opin Ther Pat* 2009;19:727-30.

[24] Taupin P. Fourteen compounds and their derivatives for the treatment of diseases and injuries characterized by reduced neurogenesis and neurodegeneration. *Expert Opin Ther Pat* 2009;19:541-7.

[25] Taupin P. Apigenin and related compounds stimulate adult neurogenesis. *Expert Opin Ther Pat* 2009;19:523-7.

[26] Taupin P. Adult neurogenesis and neural stem cells as a model for the discovery and development of novel drugs. Ex*pert Opin Drug Discov* 2010;5:921-25.

[27] 27.Taupin P. Neurogenic drugs and compounds. *Recent Pat CNS Drug Discov* 2010;5:253-7.

Chapter XVI

Antibodies against CD20 (Rituximab) for Treating Multiple Sclerosis

Abstract

Background

The application is in the field of medication and treatment for MS.

Objective

It aims at identifying and characterizing the activity and potency of antibodies against CD20 (rituximab) for treating MS and at devising treatments and dosing protocols for various forms of MS.

Methods

Various doses of antibody and different time points were assessed to devise treatments and dosing protocols for MS. Results. Rituximab depletes peripheral B cells and reduces the level of B cells in the cerebrospinal fluid of patients with relapsing-remitting MS. Various treatments and dosing protocols are proposed for improving the signs, symptoms or other indicators of patients with relapsing-remitting MS and with primary progressive MS.

Conclusion

Antibodies against CD20 and rituximab offer new opportunities to treat patients with MS. The application claims the use of antibodies against CD20 and rituximab for treating the various forms of MS. The application claims the administration of the antibodies at separate intervals, and alone or in combination with other drugs and treatments. It claims a manufacture product for the medication. It further claims the administration of antibodies against CD20 by gene therapy for treating MS.

Introduction

MS is a demyelinating disease. It is an autoimmune inflammatory disease that attacks the oligodendrocytes of the CNS, leading to demyelination and scarring in the CNS and to progressive and broad deficits and disabilities [1,2]. MS is a disease of young adults, with 70 - 80% having an onset between 20 and 40 years of age [3-5]. There are four forms of MS: primary progressive MS (PPMS, 10 - 15% of cases at onset), relapsing-remitting MS (RRMS, 80 - 85% at onset), secondary progressive MS (SPMS) and progressive relapsing MS (5% at onset). An estimated 50% of patients with RRMS will develop SPMS within 10 years and up to 90% of patients with RRMS will develop SPMS [6]. The disease affects 2.5 million individuals worldwide and 300,000 in the US. There are currently treatments available that alleviate MS-associated symptoms. Among the current treatments for MS are treatments that alleviate symptoms for RRMS, such as IFNs, glatiramer acetate, natalizumab (antibody against cellular adhesion molecule α4-integrin, Tysabry, Biogen Idec-Elan) and mitoxantrone [7].

MS is a disease difficult to diagnose, particularly at the early stage. Diagnosis of MS involves analysis of MRI scans of the brain of patients and analysis of the patient cerebrospinal fluid (CSF) and serum. MRI scans of the brain of patients with MS show scattered lesions in the central white matter [8,9]. Analysis of the CSF and serum of patients with MS shows the presence or elevated levels of CSF oligoclonal bands; anti-myelin antibodies, such as antibodies against myelin basic protein and myelin oligodendrocyte glycoprotein; IL-15; and B lymphocytes [10-13]. The presence or the elevated levels of these biomarkers in the CSF and serum of patients is predictive of the diagnosis of the disease from a clinically isolated demyelinating event to MS (RRMS). It correlates with MS attacks and may be predictive of more severe outcomes [12,14].

B lymphocytes (B cells) express and are characterized by hydrophobic transmembrane proteins or B-cell surface antigens; among them, the CD20 antigen (CD20, also called human B-lymphocyte-restricted differentiation antigen or Bp35). CD20 is a 35-kDa non-glycosylated phosphoprotein. CD20 is expressed on the surface of 90% of pre-B and mature B lymphocytes of lymphoid organs and peripheral blood. CD20 is not expressed by hematopoietic stem cells and is expressed by malignant B cells, particularly by > 90% of B-cell non-Hodgkin's lymphomas (NHL) [15]. CD20 is not expressed on pro-B cells, normal plasma cells or other normal tissues. Hence, CD 20 is a biomarker of choice to target malignant B cells and antibodies against CD20 have been generated and used for the treatment of malignant hematologic diseases, such as B-cell NHL [16]. The application claims the use of antibodies against CD20, rituximab, and treatments using antibodies against CD20 for treating MS.

Chemistry and Synthesis

Rituximab is a genetically engineered, chimeric monoclonal antibody ('C2B8', Genentech, Inc.) directed against the lineage specific antigen of B lymphocytes CD20. It binds the human complement and lyses B cells through complement-dependent cytotoxicity. The anitbody was originally developed for the treatment of B-cell NHL [16]. Ocrelizumab is a humanized 2H7 antibody variant of CD20 (Genentech).

Biology and Action

The antibody, rituximab, is administered to the patients and binds to the CD20 antigen of B cells, both normal and present in the CSF of patients with MS. It binds the human complement and lyses B cells through complement-dependent cytotoxicity, leading to the destruction of the B cells, including in the CSF [17]. The antibody is administered intravenously (i.v.), subcutaneously or intrathecally.

- Treatment of PPMS. Administrations (i.v.) of 1 g rituximab on days 1 and 15. Subsequent courses of treatment at week 24 (day 169), week 48 (day 337) and week 72 (day 505), with second infusion 14 ± 1 days after the first one.
- Treatment of RRMS. Administrations (i.v.) of 1 g rituximab on days 1 and 15. Subsequent courses of treatment at week 24 (day 169), week 48 (day 337) and week 72 (day 505), with second infusion 14 ± 1 days after 100 the first one.
- Treatment of RRMS. Administrations (i.v.) of 1 g rituximab on days 1 and 15. Subsequent courses of treatment at weeks 48 and 96, with second infusion 14 ± 1 days after the first one.

The primary efficacy outcome measure is the time to confirmed disease progression (for PPMS and RRMS) or the MRI end point of gadolinium-enhancing lesions (for RRMS). The time to confirmed disease progression is defined as an increase of >= 1 point from baseline Expanded Disability Status Scale (EDSS) [18]. If the baseline EDSS is between 2 and 5.5 points (inclusive) or an increase of >= 0.5 point if the baseline EDSS is >= 5.5 points (inclusive), for which change is not attributable to another etiology (e.g., fever, concurrent illness, MS relapse or exacerbation, or concomitant medication). Confirmation of disease progression may occur at a regularly scheduled visit that is at least 12 weeks (84 days) after the initial progression. The MRI end point of gadolinium-enhancing lesions is the total number of gadolinium-enhancing T1 lesions observed on serial MRI scans of the brain at weeks 12, 16, 20 and 24.

The application claims the treatments above for improving the signs, symptoms or other indicators of patients with PPMS or RRMS. The treatments may be combined with others, such as the administration of corticosteroids, IFN-☐, glatiramer acetate, methotrexate, cyclophosphamide and mitoxantrone, in case of relapse between the courses of the antibody treatments.

Expert Opinion

There is currently no cure for MS and current treatments approved for RRMS primarily alleviate symptoms of the diseases with limited efficacy in preventing disabilities and with a high rate of relapse [19,20]. Hence, there is a need to discover and develop new drugs and treatments for MS. Antibodies against CD20 (rituximab) have been used and show efficiency in treating a broad range of autoimmune and immune-mediated disorders, as well as malignant hematologic diseases, such as autoimmune anemia, autoimmune neuropathy, dermatomyositis, chronic lymphocytic leukemia, NHL, rheumatoid arthritis and systemic lupus erythematosus [21-26]. The antibodies have been reported to deplete peripheral B cells and reduce the level of B cells in the CSF of patients with RRMS [27]. Rituximab and antibodies against CD20 offer, therefore, an opportunity for developing new treatments for MS and improving the lives of patients with MS. This confirms the potency and efficiency of antibodies against CD20, and rituximab, for treating a broad range of autoimmune and immune-mediated disorders. The potential benefits of antibodies against CD20 and rituximab for treating MS remain to be validated in large scale studies and the extent of the recovery following the treatments remain to be fully evaluated in patients.

MS is a complex multifactorial disease. Antibodies against CD20 and rituximab address one – specific – aspect of the disease. Hence, the proposed treatments may improve certain symptoms and deficits of the disease. Treating and curing MS will involve a combination of drugs and therapies, including anti-inflammatory, immune-modulatory, neuro-protective and neuro-regenerative treatments, particularly drugs promoting the differentiation of oligodendrocyte progenitor cells and endogenous remyelination [28-30]. Future studies will involve the administration of antibodies against CD20 by gene therapy and studying and characterizing the administration of multiples drugs, in combination rituximab, for treating MS.

Declaration of Interest

P Taupin declares no conflict of interest and has received no payment in preparation of this manuscript.

Acknowledgments

Reproduced with permission from Informa Healthcare: Taupin P. Antibodies against CD20 (rituximab) for treating multiple sclerosis: US20100233121. Expert Opinion on Therapeutic Patents (2011) 21(1):111-114. Copyright 2010, Informa Healthcare (Informa UK Ltd).

Bibliography

Papers of special note have been highlighted as either of interest (*) or of considerable interest (**) to readers.

[1]   Confavreux C, Vukusic S. Natural history of multiple sclerosis: a unifying concept. *Brain* 2006;129:606-16.

[2]   Vukusic S, Confavreux C. Natural history of multiple sclerosis: risk factors and prognostic indicators. *Curr Opin Neurol* 2007;20:269-74.

[3]   Noonan CW, Kathman SJ, White MC. Prevalence estimates for MS in the United States and evidence of an increasing trend for women. *Neurology.* 2002;58:136-8.

[4]   Confavreux C, Vukusic S. Age at disability milestones in multiple sclerosis. *Brain* 2006;129:595-605.

[5]   Alonso A, Hernan MA. Temporal trends in the incidence of multiple sclerosis: a systematic review. *Neurology.* 2008;71:129-35.

[6]   Confavreux C, Vukusic S, Moreau T, Adeleine P. Relapses and progression of disability in multiple sclerosis. *N Engl J Med* 2000;343:1430-8.

[7]   Scott LJ, Figgitt DP. Mitoxantrone: a review of its use in multiple sclerosis. *CNS Drugs.* 2004;18:379-96.

[8]   Confavreux C, Vukusic S, Adeleine P. Early clinical predictors and progression of irreversible disability in multiple sclerosis: an amnesic process. *Brain* 2003;126:770-82.

[9]   Lunde Larsen LS, Larsson HB, Frederiksen JL. The value of conventional high-field MRI in MS in the light of the McDonald criteria: a literature review. *Acta Neurol Scand* 2010;122:149-58.

[10]   Angelucci F, Mirabella M, Frisullo G, et al. Serum levels of anti-myelin antibodies in relapsing-remitting multiple sclerosis patients during different phases of disease activity and immunomodulatory therapy. *Dis Markers* 2005;21:49-55.

[11]   Rentzos M, Cambouri C, Rombos A, et al. IL-15 is elevated in serum and cerebrospinal fluid of patients with multiple sclerosis. *J Neurol Sci* 2006;241:25-9.

[12]   Kuenz B, Lutterotti A, Ehling R, et al. Cerebrospinal fluid B cells correlate with early brain inflammation in multiple sclerosis. *PLoS One* 2008;3:e2559.

**   The presence of B cells in the CSF and serum of patients is predictive of the diagnosis of the disease from a clinically isolated demyelinating event to MS (RRMS). It correlates with MS attacks and may be predictive of more severe outcomes.

[13]   Tumani H, Hartung HP, Hemmer B, et al. Cerebrospinal fluid biomarkers in multiple sclerosis. *Neurobiol Dis* 2009;35:117-27.

[14]   Mandrioli J, Sola P, Bedin R, et al. A multifactorial prognostic index in multiple sclerosis. Cerebrospinal fluid IgM oligoclonal bands and clinical features to predict the evolution of the disease. *J Neurol* 2008;255:1023-31.

[15]   Clark EA, Shu G, Ledbetter JA. Role of the Bp35 cell surface polypeptide in human B-cell activation. *Proc Natl Acad Sci U S A* 1985;82:1766-70.

[16]   Keating GM. Rituximab: a review of its use in chronic lymphocytic leukaemia, low-grade or follicular lymphoma and diffuse large B-cell lymphoma. *Drugs* 2010;70:1445-76.

[17] Perosa F, Prete M, Racanelli V, Dammacco F. CD20-depleting therapy in autoimmune diseases: from basic research to the clinic. *J Intern Med* 2010;267:260-77.

[18] Kurtzke JF. Rating neurologic impairment in multiple sclerosis: an expanded disability status scale (EDSS). *Neurology* 1983;33:1444-52.

[19] Bell C, Graham J, Earnshaw S, et al. Cost-effectiveness of four immunomodulatory therapies for relapsing-remitting multiple sclerosis: a Markov model based on long-term clinical data. *J Manag Care Pharm.* 2007;13:245-61.

[20] Goldberg LD, Edwards NC, Fincher C, et al. Comparing the cost-effectiveness of disease-modifying drugs for the first-line treatment of relapsing-remitting multiple sclerosis. *J Manag Care Pharm* 2009;15:543-55.

[21] Plosker GL, Figgitt DP. Rituximab: a review of its use in non-Hodgkin's lymphoma and chronic lymphocytic leukaemia. *Drugs* 2003;63:803-43.

[22] Held G, Pöschel V, Pfreundschuh M. Rituximab for the treatment of diffuse large B-cell lymphomas. *Expert Rev Anticancer Ther* 2006;6:1175-86.

[23] Rios Fernández R, Callejas Rubio JL, Sánchez Cano D, et al. Rituximab in the treatment of dermatomyositis and other inflammatory myopathies. A report of 4 cases and review of the literature. *Clin Exp Rheumatol* 2009;27:1009-16.

[24] Tzaribachev N, Koetter I, Kuemmerle-Deschner JB, Schedel J. Rituximab for the treatment of refractory pediatric autoimmune diseases: a case series. *Cases J.* 2009;2:6609.

[25] Dalakas MC. Pathogenesis and Treatment of Anti-MAG Neuropathy. *Curr Treat Options Neurol* 2010;12:71-83.

[26] Taupin P. Transplantation of cord blood stem cells for treating hematologic diseases and strategies to improve engraftment. *Therapy* 2010;7:703-15.

[27] Piccio L, Naismith RT, Trinkaus K, et al. Changes in B- and T-lymphocyte and chemokine levels with rituximab treatment in multiple sclerosis. *Arch Neurol* 2010;67:707-14.

** Rituximab treatment depletes peripheral B cells and reduces the level of B cells in the CSF of patients with RRMS.

[28] Taupin P. Thirteen compounds promoting oligodendrocyte progenitor cell differentiation and remyelination for treating multiple sclerosis: WO2010054307. *Expert Opin Ther Pat* 2010;20:1767-1773.

* Drugs and compounds that promote the differentiation of endogenous oligodendrocyte progenitor cells and induce the remyelination of nerve cells offer new opportunities for treating MS and myelin-related disorders.

[29] Taupin P. Adult neurogenesis and neural stem cells as a model for the discovery and development of novel drugs. *Expert Opin Drug Discov* 2010;5:921-25.

[30] Taupin P. Neurogenic drugs and compounds. *Recent Pat CNS Drug Discov* 2010;5:253-7.

Conclusion 1

Neurogenic Drugs for Treating Neurological Diseases and Disorders

Neurogenesis occurs in the adult brain, and neural stem cells (NSCs) reside in the adult central nervous system of mammals [1,2]. Neurogenesis occurs primarily in two regions of the adult mammalian brain, the hippocampus and the subventricular zone, in various species including humans [3,4]. Newly generated neuronal cells in the adult brain would originate from a pool of residual stem cells. NSCs are the self-renewing multipotent cells that generate the main phenotypes of the nervous system, nerve cells, astrocytes, and oligodendrocytes. Because of their potential, NSCs represent a promising model for cellular therapy to treat and cure a broad range of neurological diseases and injuries, ranging from neurodegenerative diseases, such as Alzheimer's disease (AD) and Parkinson's disease, to cerebral strokes and traumatic brain and spinal cord injuries. The stimulation of endogenous neural progenitor or stem cells of the adult brain and the transplantation of adult-derived neural progenitor and stem cells are proposed to repair and restore the degenerated or injured nerve pathways. Adult NSCs remain elusive, and the molecular and cellular mechanisms underlying the development of adult NSCs remain to be fully elucidated and understood [5,6]. Hence, it may be decades before adult NSC-based cellular therapy is brought to therapy for the treatment of neurological diseases and disorders [7].

Neurogenesis is modulated in the adult brain, particularly in the hippocampus. It is modulated by a broad range of stimuli, physiological and pathological processes, trophic factors/cytokines, and drugs, such as learning and memory tasks, in the brain of patients with AD, in animal models of epilepsy, and in drugs used for treating AD and depression, respectively [8-13]. The hippocampus is involved in physiological and pathological processes, such as learning and memory, AD, epilepsy, and depression [14-17]. This reveals that adult neurogenesis and newly generated neuronal cells of the adult brain would contribute to conditions and processes of the nervous system, particularly associated with the hippocampus, such as learning and memory, AD, and depression [17-19]. They are the target and may mediate the activities of drugs used for treating neurological diseases and disorders, particularly AD and depression [20,21].

The cellular and molecular mechanisms underlying the activity of adult neurogenesis and newly generated neuronal cells of the adult brain on the physiological and pathological conditions and processes of the nervous system remain to be elucidated. On the cellular level, in the hippocampus, the mossy fibers (MF) are the axons of the dentate granule cells. They project to the Cornu Ammonis region 3 (CA3) of the hippocampus [22]. Newly generated neuronal cells in the adult dentate gyrus (DG) project to the CA3 region and establish synaptic contacts with their target cells, like mature granule cells [23,24]. They establish MF-like synapses with their target cells of the CA3 region [24]. The MF synapses represent a small fraction of the synapses of the adult hippocampus, less than 1 percent in mice [22]. Hence, the signals transmitted through the MF pathway, ie, the link between the granule cells of the DG and the pyramidal cells of the CA3 region of the hippocampus, are subject to saturation [22]. The generation of nerve cells in the adult DG and the modulation of adult neurogenesis, in a saturated circuit, may therefore play a critical role in the signals transmitted to the CA3 region and in the physiology and pathology of the hippocampus [24]. On the molecular level, drugs that target the NSCs of the adult brain or neurogenic drugs may act via their pharmacological activities, on messenger signaling pathways, and/or via a neurogenic activity, by modulating neurogenesis [25]. In support of this contention, AD and depression are associated with loss of nerve cells, particularly in the hippocampus [16,17]. Drug treatments that stimulate neurogenesis in the adult hippocampus may therefore be beneficial for the treatment of AD and depression particularly, by compensating for the neuronal loss in the hippocampus.

Therefore, neurogenic drugs represent a novel class of drugs for treating neurological diseases and disorders; drugs that specifically target the NSCs of the adult brain and reverse or compensate deficits and impairments [26]. They may be used for the treatment of neurological diseases and disorders to reverse or compensate deficits and impairments, particularly associated with the hippocampus, such as learning and memory deficits and impairments, AD, depression, epilepsy, schizophrenia, and sleep disorders. Neurogenic drugs may be used to reverse or compensate deficits and impairments of neurological diseases and disorders, associated with the olfactory bulb, such as anosmia in AD, by stimulating neural progenitor and stem cells in the subventricular zone. Neurogenic drugs may also be used to treat multiple diseases, alone or in combination with other drugs. They may have potential for regenerative medicine and for the treatment of brain tumors. Therefore, the discovery and development of such novel drugs open new avenues and opportunities for treating neurological disease and disorders.

However, there are controversies, limitations, and pitfalls that need to be overcome for the discovery and development of such drugs. Among them, reports indicate that antidepressants, such as fluoxetine, do not elicit proneurogenic effects [27-29]. Hence, the contribution of adult neurogenesis to the activity of antidepressants remains to be fully elucidated and understood. Others report conflicting data in studying adult neurogenesis in vivo, in animal models of and in autopsies of human brains with neurological diseases and disorders. The apparent discrepancies reported in the modulation of adult neurogenesis in neurodegenerative diseases may originate from (i) the validity of these animal models as representative of the diseases and to study adult phenotypes, such as adult neurogenesis; (ii) the limitations and pitfalls of the paradigms and protocols used to study and quantify adult neurogenesis in vivo, particularly the bromodeoxyuridine labeling paradigm and the immunohistochemistry for markers of the cells cycle; (iii) the lack of consensus on the term neurogenesis, some studies only present proliferation data, whereas others present only neuronal differentiation or survival data; and (iv) the fact that in most studies, and in particular in the human postmortem studies, only one time point along the pathology is analyzed [30-33]. Hence, studies of adult neurogenesis in animal models and in human tissues need to be carefully analyzed and discussed, as well as further confirmed and validated. Also, the current protocols established and used for isolating and propagating self-renewing multipotent NSCs in vitro yield to heterogeneous populations of neural progenitor and stem cells [34,35]. Other limitations to use NSCs for modeling in vivo neurogenesis and drug effect(s) include the accessibility of tissues, particularly in human, and the ability to establish a robust baseline for in vitro differentiation [36,37].

Thus, adult neurogenesis and NSCs offer new avenues and opportunities to discover and develop novel drugs for treating neurological diseases and disorders [33,38-40]. Drugs that specifically target the NSCs of the adult brain, or neurogenic drugs, reverse or compensate deficits and impairments associated with neurological diseases and disorders, particularly associated with the hippocampus. Adult neurogenesis and NSCs represent a promising model to discover and develop novel drugs for treating neurological diseases and disorders, such as learning and memory deficits and impairments, AD, depression, epilepsy, schizophrenia, and sleep disorders. These drugs may have potential for regenerative medicine and for the treatment of brain tumors. Adult neurogenesis and NSCs contribute, both beneficially and detrimentally, to the pathology of neurological diseases and disorders, particularly in AD [19]. Hence, the process of drug discovery and development will aim at identifying candidate drugs that limit the potential deleterious effects of the drugs on adult neurogenesis, without disrupting its regenerative capacity [41]. Controversies, limitations, and pitfalls over the study and characterization of adult NSCs in vivo and in vitro may hinder the drug discovery and development process of neurogenic drugs as well as their potency and specificity that may limit their therapeutic potential and applications. Hence, although adult NSCs represent a model of choice to discover and develop novel drugs for treating neurological diseases and disorders, more stringent and more specific assays that specifically target the NSCs of the adult brain in vitro, ex vivo, and in vivo need to be designed and developed to discover and develop more quickly novel drugs that are more potent and more specific for treating neurological disease and disorders. The contribution of adult neurogenesis and NSCs to the activities of these drugs, as well as their mechanisms of action, will need to be characterized and determined.

Acknowledgments

Reproduced from: Taupin P. Neurogenic drugs for treating neurological diseases and disorders. Journal of Neurodegeneration and Regeneration (2010) 3(1):1-3 (in press), with permission of Weston Medical Publishing, LLC.

References

[1]   Taupin P, Gage FH: Adult neurogenesis and neural stem cells of the central nervous system in mammals. *J Neurosci Res*. 2002; 69(6): 745-749.

[2] Duan X, Kang E, Liu CY, et al.: Development of neural stem cell in the adult brain. *Curr Opin Neurobiol.* 2008; 18(1): 108-115.

[3] Eriksson PS, Perfilieva E, Bjork-Eriksson T, et al.: Neurogenesis in the adult human hippocampus. *Nat Med.* 1998; 4(11): 1313-1317.

[4] Curtis MA, Kam M, Nannmark U, et al.: Human neuroblasts migrate to the olfactory bulb via a lateral ventricular extension. *Science.* 2007; 315(5816): 1243-1249.

[5] Taupin P: Adult neural stem cells, neurogenic niches and cellular therapy. *Stem Cell Rev.* 2006; 2(3): 213-220.

[6] Mitsiadis TA, Barrandon O, Rochat A, et al.: Stem cell niches in mammals. *Exp Cell Res.* 2007; 313(16): 3377-3385.

[7] Taupin P: Adult neural stem cells from promise to treatment: The road ahead. *J Neurodegener Regene.* 2008; 1(1): 7-8.

[8] Parent JM, Yu TW, Leibowitz RT, et al.: Dentate granule cell neurogenesis is increased by seizures and contributes to aberrant network reorganization in the adult rat hippocampus. *J Neurosci.* 1997; 17(10): 3727-3738.

[9] Gould E, Beylin A, Tanapat P, et al.: Learning enhances adult neurogenesis in the hippocampal formation. *Nat Neurosci.* 1999; 2(3): 260-265.

[10] Malberg JE, Eisch AJ, Nestler EJ, et al.: Chronic antidepressant treatment increases neurogenesis in adult rat hippocampus. *J Neurosci.* 2000; 20(24): 9104-9110.

[11] Jin K, Peel AL, Mao XO, et al.: Increased hippocampal neurogenesis in Alzheimer's disease. *Proc Natl Acad Sci USA.* 2004; 101(1): 343-347.

[12] Jin K, Xie L, Mao XO, et al.: Alzheimer's disease drugs promote neurogenesis. *Brain Res.* 2006; 1085(1): 183-188.

[13] Perera TD, Coplan JD, Lisanby SH, et al.: Antidepressant-induced neurogenesis in the hippocampus of adult nonhuman primates. *J Neurosci.* 2007; 27(18): 4894-4901.

[14] Holmes GL, Ben-Ari Y: The neurobiology and consequences of epilepsy in the developing brain. *Pediatr Res.* 2001; 49(3): 320-325.

[15] Burns A, Byrne EJ, Maurer K: Alzheimer's disease. *Lancet* 2002; 360(9327): 163-165.

[16] Campbell S, Marriott M, Nahmias C, et al.: Lower hippocampal volume in patients suffering from depression: a meta-analysis. *Am J Psychiatry.* 2004; 161(4): 598-607.

[17] Taupin P: Neurogenesis and the Effects of Antidepressants. *Drug Target Insights* 2006; 1: 13-17.

[18] Shors TJ, Miesegaes G, Beylin A, et al.: Neurogenesis in the adult is involved in the formation of trace memories. *Nature.* 2001; 410(6826): 372-376. Erratum in: *Nature.* 2001; 414(6866): 938.

[19] Taupin P: Adult neurogenesis, neural stem cells and Alzheimer's disease: Developments, limitations, problems and promises. *Curr Alzheimer Res.* 2009; 6(6): 461-470.

[20] Santarelli L, Saxe M, Gross C, et al.: Requirement of hippocampal neurogenesis for the behavioral effects of antidepressants. *Science.* 2003; 310(5634): 805-809.

[21] Taupin P: Adult neurogenesis pharmacology in neurological diseases and disorders. *Exp Rev Neurother.* 2008; 8(2): 311-320.

[22] Braitenberg V, Schüz A: Some anatomical comments on the hippocampus. In W Seifert, editor. *Neurobiology of the hippocampus.* Academic Press 21-37 (1983).

[23] Toni N, Teng EM, Bushong EA, et al.: Synapse formation on neurons born in the adult hippocampus. *Nat Neurosci.* 2007; 10(6): 727-734.

[24] Taupin P: Characterization and isolation of synapses of newly generated neuronal cells of the adult hippocampus at early stages of neurogenesis. *J Neurodegener Regene.* 2009; 2(1): 9-17.

[25] Taupin P: Adult neurogenesis and drug therapy. *Cent Nerv Syst. Agents Med Chem.* 2008; 8: 198-202.

[26] Taupin P: Neurogenic drugs and compounds. *Recent Pat CNS Drug Discov.* 2010; 5(3): 253-257.

[27] Holick KA, Lee DC, Hen R, et al.: Behavioral Effects of Chronic Fluoxetine in BALB/cJ Mice Do Not Require Adult Hippocampal Neurogenesis or the Serotonin 1A Receptor. *Neuropsychopharmacology.* 2008; 33(2): 406-417.

[28] Couillard-Despres S, Wuertinger C, Kandasamy M, et al.: Ageing abolishes the effects of fluoxetine on neurogenesis. *Mol Psychiatry.* 2009; 14(9): 856-864.

[29] Lucassen PJ, Stumpel MW, Wang Q, et al: Decreased numbers of progenitor cells but no response to antidepressant drugs in the hippocampus of elderly depressed patients. *Neuropharmacology.* 2010; 58(6): 940-949.

[30] Nowakowski RS, Hayes NL: New neurons: Extraordinary evidence or extraordinary conclusion? *Science.* 2000; 288(5467): 771.

[31] Rakic P: Adult neurogenesis in mammals: an identity crisis. *J Neurosci.* 2002; 22(3): 614-618.

[32] Taupin P: BrdU Immunohistochemistry for Studying Adult Neurogenesis: Paradigms, pitfalls, limitations, and validation. *Brain Res Rev.* 2007; 53(1): 198-214.

[33] Taupin P: Adult neurogenesis and neural stem cells as a model for the discovery and development of novel drugs. *Expert Opin Drug Discov.* 2010; 5(10): 921-925.

[34] Chin VI, Taupin P, Sanga S, et al.: Microfabricated platform for studying stem cell fates. *Biotechnol Bioeng.* 2004; 88(3): 399-415.

[35] Reynolds BA, Rietze RL: Neural stem cells and neurospheres--re-evaluating the relationship. *Nat Methods.* 2005; 2(5): 333-336.

[36] Crook JM, Kobayashi NR: Human stem cells for modeling neurological disorders: accelerating the drug discovery pipeline. *J Cell Biochem.* 2008;105(6): 1361-1366.

[37] Kobayashi NR, Sui L, Tan PS, et al: Modelling disrupted-in-schizophrenia 1 loss of function in human neural progenitor cells: tools for molecular studies of human neurodevelopment and neuropsychiatric disorders. *Mol Psychiatry.* 2010; 15(7): 672-675.

[38] Taupin P: Nootropic agents stimulate neurogenesis. *Expert Opin Ther Pat.* 2009; 19(5): 727-730.

[39] Taupin P: Fourteen compounds and their derivatives for the treatment of diseases and injuries characterized by reduced neurogenesis and neurodegeneration. *Expert Opin Ther Pat.* 2009; 19(4): 541-547.

[40] Taupin P: Apigenin and related compounds stimulate adult neurogenesis. *Expert Opin Ther Pat.* 2009; 19(4): 523-527.

[41] Taupin P: Aneuploidy and adult neurogenesis in Alzheimer's disease: therapeutic strategies. *Drug Discov Today.* 2010; 15(23/24):983-984.

Conclusion 2

Aneuploidy and Adult Neurogenesis in Alzheimer's Disease: Therapeutic Strategies

The confirmation, that neurogenesis occurs in the adult brain and neural stem cells (NSCs) reside in the adult central nervous system (CNS) of mammals reveals that the adult brain has the potential for self-repair. Neurogenesis occurs in discrete regions of the adult mammalian brain, the subventricular zone and the dentate gyrus (DG) of the hippocampus, in various species, including humans. Newly generated neuronal cells in the adult brain originate from a pool of residual NSCs. Adult NSCs contribute to the physiology and pathology of the nervous system [1]. Recent studies show that neurogenesis is enhanced in the brain of patients with Alzheimer's disease (AD) [2]. Enhanced neurogenesis in the brain of AD patients would contribute to regenerative attempts in the CNS, to compensate for the neuronal loss.

AD is a neurodegenerative disease associated with learning and cognitive deficits, and for which aging is the main risk factor. The hippocampus is the main region of the brain affected by the disease. There are two forms of the disease: the late onset form (LOAD) diagnosed after age 65 and the early onset form (EOAD) diagnosed at a younger age. Genetic background and acquired and environmental risk factors are causative factors for LOAD, whereas EOAD is primarily an inherited disease. The presence of the apolipoprotein E varepsilon 4 allele (ApoE4) in the genetic makeup of the individuals is the best-established genetic risk factor for LOAD. Mutations in the amyloid precursor protein (APP), the presenilin-1 (PSEN-1) and the presenilin-2 (PSEN-2) genes have been identified as causative for EOAD. Amyloid plaques, composed of deposits of amyloid proteins, and neurofibrillary tangles, composed of aggregated hyperphosphorylated Tau proteins, are the histopathological hallmarks of AD [3].

ADis also characterized by neurodegeneration and aneuploidy in the adult brain [4].The increase of aneuploid nerve cells in regions of degeneration in the ADbrain contributes to the development of the disease. In regions of degeneration, cell cycle re-entry and DNA duplication, without cell division, are at the origin of aneuploid nerve cells in thebrain ofpatients with AD [5].These cells are fated to die and may undergo a slow death process, underlying the process of neurodegeneration in AD [6]. The ApoE, PSEN-1, PSEN-2 and

TAU genes are located on chromosomes 19, 14, 1 and 17, respectively. Aneuploidy for chromosomes carrying genes involved in AD promotes the formation of amyloid plaques, neurofibrillary tangles and neurodegeneration in the brain of patients with AD, LOAD or EOAD depending on the genetic and/or risk factors involved.

Dividing cells are the most likely to generate aneuploid cells [7]. Hence, neurogenesis holds the potential to generate new neuronal cells that are aneuploid in the neurogenic regions of the adult brain. Aneuploid new neuronal cells and aneuploid newly generated neuronal cells that would not proceed with their developmental program in the adult brain would be a contributing factor of the pathogenesis of AD in the neurogenic regions. Aneuploidy, for chromosomes carrying genes involved in AD, in newly generated neuronal cells of the adult brain would further promote the pathological process of AD, particularly in the hippocampus [8].

Adult neurogenesis is a relatively low frequency event in the adult brain; it is estimated that 0.004% of the granule cell population is generated per day in the DG of adult macaque monkeys [1]. The hippocampus is one of the neurogenic regions of the adult brain and one of the regions of the brain the most affected in AD. Aneuploid newly generated neuronal cells originating from the nondisjunction of chromosomes during cell division may have their lifespan shortened or may survive for extended period of time. They would contribute to the pathogenesis of AD by promoting the formation of amyloid plaques, neurofibrillary tangles, neurodegeneration and aneuploidy, locally. This suggests that, despite being a low frequency event, the generation of aneuploid new neuronal cells in the hippocampus, in particular, may play a critical contribution to the pathology of AD.

d forms of PSEN-1 are detected in interphase kinetochores and centrosomes of dividing cells, where they may be involved in the segragation and migration of chromosomes during cell division [9]. The hyperphosphorylation of Tau by kinases leads to the dissociation of Tau and tubulin and to the breakdown of microtubles causing the disruption in the mitotic spindle, which promotes aneuploidy during mitosis [10]. Hence, genetic and/or risk factors involved in AD would promote the generation of aneuploid new neuronal cells in the adult brain. Enhanced neurogenesis in the hippocampus of patients with AD, and more generally conditions that promote neurogenesis, would contribute to an increase of aneuploidy newly generated neuronal cells in the adult brain. This reveals that adult neurogenesis may be involved in the pathogenesis of AD.

In all, adult neurogenesis may contribute not only to regenerative attempts in the nervous system, but also to the pathogenesis of neurological diseases and disorders, particularly in AD. The contribution of aneuploid newly generated neuronal cells of the adult hippocampus to the pathogenesis of AD opens new avenues and perspectives for our understanding of and for treating the disease. Therapeutic strategies will aim at specifically targeting aneuploid newly generated neuronal cells of the adult brain, to limit their potential deleterious effects in patients with AD, without disrupting the regenerative capacity of adult neurogenesis.

Acknowledgments

Reproduced from: Taupin P. Aneuploidy and adult neurogenesis in Alzheimer's disease: therapeutic strategies. Drug Discovery Today (2010) 15(23/24):983-984. Copyright (2010), with permission from Elsevier.

References

[1]   Taupin, P. (2006) Neurogenesis in the adult central nervous system. C. R. Biol. 329, 465-475.

[2]   Jin, K. et al. (2004) Increased hippocampal neurogenesis in Alzheimer's disease. Proc. Natl. Acad. Sci. U. S. A. 101, 343-347.

[3]   Querfurth, H.W. et al. (2010) Alzheimer's disease. N. Engl. J. Med. 362, 329-344.

[4]   Kingsbury, M.A. et al. (2006) Aneuploidy in the normal and diseased brain. Cell. Mol. Life. Sci. 63, 2626-2641.

[5]   Yang, Y. et al. (2003) Neuronal cell death is preceded by cell cycle events at all stages of Alzheimer's disease. J. Neurosci. 23, 2557-2563.

[6]   Yang, Y. et al. (2007) Cell division in the CNS: protective response or lethal event in post-mitotic neurons? Biochim. Biophys. Acta 1772, 457-466.

[7]   Torres, E.M. et al. (2008) Aneuploidy: cells losing their balance. Genetics 179, 737-746.

[8]   Taupin, P. (2009) Adult neurogenesis, neural stem cells and Alzheimer's disease: developments, limitations, problems and promises. Curr. Alzheimer Res. 6, 461-470.

[9]   Li, J. et al. (1997) Alzheimer presenilins in the nuclear membrane, interphase kinetochores, and centrosomes suggest a role in chromosome segregation. Cell 90, 917-927.

[10] Kim, H. et al. (1986) The binding of MAP-2 and tau on brain microtubules in vitro: implications for microtubule structure. Ann. N. Y. Acad. Sci. 466, 218-239.

Conclusion 3

Ex Vivo Fucosylation to Improve the Engraftment Capability and Therapeutic Potential of Human cord Blood Stem Cells

Hematopoietic stem cells (HSCs) are the self-renewing multipotent cells that give rise to the differentiated phenotypes of the blood and immune systems. The transplantation of HSCs is used to treat patients with malignant and non-malignant hematologic diseases, like leukemia, lymphoma, myeloma, Fanconi anemia and sickle cell anemia [1]. In adults, the bone marrow (BM) is the primary source of HSCs. The limited access of HSCs of the BM is the main obstacle for their use in therapy. The umbilical cord blood (CB) contains three to six times more repopulating HSCs than the BM or mobilized peripheral blood [2]. It offers an alternative source of tissue for the transplantation of HSCs, with ease of access and higher potential to reconstitute the BM [3,4].

Since the first successful transplantation of CB stem cells in children with Fanconi anemia - a rare genetic disease characterized by genomic instability and BM failure -, CB tissues have been widely used not only for pediatric transplants, but also for transplantations in adults [5,6]. The main limitations with the use of CB tissues for HSC transplantation are the low cell dose available, the delayed and poor engraftment of the CB stem cells to the BM [7]. Several strategies are being considered and proposed to overcome these issues: the transplantation of double dose or unit of CB and the propagation of CB stem cells *in vitro*, to generate higher number of cells for grafting. The transplantation of double dose of CB is currently proposed for therapy, particularly in adults [8]. On the one hand, the transplantation of double dose of CB does not resolve the efficiency of the therapeutic transplantation and limits the availability of CB tissues for treating patients. On the other hand, the propagation of CB stem cells *in vitro* carries the risk of altering the developmental and therapeutic potential of the cells and optimal culture conditions remain to be established [9]. In adults, the mortality rate of patients treated with CB stem cells for HSC transplantation remains high [10]. Further improvements in engraftment are mandated to achieve higher rate of success for CB transplantation and alternative strategies must be sought.

HSCs migrate to their niches in the BM, a process known as homing, from where they give rise to the differentiated lineages of the blood and immune systems. During homing, the HSCs migrate through the blood and across the endothelial vasculature to reach their niches, particularly in the BM [11]. HSCs have been identified and characterized as a population of cells enriched in $CD34^+$ $CD38^{-/low}$ or $CD34^+$ cells. The rolling and migration of HSCs on endothelial cells involve complex molecular and cellular interactions. Among them, is the interaction between the P- and E-selectins and their ligands, the selectin glycoprotein ligands (SGLs). P- and E-selectins are expressed constitutively on endothelial cells, whereas SGLs are expressed on CD34+ HSCs of the BM and CB in mice and in humans. The interaction P- and E-selectins on endothelial cells with SGLs on HSCs underlies the rolling and migration of HSCs to the BM [12]. HSCs isolated from human BM, but not from CB, migrate efficiently to the BM when transplanted in irradiated non-obese diabetic/severe combined immune deficiency mice [13]. The failure of CB HSCs to migrate efficiently to the BM is due to a defect in binding of P- and E-selectin to the SGLs on their surface. Hence, human CB HSCs express a form of SGL that does not bind to P- and E-selectin and as a result elicit poor homing capabilities, in contrast to their BM counterpart.

SGLs display a glycan determinant on their N-terminal region, a sialylated Lewis x (sLex). The sLex determinant, on the N-terminal region, of SGLs of human BM HSCs, but not of CB HSCs, carries a α2–3-linked sialic acid and a a1–3-linked fucose component [14].

The lack of a1–3-fucosylation of the sLex determinant of CB HSCs causes defective binding of P-selectin and E-selectin to SGLs [15,16]. Hence, proper sLex determinant on the surface of HSCs, a post-translational event, underlies their binding to P-selectin and E-selectin on endothelial cells and their homing capability to the BM. *Ex vivo* membrane fucosylation of CB CD34+ HSCs, by α1-3-fucosyltransferase VI, augments the homing to and engraftment of the cells to the BM in rodents [17]. α1–3-fucosylation of sLex would enhance the binding capabilities of P- and E-selectin to SGLs of CB HSCs and the efficiency of their migration and homing to the BM, through the interaction of P- and E-selectin with SGLs.

Homing is an important step in transplantation therapies involving HSCs [11]. CB transplantation has a tremendous potential for treating hematologic and BM diseases. However, it is limited by the low cell dose in CB tissues, the delayed and poor engraftment of CB stem cells to the BM. Strategies aiming at improving the engraftment of CB stem cells to the BM may overcome these limitations. It would improve the homing of CB stem cells to the BM, reduce the delayed engraftment of the cells and improve the success of therapy with lower cell doses, reducing the need for double CB dose for transplantation. This would result in higher efficiency of the therapeutic transplantation, particularly in adults, and more CB tissues available for patients. To this aim, *ex vivo* fucosylation of human CB stem cells, prior transplantation may provide an alternative and promising strategy for the transplantation of CB tissues. It may improve the engraftment capability of human CB stem cells to the BM and the therapeutic potential of CB tissues, particularly for adults.

Acknowledgments

Reproduced from: Taupin P. *Ex vivo* fucosylation to improve the engraftment capability and therapeutic potential of human cord blood stem cells. Drug Discovery Today (2010) 15(17/18):698-699. Copyright (2010), with permission from Elsevier.

References

[1] Thomas, E.D. (1995) History, current results, and research in marrow transplantation. Perspect. *Biol. Med.* 38, 230-237.

[2] Wang, J.C. et al. (1997) Primitive human hematopoietic cells are enriched in cord blood compared with adult bone marrow or mobilized peripheral blood as measured by the quantitative in vivo SCID-repopulating cell assay. *Blood* 89, 3919-3924.

[3] Broxmeyer, H.E. et al. (1992) Growth characteristics and expansion of human umbilical cord blood and estimation of its potential for transplantation in adults. *Proc. Natl. Acad. Sci. U. S. A.* 89, 4109-4113.

[4] Kurtzberg, J. et al. (1996) Placental blood as a source of hematopoietic stem cells for transplantation into unrelated recipients. *N. Engl. J. Med.* 335, 157-166

[5] Gluckman, E. et al. (1989) Hematopoietic reconstitution in a patient with Fanconi's anemia by means of umbilicalcord blood from an HLA-identical sibling. *N. Engl. J. Med.* 321, 1174-1178.

[6] Ballen, K. (2010) Challenges in umbilical cord blood stem cell banking for stem cell reviews and reports. *Stem Cell Rev.* 6, 8-14.

[7] Barker, J.N. et al. (2003) Umbilical cord blood transplantation: current practice and future innovations. *Crit. Rev. Oncol. Hematol.* 48, 35-43.

[8] Kelly, S.S. et al. (2010) Overcoming the barriers to umbilical cord blood transplantation. *Cytotherapy* 12, 121-130.

[9] McNiece, I.K. et al. (2002) Ex vivo expanded cord blood cells provide rapid engraftment in fetal sheep but lack long-term engrafting potential. *Exp. Hematol.* 30, 612-616.

[10] Long, G.D. et al. (2003) Unrelated umbilical cord blood transplantation in adult patients. *Biol. Blood Marrow Transplant.* 9, 772-780.

[11] Lapidot, T. et al. (2005)Howdo stem cells find their way home?*Blood* 106, 1901-1910.

[12] Katayama, Y. et al. (2003) PSGL-1 participates in Eselectin-mediated progenitor homing to bone marrow: evidence for cooperation between Eselectin ligands and 4 integrin. *Blood* 102, 2060-2067.

[13] Hidalgo, A. et al. (2002) Functional selectin ligands mediating human CD34+ cell interactions with bone marrow endothelium are enhanced postnatally. *J. Clin. Invest.* 110, 559-569.

[14] McEver, R.P. (2002) Selectins: lectins that initiate cell adhesion under flow. *Curr. Opin. Cell. Biol.* 14, 581-586.

[15] Fuhlbrigge, R.C. et al. (1997) Cutaneous lymphocyte antigen is a specialized form of PSGL-1 expressed on skin-homing T cells. *Nature* 389, 978-981.

[16] Wagers, A.J. et al. (1998) Interleukin 12 and interleukin 4 control cell adhesion to endothelial selectins through opposite effects on 1,3-fucosyltransferase VII gene expression. *J. Exp. Med.* 188, 2225-2231.

[17] Xia, L. et al. (2004) Surface fucosylation of human cord blood cells augments binding to P-selectin and E-selectin and enhances engraftment in bone marrow. *Blood* 104, 3091-3096.

Index

A

acetylcholine, 44, 75, 125
acetylcholinesterase, 60, 116
acid, 5, 6, 12, 13, 19, 40, 48, 91, 112, 135, 152
acute leukemia, 156, 163, 166, 176, 184
acute myeloid leukemia, 154, 166
adhesion, 2, 21, 78, 90, 114, 164, 165, 185, 200, 217, 218
adolescents, 92
adult stem cells, 104, 144
adulthood, 34, 73, 87, 113, 123, 133, 188, 194
adults, 75, 92, 107, 149, 150, 153, 155, 156, 157, 158, 161, 162, 163, 164, 166, 167, 168, 172, 176, 177, 180, 183, 184, 215, 216, 217
adverse effects, 21, 42, 100, 102, 114
aetiology, 109
aggregation, 19, 20, 21, 24, 26, 39, 40, 82, 113, 117, 121
agonist, 60, 66, 77, 125, 135
allele, 20, 24, 32, 33, 40, 51, 75, 112, 211
alters, 22, 68, 101
alveoli, 174
amino, 19, 20, 40, 48, 113, 135, 189, 191
amino acid(s), 19, 20, 40, 48, 113
amygdala, 13
amyloid beta, 10, 11
amyloid deposits, 19, 22, 23, 25, 26, 27, 34, 39, 40
amyloid precursor protein, 2, 11, 29, 33, 39, 52, 75, 90, 112, 121, 124, 211
amyloid protein precursor (APP), 57
amyloidosis, 31, 32, 85, 129
amyotrophic lateral sclerosis, 99, 104
ANC, 175
anemia, 150, 163, 180, 202, 215, 217

aneuploid, 20, 23, 24, 25, 26, 27, 33, 34, 37, 41, 43, 44, 45, 113, 114, 115, 116, 117, 118, 124, 211, 212
aneuploidy, 20, 21, 22, 23, 24, 26, 27, 28, 31, 34, 36, 38, 39, 41, 43, 44, 51, 53, 111, 114, 115, 116, 117, 118, 124, 127, 211, 212
antibody, 158, 199, 200, 201
antidepressant(s), 14, 60, 61, 65, 66, 67, 68, 69, 70, 71, 76, 77, 78, 81, 83, 84, 92, 105, 107, 125, 129, 130, 139, 140, 206, 208, 209
antidepressant medication, 67, 70, 76, 77, 78
antigen, 3, 36, 57, 79, 94, 116, 121, 143, 145, 153, 155, 165, 167, 177, 184, 200, 201, 217
anti-inflammatory drugs, 75
antioxidant, 112, 118
apolipoprotein E varepsilon 4 allele, 20, 33, 40, 75, 211
apoptosis, 5, 25, 29, 36, 52, 112, 113, 114, 116, 117, 118, 121, 127
arterioles, 174
artery, 59
aspartate, 44, 58, 60, 75, 82, 116, 125
astrocytes, 6, 14, 18, 35, 47, 89, 98, 102, 103, 105, 106, 107, 130, 138, 147, 196, 205
astroglial, vii, 11, 38, 113
atrophy, 68, 78, 85, 92, 107
autoimmune diseases, 100, 204
autopsy, 61, 124
axonal degeneration, 189
axons, 3, 5, 6, 137, 206

B

basal forebrain, 18, 23
base, 113
basic research, 161, 204
BBB, 98, 101, 194

behavioral change, 4, 17
behavioral models, 70
beneficial effect, 8, 28, 97, 108
benefits, 83, 118, 157, 174
beta-amyloid precursor protein (APP), 17
bioavailability, 101
biochemistry, 118
biological activities, 136
biological activity, 126
biomarkers, 200, 203
biosynthesis, 164
blood, 20, 36, 40, 48, 61, 68, 98, 103, 105, 114, 144, 145, 146, 147, 148, 149, 150, 151, 152, 154, 158, 159, 163, 164, 165, 166, 167, 168, 169, 170, 171, 172, 174, 176, 177, 179, 180, 182, 184, 185, 186, 190, 194, 204, 215, 216, 217, 218
blood flow, 48
blood group, 158
blood plasma, 190, 194
blood stream, 98
blood vessels, 152, 182
blood-brain barrier, 36, 48, 61, 103, 105, 114, 194
body weight, 154, 173, 181
bone, 28, 144, 145, 146, 147, 148, 149, 150, 154, 159, 163, 164, 165, 166, 168, 169, 170, 172, 176, 177, 179, 180, 184, 185, 186, 215, 217, 218
bone marrow, 144, 145, 146, 147, 148, 149, 150, 154, 159, 163, 164, 165, 166, 168, 169, 170, 172, 176, 177, 179, 180, 184, 185, 186, 215, 217, 218
bone marrow transplant, 176, 184
brain damage, 2, 12, 74, 90
brain functions, 1
brain tumor, 101, 123, 128, 133, 137, 206, 207
breakdown, 19, 26, 39, 40, 43, 113, 117, 212
breast cancer, 71, 83
Bromodeoxyuridine, 33, 36, 126

C

calcium, 4
cancer, 71, 83, 155, 156, 185
cancer cells, 155, 156
candidates, 66, 89, 118, 126, 127
carboxylic acid, 135
caspases, 95
cation, 30
CD8+, 157, 167
cDNA, 29, 52, 122
cell biology, 30, 51
cell cycle, 3, 20, 21, 22, 23, 27, 28, 29, 30, 32, 36, 41, 42, 51, 52, 57, 60, 68, 76, 78, 79, 91, 94, 101, 104, 113, 114, 115, 116, 117, 118, 120, 121, 122, 127, 211, 213

cell death, 4, 5, 7, 11, 19, 22, 23, 24, 26, 27, 28, 30, 32, 39, 40, 41, 51, 52, 74, 84, 95, 101, 104, 107, 109, 111, 112, 113, 116, 120, 188, 191, 213
cell differentiation, 190, 194, 195, 204
cell division, 13, 21, 22, 23, 24, 25, 27, 36, 39, 40, 41, 43, 60, 114, 115, 116, 117, 118, 121, 127, 211, 212
cell fate, 47, 130, 141, 209
cell fusion, 22, 144
cell line, 95, 97, 103, 107, 146, 147, 157, 161, 162, 172
cell lines, 146, 157, 161, 162
cell signaling, 112
cell surface, 152, 181, 200, 203
cerebral cortex, 49, 105, 106
cerebrospinal fluid, 199, 200, 203
cerebrum, 189
chemicals, 98, 99
chemokine receptor, 160
chemokines, 104, 153, 165
chemotherapy, 155, 158
chimera, 168
cholesterol, 20, 40, 51, 75
chondroitin sulfate, 188
chromosome, 20, 23, 24, 27, 28, 30, 31, 41, 43, 51, 52, 53, 115, 116, 117, 119, 121, 213
chronic lymphocytic leukemia, 202
chronic myelogenous, 169
circulation, 168
clinical depression, 66, 68, 78, 92
clinical diagnosis, 114
clinical trials, 53, 194, 195
clusters, 112
coding, 20, 40, 41
cognitive abilities, 38
cognitive deficit, 34, 38, 211
cognitive deficits, 34, 38, 211
cognitive function, 8, 75
cognitive impairment, 17, 39, 49, 107, 112, 119
comparative analysis, 176, 184
compatibility, 172, 173, 180
complement, 102, 201
complexity, 105, 120
composition, 136, 173
compounds, 8, 53, 126, 130, 131, 133, 134, 135, 136, 137, 140, 187, 188, 189, 190, 191, 193, 194, 195, 197, 204, 209
conditioning, 155, 158, 161, 162, 166, 168
conflict, 2, 128, 138, 146, 162, 176, 183, 195, 202
conflict of interest, 128, 138, 146, 176, 183, 195, 202
consensus, 124, 206
contamination, 144
control group, 136

Index 221

control measures, 102

controversies, 7, 19, 40, 56, 67, 71, 73, 77, 80, 88, 144, 206

cooperation, 164, 185, 217

coordination, 4

copper, 170

copyright, viii, 10, 28, 45, 55, 69, 81, 111, 128, 133, 146, 176, 183, 195, 202, 213, 217

corpus callosum, 196

correlation, 19, 40, 48, 99

cortex, 10, 18, 23, 29, 38, 50, 105, 119, 120

cortical neurons, 115

corticosteroids, 201

CSF, 118, 160, 161, 200, 201, 202, 203, 204

culture, 11, 35, 47, 84, 106, 127, 130, 139, 147, 160, 161, 165, 173, 177, 181, 197, 215

culture conditions, 161, 173, 177, 181, 215

curcumin, 116, 117

cure, vii, 1, 8, 9, 17, 36, 39, 74, 79, 81, 90, 95, 124, 134, 188, 189, 195, 202, 205

cures, 17, 28, 73, 189

cycles, 47, 147

cycling, 167

cyclophosphamide, 201

cytokines, 27, 36, 37, 58, 59, 65, 66, 74, 80, 96, 97, 100, 104, 133, 134, 160, 161, 205

cytometry, 182

cytoplasm, 145

cytotoxicity, 195, 201

dermatomyositis, 202, 204

developing brain, 140, 208

diabetes, 20, 112, 145, 173, 175, 183

disability, 203, 204

disease activity, 203

disease progression, 201

disorder, 4, 31, 61, 65, 79, 85, 93, 98, 128, 188

DNA, 21, 22, 23, 24, 27, 32, 36, 41, 51, 60, 68, 91, 101, 109, 112, 113, 114, 115, 117, 118, 120, 127, 167, 190, 196, 211

DNA damage, 112, 115, 117

DNA repair, 22

donors, 150, 151, 157, 165, 166, 167, 168, 172, 173, 176, 180, 184

dopamine, 3, 7, 57, 94, 95

dopaminergic, 4, 7, 11, 58, 94, 95, 104

dosing, 199

Down syndrome, 31, 121

drug design, 61

drug discovery, 126, 127, 128, 131, 133, 207, 209

drug therapy, 22, 32, 53, 55, 71, 73, 76, 85, 90, 92, 103, 121, 129, 134, 141, 209

drug treatment, 56, 61, 68, 101, 136

drugs, 27, 28, 33, 36, 37, 44, 45, 53, 55, 60, 61, 65, 69, 70, 73, 74, 75, 76, 77, 78, 80, 83, 92, 104, 118, 122, 123, 124, 125, 126, 127, 129, 130, 133, 134, 135, 136, 137, 139, 158, 188, 189, 194, 195, 197, 199, 202, 204, 205, 206, 207, 208, 209

drusen, 28, 50, 119

D

deep brain stimulation, 94

deficiency, 152, 179, 181, 216

degradation, 112

dementia, 2, 18, 19, 23, 29, 31, 51, 74, 90, 105, 107, 111, 112, 119

demyelinating disease, 188, 200

demyelination, 187, 188, 189, 190, 191, 200

dendrites, 5, 93

dendritic cell, 160, 161

dentate gyrus, vii, 2, 12, 13, 14, 15, 18, 29, 31, 33, 34, 46, 47, 48, 52, 56, 58, 65, 69, 70, 73, 81, 82, 84, 88, 102, 103, 104, 106, 107, 108, 113, 120, 123, 129, 130, 134, 138, 140, 206, 211

deposits, 2, 19, 23, 24, 26, 28, 39, 40, 50, 74, 90, 113, 119, 211

depression, vii, 7, 8, 14, 15, 44, 53, 57, 60, 61, 65, 66, 67, 68, 69, 70, 71, 73, 74, 75, 76, 77, 78, 80, 81, 82, 83, 84, 85, 87, 90, 91, 92, 93, 99, 100, 104, 105, 107, 109, 123, 124, 125, 126, 127, 129, 130, 133, 134, 136, 137, 140, 205, 206, 207, 208

derivatives, 53, 130, 135, 136, 140, 197, 209

E

early-onset AD (EOAD), 17, 112

EDSS, 201, 204

electron, 143, 145

electron microscopy, 143, 145

elucidation, 61, 124

embryonic stem cells, 143, 147, 162, 181, 183

employment, 162

encephalitis, 194

encoding, 29, 52, 122

endoderm, 144

endothelial cells, 152, 153, 154, 164, 165, 182, 183, 185, 216

endothelium, 164, 174, 185, 217

engineering, 148, 161

entorhinal cortex, 19, 39, 80, 113

environment, 15, 36, 47, 56, 98, 105, 139

environmental conditions, 55

environmental factors, 19

environmental stimuli, 36, 59

enzyme(s), 19, 20, 24, 40, 111, 112, 152, 155, 159, 181

ependymal, 103, 106
epilepsy, 4, 5, 6, 8, 12, 13, 15, 36, 57, 58, 74, 76, 79, 87, 90, 91, 93, 100, 123, 124, 125, 126, 134, 136, 137, 140, 205, 206, 207, 208
epileptogenesis, 7, 12, 13, 14, 15, 57, 58, 79, 93
Epstein-Barr virus, 168
equilibrium, 7
erythropoietin, 96, 160
ester, 41, 51
etiology, 22, 58, 61, 68, 69, 81, 84, 90, 92, 94, 101, 201
euchromatin, 145
evolution, 88, 203
excitability, 12
exercise, 48, 101, 107, 130, 136
experimental autoimmune encephalomyelitis, 197

F

familial Alzheimer's disease (FAD), 10, 17, 20, 21, 23, 32, 33, 40, 41, 52, 75, 85, 109, 112
families, 17, 38
family history, 17, 41
fascia, 12
feedback inhibition, 12
fibroblast growth factor, 15, 58, 59, 104, 136, 145, 189
fibroblasts, 122
filament, 35, 47
fluid, 158, 181, 182, 203
fluorescence, 181, 189, 190
fluoxetine, 60, 76, 77, 78, 83, 92, 106, 123, 124, 125, 129, 130, 134, 137, 206, 209
forebrain, 10, 11, 46, 103, 105, 120, 129
formation, 2, 3, 4, 6, 7, 13, 14, 18, 19, 22, 23, 24, 25, 26, 27, 30, 39, 40, 41, 43, 44, 46, 48, 57, 75, 79, 85, 93, 94, 101, 108, 113, 115, 116, 117, 130, 138, 139, 141, 145, 208, 212
free radicals, 112
functional activation, 167
functional analysis, 191

G

GABA, 12
gadolinium, 201
gastrulation, 146
GDP, 158, 159, 181
gene expression, 165, 218
gene therapy, 161, 200, 202
genes, 2, 11, 17, 20, 21, 24, 26, 39, 40, 41, 42, 90, 94, 112, 116, 117, 124, 211, 212

genetic disease, 215
genetic disorders, 20
genetic factors, 17
genetic mutations, 2, 17, 20, 24, 40, 41, 114
genetics, 50, 85, 108
genome, 113, 118, 120
genomic instability, 215
genotype, 31, 51, 84, 107
germ layer, 144
glatiramer acetate, 200, 201
glia, 6, 13, 14, 46, 82, 102, 144
glial cells, 35, 98
glutamate, 44, 60, 75, 98, 116, 125, 135
glutamate receptor antagonists, 44, 60, 75
glutamine, 3, 79, 94
glutathione, 112
glycans, 159
glycoproteins, 159
granule cell axons, 5
growth, 5, 15, 35, 58, 59, 70, 95, 97, 103, 105, 106, 118, 122, 127, 134, 149, 160, 161, 188, 196
growth arrest, 118, 122
growth factor, 15, 58, 59, 70, 95, 97, 103, 105, 106, 134, 160, 161, 188, 196
guidelines, 165, 176, 184
Guillain-Barre syndrome, 188

H

heart disease, 145, 173, 175, 183
hematopoietic stem cells, 149, 150, 154, 159, 164, 168, 169, 184, 200, 217
hematopoietic system, 98
hemisphere, 18, 23
hemostasis, 164
hepatocytes, 28
heterogeneity, 35, 38, 108, 127, 137
histochemistry, 114
histology, 190
histone, 36, 118
histone deacetylase, 118
HLA, 150, 151, 155, 156, 157, 163, 167, 168, 172, 173, 178, 180, 217
homeostasis, 10
hormone(s), 8, 56, 58, 60, 66, 67, 77
host, 30, 96, 97, 98, 100, 155, 166, 172, 173, 174, 175, 180, 183
human brain, 31, 47, 84, 106, 130, 139, 147, 197, 206
human chorionic gonadotropin, 96
human leukocyte antigen, 146, 172, 180
hydrogen, 111, 189, 191
hydrogen peroxide, 111

hydroxyl, 111, 135, 191
hypertension, 20, 40, 75, 112
hypothalamus, 59
hypothesis, 5, 10, 19, 23, 30, 31, 40, 50, 70, 83, 84, 107, 116, 120, 121, 122, 148

I

identification, 144, 167, 191, 194, 196
identity, 141, 209
IFN, 201
immune disorders, 166
immune response, 99, 151
immune system, 106, 151, 155, 156, 172, 180, 215, 216
immunocytology, 126, 143, 189
immunodeficiency, 168
immunofluorescence, 3
immunogenicity, 151
immunoglobulin, 85
immunohistochemistry, 21, 31, 32, 36, 42, 48, 60, 71, 78, 91, 106, 108, 114, 131, 138, 190, 206
immunomodulation, 189, 196
immunomodulatory, 100, 107, 188, 203, 204
immunoreactivity, 2, 70, 157
immunotherapy, 85
impairments, 1, 18, 80, 123, 125, 126, 127, 133, 137, 206, 207
improvements, 75, 97, 215
in vitro, 3, 8, 10, 18, 30, 35, 38, 48, 50, 56, 59, 65, 70, 80, 87, 89, 95, 96, 97, 116, 126, 127, 128, 134, 135, 136, 138, 145, 149, 150, 151, 153, 157, 158, 160, 161, 162, 169, 173, 175, 177, 179, 181, 182, 187, 188, 189, 191, 194, 196, 207, 213, 215
in vivo, 3, 10, 12, 15, 35, 48, 56, 58, 59, 67, 68, 70, 77, 101, 106, 107, 126, 127, 128, 130, 135, 136, 138, 147, 153, 158, 160, 163, 176, 182, 183, 184, 185, 187, 188, 189, 194, 196, 206, 207, 217
induction, 7, 13, 30, 57, 79, 93, 114, 124, 136
infection, 155, 174
inflammation, 83, 99, 100, 101, 102, 106, 108, 153, 164, 189, 196, 203
inflammatory demyelination, 188
inflammatory disease, 50, 107, 188, 194, 200
inflammatory responses, 100
inherited disorder, 188
inhibition, 5, 12, 58, 81
inhibitor, 5, 39, 44, 116, 125
injections, 58, 171, 181
injuries, vii, 9, 18, 25, 27, 33, 36, 37, 38, 45, 53, 55, 56, 59, 60, 74, 79, 80, 95, 97, 98, 100, 101, 124, 130, 134, 135, 136, 137, 140, 145, 146, 151, 161, 172, 173, 175, 182, 183, 188, 197, 205, 209

insulin, 58, 59, 134
integration, 97, 98, 129
integrin, 164, 185, 200, 217
integrins, 153, 160, 165
intellectual property, 196
interface, 106
interneuron(s), 5, 12, 18, 34, 74, 88, 114
interphase, 26, 30, 39, 43, 53, 212, 213
intervention, 59, 70, 95
intravenously, 38, 80, 97, 152, 162, 173, 174, 175, 179, 180, 182, 183, 201
iodine, 53, 121
irradiation, 6, 7, 14, 57, 77, 79, 84, 93, 100, 106, 151
ischemia, 8, 14, 48, 59, 104, 169
isolation, 16, 32, 35, 46, 65, 79, 85, 120, 131, 138, 144, 147, 196, 209
issues, 9, 215

L

labeling, 4, 21, 36, 42, 60, 68, 75, 91, 94, 114, 126, 127, 138, 206
late-onset AD (LOAD), 17, 112
lead, vii, 17, 20, 24, 25, 28, 35, 40, 43, 55, 68, 73, 80, 112, 116, 117, 126, 127, 150, 162, 191, 194
lesions, 79, 95, 96, 106, 108, 113, 140, 200, 201
leucocyte, 167, 177, 184
leukemia, 150, 155, 156, 163, 166, 167, 168, 169, 215
life expectancy, 17, 188
ligand, 152, 154, 159, 160, 161, 164, 165, 169
light, 12, 22, 61, 68, 100, 114, 203
lipid peroxidation, 112
lipids, 20, 40, 112
lithium, 8, 15
liver, 144, 146, 160, 173, 174, 175, 181, 183
liver disease, 173, 175, 183
localization, 29, 30, 52, 122
locomotor, 103
locus, 18, 23, 31, 52, 119, 172
loss of consciousness, 4, 93
low risk, 156, 166, 172, 180
lymphocytes, 20, 31, 41, 51, 98, 118, 121, 156, 166, 200, 201
lymphoid, 153, 160, 163, 169, 200
lymphoid organs, 200
lymphoid tissue, 153
lymphoma, 150, 163, 168, 180, 203, 204, 215

M

macromolecules, 112

macrophages, 98, 108, 174

macular degeneration, vii, 28, 50, 119

magnetic resonance, 68

magnetic resonance imaging, 68

major depression, 66, 67, 70, 82, 85, 102, 103, 107

mammalian brain, 24, 25, 29, 30, 34, 46, 56, 65, 69, 73, 83, 88, 103, 105, 113, 123, 134, 205, 211

mammals, 17, 27, 29, 33, 43, 47, 49, 56, 68, 69, 73, 79, 83, 87, 88, 89, 95, 108, 111, 113, 126, 133, 138, 139, 141, 144, 147, 148, 197, 205, 207, 208, 209, 211

marrow, 28, 146, 147, 148, 150, 154, 159, 161, 163, 166, 169, 176, 183, 217

mass spectrometry, 190, 194

MBP, 155, 188, 189, 190

medicine, 4, 45, 123, 124, 128, 133, 134, 137, 143, 145, 146, 148, 149, 150, 151, 161, 162, 170, 206, 207

meiosis, 22

melanin, 67

memory, vii, 2, 4, 7, 8, 10, 15, 18, 34, 36, 38, 43, 51, 53, 74, 75, 82, 90, 103, 113, 120, 125, 126, 129, 134, 135, 136, 137, 140, 155, 205, 206, 207

memory function, 8

memory performance, 136

mesencephalon, 16

mesenchymal stem cells, 146, 162, 169, 173, 181, 183

mesoderm, 144

meta-analysis, 70, 71, 83, 105, 208

metabolism, 48, 69, 84, 112, 118, 195

metabolites, 70

microenvironments, vii, 38, 77, 80, 123, 134

microscope, 189, 190

microscopy, 56, 57, 94, 114, 126, 189, 190

midbrain, 3

migration, 3, 6, 7, 9, 16, 26, 29, 30, 31, 37, 39, 43, 46, 48, 49, 56, 57, 71, 79, 83, 94, 105, 106, 121, 130, 153, 164, 165, 182, 212, 216

mitochondria, 118

mitochondrial DNA, 113

mitogen, 67

mitosis, 22, 23, 26, 212

Mitoxantrone, 203

models, 2, 4, 5, 6, 7, 9, 10, 11, 13, 21, 29, 31, 36, 37, 42, 50, 52, 57, 60, 68, 70, 73, 74, 76, 78, 79, 80, 82, 87, 90, 91, 93, 95, 97, 100, 114, 123, 124, 126, 127, 133, 137, 187, 191, 194, 195, 196, 205, 206

modifications, 42, 152, 154

MOG, 188, 190

molecular biology, 126

molecular mass, 190

molecules, 3, 31, 50, 52, 55, 58, 126, 127, 160, 187, 189, 190, 191, 194

monoamine oxidase inhibitors, 60, 76

monoclonal antibody, 158, 201

mood disorder, 71, 81, 140

morbidity, 149, 150, 153, 156, 163, 172, 180

morphology, 145

mortality, 149, 150, 153, 155, 156, 163, 172, 177, 180, 184, 215

mortality rate, 215

mossy fiber (MF)-like processes, 57

motor system, 4

MRI, 196, 200, 201, 203

mRNA, 3

MTI, 127

mucin, 152

multiple sclerosis, 9, 16, 38, 49, 84, 97, 99, 107, 178, 186, 188, 195, 196, 197, 202, 203, 204

multipotent, vii, 18, 25, 35, 38, 45, 56, 74, 88, 89, 95, 107, 113, 124, 127, 134, 144, 160, 172, 180, 196, 205, 207, 215

muscle spasms, 93

mutant, 2, 10, 21, 23, 32, 52, 85, 90, 109, 114, 124

mutation(s), 2, 3, 15, 17, 19, 21, 23, 39, 40, 41, 42, 57, 75, 76, 78, 79, 90, 91, 94, 111, 112, 114, 118, 120, 124, 165, 185

myelin, 188, 189, 190, 194, 195, 200, 203, 204

myelin basic protein, 188, 200

myelin oligodendrocyte glycoprotein, 188, 200

myelodysplasia, 150, 180

myocardial infarction, 148, 178, 186

N

natural killer cell, 150, 169

necrosis, 13, 112

neocortex, 18, 23, 35, 38, 47, 56, 80, 88, 104, 105, 113

neonates, 168

nerve, vii, 2, 4, 17, 18, 19, 21, 23, 30, 35, 37, 38, 39, 40, 41, 45, 55, 59, 60, 68, 74, 78, 80, 87, 90, 91, 96, 104, 113, 114, 115, 116, 117, 120, 124, 128, 134, 137, 187, 188, 189, 191, 194, 195, 204, 205, 206, 211

nervous system, vii, viii, 1, 18, 25, 30, 33, 34, 35, 36, 37, 45, 55, 56, 61, 65, 66, 68, 73, 74, 81, 87, 88, 89, 90, 91, 95, 97, 101, 106, 108, 113, 122, 123, 124, 125, 134, 137, 187, 191, 205, 206, 211, 212

Neural stem cells (NSCs), vii, 88, 89

neurobiology, 140, 208

neuroblasts, 3, 14, 29, 46, 57, 69, 79, 82, 94, 103, 147, 208 neurodegeneration, 18, 21, 22, 23, 25, 26, 27, 34, 37, 38, 39, 41, 43, 50, 53, 75, 80, 99, 116, 117, 118, 126, 130, 140, 188, 189, 196, 197, 209, 211, 212

neurodegenerative diseases, 1, 6, 8, 9, 22, 25, 27, 30, 36, 70, 71, 74, 76, 79, 83, 97, 99, 106, 111, 112, 124, 128, 134, 136, 137, 145, 173, 183, 196, 205, 206

neurodegenerative disorders, 7

neurofibrillary tangles, 2, 10, 18, 19, 22, 24, 25, 26, 27, 30, 34, 38, 39, 40, 41, 43, 50, 74, 90, 99, 112, 113, 115, 117, 211, 212

neuroinflammation, 20, 75, 77, 98, 99, 100, 101, 102, 103, 104, 105, 106, 111, 112

neurological disease, vii, 1, 2, 6, 7, 8, 9, 10, 18, 21, 22, 25, 27, 32, 33, 36, 37, 38, 44, 45, 48, 55, 57, 58, 60, 61, 66, 68, 71, 73, 74, 76, 77, 78, 79, 80, 85, 87, 90, 91, 94, 97, 98, 99, 100, 101, 114, 121, 123, 124, 125, 126, 127, 129, 133, 134, 135, 136, 137, 139, 145, 161, 173, 175, 183, 188, 195, 205, 206, 207, 208, 212

neuronal apoptosis, 50

neuronal cells, vii, 1, 2, 3, 4, 5, 6, 7, 9, 18, 19, 21, 22, 24, 25, 26, 27, 32, 33, 34, 35, 36, 37, 42, 43, 44, 45, 46, 55, 56, 57, 59, 60, 61, 69, 73, 74, 77, 78, 79, 80, 85, 88, 90, 91, 93, 95, 101, 111, 112, 113, 114, 115, 117, 118, 120, 123, 125, 126, 131, 133, 134, 135, 136, 137, 138, 190, 205, 209, 211, 212

neuronal stem cells, 140, 175

neurons, 2, 3, 4, 5, 6, 7, 8, 11, 13, 14, 15, 20, 21, 23, 28, 29, 31, 32, 46, 47, 52, 55, 57, 59, 79, 81, 82, 84, 85, 88, 93, 94, 102, 104, 105, 106, 107, 108, 113, 114, 116, 118, 121, 129, 130, 138, 139, 141, 144, 147, 196, 208, 209, 213

neuropathy, 202

neuropeptides, 59

neuroprotection, 99, 100, 103, 107, 196

neurotoxicity, 121

neurotransmission, 75

neurotransmitter, 3, 4, 55, 66

neurotransmitters, 36, 55

neutrophils, 167, 177

nitric oxide, 58, 98, 99, 112

nondisjunction, 22, 24, 25, 26, 31, 41, 43, 111, 115, 116, 117, 121, 212

non-Hodgkin's lymphoma, 200

norepinephrine, 60, 76

nuclear membrane, 30, 53, 213

nucleic acid, 112

nucleus, 3, 56, 79, 94, 145

O

occlusion, 59

odor memory, 14

olfaction, 42

olfactory bulb (OB), 88

oligodendrocytes, 18, 35, 188, 189, 194, 200, 205

oligodendroglial, vii, 113

oncogenes, 116

oxidation, 112, 113, 118

oxidative damage, 112

oxidative stress, 20, 29, 32, 40, 43, 51, 53, 75, 82, 111, 112, 115, 116, 117, 118

oxygen, 111

P

p53, 31, 53, 121, 122

parenchyma, 59

parents, 162

parietal lobe, 19, 39, 113

parkinsonism, 103

patents, 133, 135

pathogenesis, 5, 11, 18, 21, 22, 23, 24, 25, 26, 27, 29, 32, 33, 34, 39, 41, 42, 43, 45, 50, 51, 53, 61, 75, 81, 82, 83, 87, 90, 94, 99, 100, 101, 103, 105, 111, 112, 113, 115, 116, 117, 122, 124, 212

pathology, 4, 7, 12, 16, 18, 19, 22, 23, 25, 27, 31, 33, 34, 39, 41, 42, 45, 51, 56, 61, 65, 71, 73, 74, 80, 84, 85, 87, 93, 101, 103, 107, 111, 112, 118, 121, 123, 124, 128, 134, 137, 188, 196, 206, 207, 211, 212

pathophysiology, 69, 82, 84, 102, 108

pathways, vii, 4, 13, 18, 29, 37, 38, 45, 65, 69, 74, 75, 80, 84, 87, 105, 118, 124, 128, 134, 165, 195, 205

PCR, 126, 145

PEPA, 135

peptide(s), 10, 11, 19, 30, 39, 40, 52, 113, 121, 122

perfusion, 161

peripheral blood, 31, 51, 121, 145, 148, 150, 163, 166, 167, 172, 176, 178, 180, 184, 200, 215, 217

permeability, 36, 48, 101, 114

peroxidation, 112

peroxide, 112

peroxynitrite, 112

pharmacology, 22, 27, 32, 36, 45, 48, 56, 61, 65, 68, 71, 73, 74, 77, 79, 81, 85, 121, 129, 139, 208

phencyclidine, 58

phenotype, 11, 21, 52, 95, 145, 151, 167

phenotypes, vii, 18, 21, 25, 36, 42, 56, 74, 78, 88, 89, 91, 113, 114, 124, 134, 144, 146, 147, 151, 161, 180, 205, 206, 215

phosphate, 173

phosphorylation, 50, 102

physical activity, 36

physical exercise, 15
physiology, 87, 101, 206, 211
physiopathology, viii, 18, 25, 59, 73, 81
plaque, 2, 74, 90
plasma cells, 200
plasticity, vii, 1, 6, 9, 12, 25, 36, 59, 68, 76, 78, 91, 93, 101, 134
platelets, 164
platform, 47, 130, 136, 141, 209
PLP, 188, 189, 190
polymerization, 26
polymorphism, 29, 50, 51
polymorphisms, 41, 167
polypeptide, 58, 60, 203
post-transplant, 156, 161
potential benefits, 202
precipitation, 66, 78, 92
precursor cells, 11, 16, 43
preparation, iv, 128, 138, 146, 174, 176, 183, 195, 196, 202
presenilin-1, 10, 20, 32, 34, 40, 50, 52, 75, 85, 91, 103, 109, 112, 120, 124, 129, 211
presenilin-2, 20, 34, 40, 75, 112, 211
preservation, 168
prevention, 31, 120
primate, 105, 147
probability, 17, 20, 41, 112, 157, 168, 175
progenitor cells, 2, 8, 11, 12, 16, 24, 25, 26, 27, 34, 35, 42, 47, 48, 57, 58, 59, 67, 77, 80, 84, 88, 89, 94, 98, 104, 107, 115, 117, 118, 122, 125, 129, 130, 131, 134, 138, 139, 146, 149, 160, 161, 162, 167, 168, 169, 170, 187, 188, 189, 190, 191, 194, 195, 196, 202, 204, 209
proliferation, 2, 3, 5, 6, 9, 11, 13, 14, 15, 16, 22, 30, 31, 36, 38, 42, 48, 56, 57, 59, 60, 67, 68, 69, 70, 71, 77, 79, 82, 83, 84, 91, 94, 95, 96, 101, 103, 105, 106, 107, 108, 114, 115, 116, 118, 121, 122, 124, 126, 127, 129, 130, 134, 139, 140, 194, 196, 206
prolonged status epilepticus (SE), 5
propagation, 4, 12, 149, 150, 151, 157, 160, 161, 162, 173, 177, 181, 215
protection, 75, 174, 196
protein kinase C, 118
protein kinases, 118
protein synthesis, 5
proteins, 19, 20, 21, 24, 26, 28, 30, 39, 40, 41, 43, 51, 52, 91, 112, 113, 114, 116, 117, 120, 190, 200, 211
proteolipid protein, 188
psychiatric disorders, 83, 105
psychiatry, 14, 70, 83, 104
psychosocial stress, 14

public health, 75, 92
pulmonary circulation, 174
purines, 112
pyramidal cells, 5, 13, 93, 137, 206

Q

quantification, 76
quinolinic acid, 3, 11, 57, 76, 79, 85, 94, 108

R

radiation, 6, 155, 158
radicals, 112, 122
reactive oxygen, 98, 118
receptors, 60, 87, 100, 135, 153, 196
recovery, 1, 6, 7, 8, 9, 16, 37, 44, 49, 59, 66, 76, 78, 80, 84, 92, 96, 97, 98, 100, 103, 107, 155, 161, 166, 167, 175, 177, 178, 186, 202
recovery process(es), 37, 97
regenerate, 8, 55, 88, 113, 182
regeneration, 8, 12, 35, 55, 60, 80, 95, 97, 103, 134, 146, 169, 196
regenerative capacity, 37, 45, 111, 118, 128, 207, 212
registries, 150, 172, 180
rejection, 157, 167, 173
relapsing-remitting multiple sclerosis, 203, 204
relevance, 12, 121
remyelination, 187, 188, 189, 190, 191, 194, 195, 202, 204
repair, vii, 7, 12, 18, 27, 36, 37, 38, 45, 56, 59, 60, 65, 74, 80, 95, 96, 99, 101, 111, 112, 118, 124, 128, 134, 145, 182, 187, 188, 194, 205
replication, 23, 32, 51, 60, 91, 109, 115, 120
repression, 48
RES, 174, 175
researchers, 1, 9
residues, 152
response, 7, 52, 104, 105, 122, 130, 165, 167, 209, 213
rheumatoid arthritis, 202
risk factors, 17, 20, 23, 39, 40, 75, 90, 111, 112, 163, 203, 211, 212
rituximab, 158, 168, 199, 200, 201, 202, 204
RNA, 35, 47
rodents, 4, 5, 7, 8, 34, 36, 44, 56, 57, 58, 60, 66, 67, 68, 74, 75, 76, 77, 78, 79, 88, 94, 116, 117, 125, 126, 135, 136, 143, 144, 151, 175, 216
rostro-migratory stream (RMS), 18, 34, 59, 74, 80, 88, 114

S

safety, 169
saturation, 137, 206
schema, 161
schizophrenia, 58, 70, 84, 107, 124, 129, 131, 137, 206, 207, 209
sclerosis, 9, 13, 97
segregation, 30, 53, 213
seizure, 4, 5, 6, 7, 12, 13, 14, 57, 79, 84, 93, 106
selective serotonin reuptake inhibitor, 60, 66, 76, 77, 92
self-renewing multipotent cells, vii, 18, 25, 35, 56, 74, 88, 89, 113, 124, 134, 160, 172, 180, 205, 215
self-repair, vii, 7, 8, 34, 35, 79, 211
senescence, 122
senile dementia, 34, 38
septum, 59
serine, 39
serotonin, 66, 69, 70, 75, 83, 130
serum, 161, 200, 203
sheep, 170, 177, 185, 217
sialic acid, 152, 216
sickle cell, 150, 215
sickle cell anemia, 150, 215
signaling pathway, 44, 61, 65, 67, 69, 78, 125, 137, 206
skin, 144, 164, 165, 217
somatic cell, 23, 41, 43, 116, 117
species, 34, 35, 56, 73, 88, 98, 111, 113, 118, 123, 126, 133, 144, 151, 205, 211
spinal cord, vii, 27, 35, 36, 56, 74, 89, 95, 97, 98, 103, 107, 109, 124, 134, 136, 137, 145, 173, 183, 205
spinal cord injury, 97, 103
spindle, 26, 39, 43, 212
spleen, 145, 146, 174
sprouting, 5, 6, 13, 57, 79, 93
status epilepticus, 5, 13, 15, 103
stem cell lines, 16, 49, 81, 102, 147, 178, 186
steroids, 8, 15, 70, 82
stress, 7, 27, 29, 30, 43, 65, 66, 68, 69, 77, 82, 83, 84, 104, 106, 111, 112, 115, 116, 117, 118, 119, 122, 129, 151
striatum, 3, 11, 16, 35, 47, 49, 57, 59, 79, 85, 94, 95, 96, 102, 105, 108
stroke, 7, 8, 49, 81, 96, 102, 106, 148
stroma, 161
stromal cells, 160
structure, 30, 40, 50, 145, 213
subcortical nuclei, 71, 81, 140
subcutaneous injection, 59
subgranular zone (SGZ), 18, 34, 73, 88

substrates, 152, 181
success rate, 150
surgical technique, 4
survival, 3, 32, 55, 85, 103, 124, 126, 129, 154, 155, 157, 165, 174, 176, 178, 184, 186, 206
survival rate, 174
survivors, 71, 83
symptoms, 1, 4, 8, 17, 19, 39, 40, 44, 75, 93, 94, 188, 199, 200, 201, 202
synaptic vesicles, 46, 106
syndrome, 23, 29, 50, 167
synthesis, 22, 36, 40, 60, 68, 101, 114, 127, 190, 196
system analysis, 148
systemic lupus erythematosus, 202

T

T cell, 151, 155, 157, 161, 164, 165, 167, 169, 217
T lymphocytes, 150, 151, 155, 166, 172, 180
tau, 10, 19, 24, 26, 27, 28, 30, 50, 52, 120, 122, 124, 213
techniques, 56, 80, 126
technologies, 127, 162
temporal lobe, 4, 12, 93, 104, 108
temporal lobe epilepsy, 4, 12, 93, 104
testing, 195
TGF, 58
Th cells, 164
thalamus, 59
thalassemia, 180
therapeutic approaches, 37
therapeutic benefits, 76
therapeutic interventions, 8
therapeutic targets, 67
therapeutic use, 35, 161
therapeutics, 10, 30, 108, 120
threonine, 152
thrombopoietin, 160, 161
thymus, 146, 169
tissue, 35, 80, 87, 96, 97, 98, 134, 144, 146, 148, 171, 172, 173, 174, 175, 177, 180, 181, 182, 183, 184, 190, 215
tissue homeostasis, 146
toxicity, 112, 158, 161, 190
toxin, 97
trafficking, 20, 164
transcription factors, 35
transformation, 144
transforming growth factor, 58, 59, 98, 108
transfusion, 174
transplant, 150, 153, 155, 156, 157, 161, 162, 163, 165, 166, 167, 172, 173, 176, 177, 180, 184
traumatic brain injury, 7, 15, 48, 104

tremor, 4
trial, 15, 96, 98, 127, 140, 161, 169, 170
tricyclic antidepressant, 60, 76
tricyclic antidepressants, 60, 76
triggers, 12, 22, 30, 101, 104, 120
trisomy, 23, 29, 121
trisomy 21, 29, 121
tropism, 16
tryptophan, 69, 84
tyrosine, 95, 102, 160, 165
tyrosine hydroxylase, 95, 102

U

umbilical cord, 143, 146, 163, 164, 165, 166, 167, 168, 169, 170, 172, 176, 177, 179, 180, 184, 215, 217
urea, 135

V

vascular cell adhesion molecule, 153, 164, 185
vascular endothelial growth factor (VEGF), 67

vasculature, 152, 182, 216
ventricle, 56, 59
vessels, 152, 153, 154, 158, 182, 183
viral infection, 155

W

western blot, 189, 190
white blood cells, 98
white matter, 200
wild type, 3, 10, 23, 32, 52, 85, 109
Wiskott-Aldrich syndrome, 167
working memory, 140
worldwide, 39, 74, 113, 150, 188, 200

X

X-irradiation, 14, 60, 66, 67, 68, 77, 108